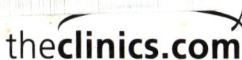

theclinics.com

GASTROINTESTINAL ENDOSCOPY CLINICS OF NORTH AMERICA

Endoscopy and Oncology

GUEST EDITORS
Michael L. Kochman, MD, FACP
Janak N. Shah, MD

CONSULTING EDITOR
Charles J. Lightdale, MD

July 2005 • Volume 15 • Number 3

SAUNDERS

An Imprint of Elsevier, Inc.
PHILADELPHIA   LONDON   TORONTO   MONTREAL   SYDNEY   TOKYO

W.B. SAUNDERS COMPANY
A Division of Elsevier Inc.

Elsevier Inc. • 1600 John F. Kennedy Blvd. • Philadelphia, Pennsylvania 19103-2899

http://www.theclinics.com

GASTROINTESTINAL ENDOSCOPY CLINICS
OF NORTH AMERICA   Volume 15, Number 3
July 2005   ISSN 1052–5157
Editor: Kerry Holland   ISBN 1-4160-2692-4

Reprints. For copies of 100 or more, of articles in this publication, please contact the Commercial Reprints Department, Elsevier Inc., 360 Park Avenue South, New York, New York 10010-1710. Tel. (212) 633-3813 Fax: (212) 462-1935 email: reprints@elsevier.com

The ideas and opinions expressed in *Gastrointestinal Endoscopy Clinics of North America* do not necessarily reflect those of the Publisher. The Publisher does not assume any responsibility for any injury and/or damage to persons or property arising out of or related to any use of the material contained in this periodical. The reader is advised to check the appropriate medical literature and the product information currently provided by the manufacturer of each drug to be administered to verify the dosage, the method and duration of administration, or contraindications. It is the responsibility of the treating physician or other health care professional, relying on independent experience and knowledge of the patient, to determine drug dosages and the best treatment for the patient. Mention of any product in this issue should not be construed as endorsement by the contributors, editors, or the Publisher of the product or manufacturers' claims.

Gastrointestinal Endoscopy Clinics of North America (ISSN 1052-5157) is published quarterly by W.B. Saunders Company. Corporate and editorial offices: Elsevier Inc., 1600 John F. Kennedy Blvd., Philadelphia, PA, 19103-2899. Accounting and circulation offices: 6277 Sea Harbor Drive, Orlando, FL 32887-4800. Periodicals postage paid at Orlando, FL 32862, and additional mailing offices. Subscription prices are $190.00 per year for US individuals, $276.00 per year for US institutions, $95.00 per year for US students and residents, $206.00 per year for Canadian individuals, $327.00 per year for Canadian institutions, $245.00 per year for international individuals, $327.00 per year for international institutions and $123.00 per year for Canadian and foreign students/residents. To receive student/resident rate, orders must be accompanied by name of affiliated institution, date of term, and the *signature* of program/residency coordinator on institution letterhead. Orders will be billed at individual rate until proof of status is received. Foreign air speed delivery is included in all *Clinics* subscription prices. All prices are subject to change without notice. POSTMASTER: Send address changes to *Gastrointestinal Endoscopy Clinics of North America*, W.B. Saunders Company, Periodicals Fulfillment, Orlando, FL 32887-4800. **Customer Service: 1-800-654-2452 (US). From outside of the US, call 1-407-345-4000. E-mail: hhspcs@harcourt.com**

Gastrointestinal Endoscopy Clinics of North America is covered in *Excerpta Medica, Index Medicus, and MEDLINE/MEDLARS.*

Printed in the United States of America.

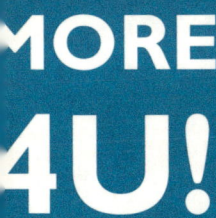

MORE 4U!

theclinics.com

This Clinics series is available online.

ere's what ou get:

- Full text of EVERY issue from 2002 to NOW
- Figures, tables, drawings, references and more
- Searchable: find what you need fast

  Search | All Clinics ▼ | for [ ] | GO |

- Linked to MEDLINE and Elsevier journals
- E-alerts

NDIVIDUAL JBSCRIBERS

LOG ON TODAY. IT'S FAST AND EASY.

lick Register nd follow struction

ou'll need your ccount number

Your subscriber account number → is on your mailing label

| This is your copy of: |
| THE CLINICS OF NORTH AMERICA |
| CXXX   **2296532-2**   2   Mar 05 |
| J.H. DOE, MD |
| 531 MAIN STREET |
| CENTER CITY, NY 10001-001 |

BOUGHT A SINGLE ISSUE? Sorry, you won't be able to access full text online. Please subscribe today to get complete content by contacting customer service at 800 645 2452 (US and Canada) or 407 345 4000 (outside US and Canada) or via email at elsols@elsevier.com.

NEW!

Now also available for INSTITUTIONS

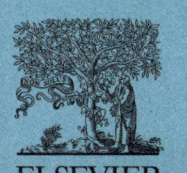

ELSEVIER

Works/Integrates with MD Consult
Available in a variety of packages: Collections containing 14, 31 or 50 Clinics titles
Or Collection upgrade for existing MD Consult customers

Call today! 877-857-1047 or e-mail: mdc.groupinfo@elsevier.com

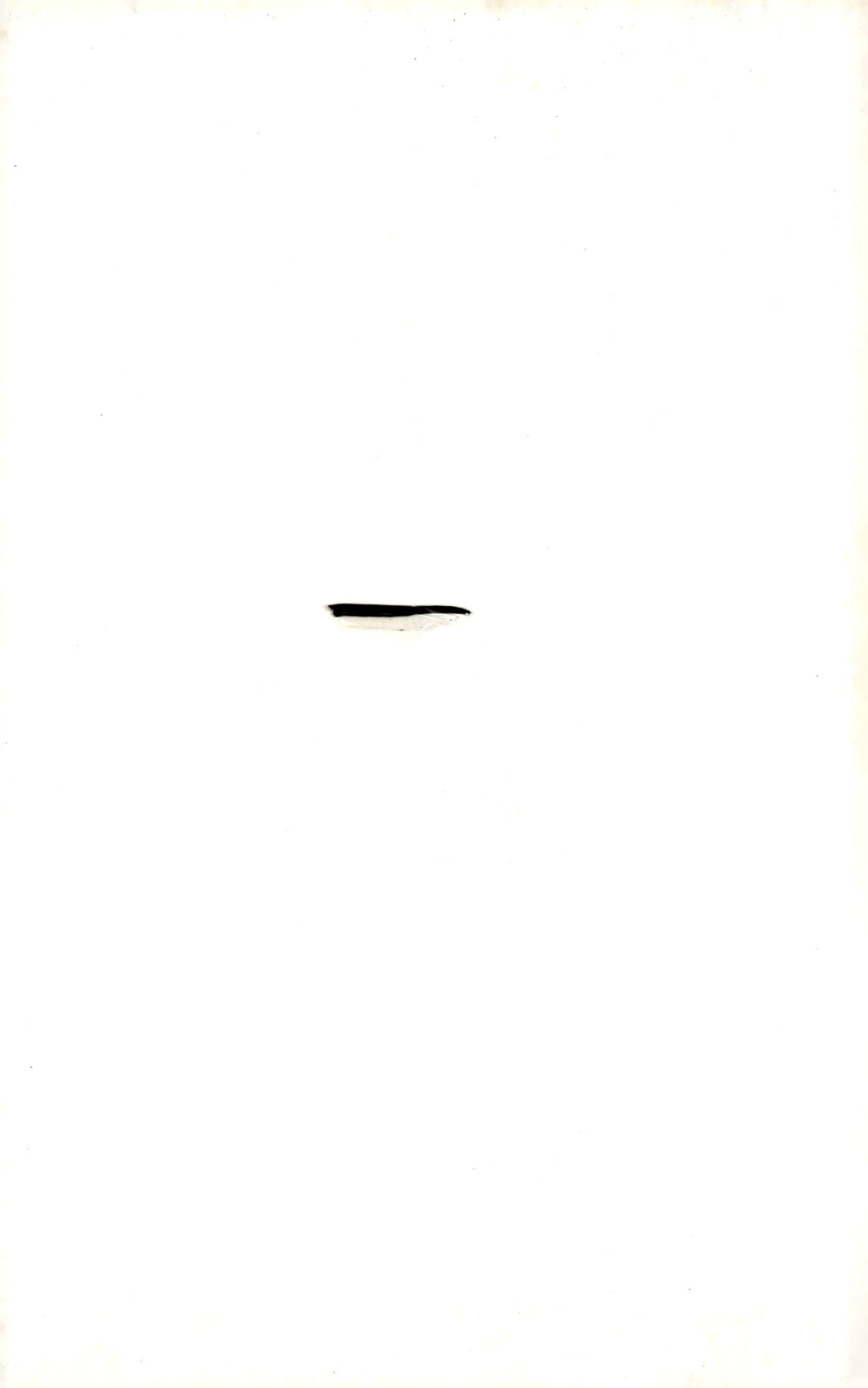

CONSULTING EDITOR

CHARLES J. LIGHTDALE, MD, Professor, Department of Medicine, Columbia University Medical Center, New York, New York

GUEST EDITORS

MICHAEL L. KOCHMAN, MD, FACP, Professor of Medicine, Co-Director Gastrointestinal Oncology, Endoscopy Training Director, Gastroenterology Division, Hospital of the University of Pennsylvania, Philadelphia, Pennsylvania

JANAK N. SHAH, MD, Assistant Clinical Professor of Medicine, University of California, San Francisco; Director of Therapeutic Endoscopy, Veterans Affairs Medical Center, San Francisco, California

CONTRIBUTORS

MATTHEW A. BARISH, MD, Director, 3D and Image Processing Center, Division of Abdominal Imaging and Intervention, Department of Radiology, Brigham and Women's Hospital, Harvard Medical School, Boston, Massachusetts

TODD H. BARON, MD, FACP, Consultant, Professor of Medicine, Division of Gastroenterology and Hepatology, Mayo Clinic College of Medicine, Rochester, Minnesota

WILLIAM R. BRUGGE, MD, Associate Professor of Medicine, Harvard Medical School; Director, Gastrointestinal Endoscopy, Gastrointestinal Unit, Massachusetts General Hospital, Boston, Massachusetts

MOHAMAD A. ELOUBEIDI, MD, MHS, Associate Professor of Medicine, Director, Endoscopic Ultrasound Program, Co-Director Pancreatico-biliary Center, Division of Gastroenterology and Hepatology, University of Alabama at Birmingham, Birmingham, Alabama

SUKRU MEHMET ERTURK, MD, Research Fellow, Division of Abdominal Imaging and Intervention, Department of Radiology, Brigham and Women's Hospital, Harvard Medical School, Boston, Massachusetts

CHARLES J. KAHI, MD, MSc, Assistant Professor of Medicine, Department of Gastroenterology and Hepatology, Indiana University School of Medicine, Roudebush VA Medical Center, Indianapolis, Indiana

ALBERTO LARGHI, MD, PhD, Instructor of Medicine, Interventional Fellow, Department of Endoscopy and Therapeutics, The University of Chicago, Chicago, Illinois

LINDA S. LEE, MD, Clinical Fellow in Gastroenterology, Brigham and Women's Hospital, Harvard Medical School, Boston, Massachusetts

MICHAEL J. LEVY, MD, Consultant, Developmental Endoscopy Unit, Division of Gastroenterology and Hepatology, Mayo Clinic, Rochester, Minnesota

KOENRAAD J. MORTELÉ, MD, Assistant Professor, Department of Radiology, Harvard Medical School, Boston; Associate Director, Division of Abdominal Imaging and Intervention; Director, Abdominal and Pelvic MRI; Director, CME, Brigham and Women's Hospital, Boston, Massachusetts

V. RAMAN MUTHUSAMY, MD, Assistant Clinical Professor of Medicine, University of California; Director of Endoscopic Ultrasound-Moffit-Long/Mt. Zion Hospitals, San Francisco, California

NICHOLAS NICKL, MD, Professor of Medicine, Department of Medicine, University of Kentucky Medical Center, Lexington, Kentucky

KYUNG W. NOH, MD, Fellow, Division of Gastroenterology and Hepatology, Mayo Clinic, Jacksonville, Florida

M. RAQUEL OLIVA, MD, Clinical Fellow, Division of Abdominal Imaging and Intervention, Department of Radiology, Brigham and Women's Hospital, Harvard Medical School, Boston, Massachusetts

JOHN M. PONEROS, MD, Instructor in Medicine, Gastroenterology Division, Brigham and Women's Hospital, Harvard Medical School, Boston, Massachusetts

RAGHURAM P. REDDY, MD, Fellow, Developmental Endoscopy Unit, Division of Gastroenterology and Hepatology, Mayo Clinic, Rochester, Minnesota

DOUGLAS K. REX, MD, Professor of Medicine, Director of Endoscopy, Indiana University School of Medicine Indiana, University Medical Center, Indianapolis, Indiana

JANAK N. SHAH, MD, Assistant Clinical Professor of Medicine, University of California, San Francisco; Director of Therapeutic Endoscopy, Veterans Affairs Medical Center, San Francisco, California

DIA T. SIMMONS, MD, Fellow, Instructor of Medicine, Division of Gastroenterology and Hepatology, Mayo Clinic College of Medicine, Rochester, Minnesota

JONATHAN P. TERDIMAN, MD, Associate Professor of Clinical Medicine, Division of Gastroenterology, Department of Medicine, University of California, San Francisco, California

GEORGE TRIADAFILOPOULOS, MD, Clinical Professor of Medicine, Division of Gastroenterology and Hepatology, Stanford University School of Medicine, Stanford, California

SHYAM VARADARAJULU, MD, Assistant Professor of Medicine, Division of Gastroenterology and Hepatology, University of Alabama at Birmingham, Birmingham, Alabama

MICHAEL B. WALLACE, MD, MPH, Associate Professor of Medicine, Division of Gastroenterology and Hepatology, Mayo Clinic, Jacksonville, Florida; Director, Endoscopic Research, Mayo Clinic, Jacksonville, Florida

IRVING WAXMAN, MD, Professor of Medicine and the Cancer Center Research Center; Director of Endoscopy, Department of Endoscopy and Therapeutics, The University of Chicago, Chicago, Illinois

MAURITS J. WIERSEMA, MD, GI Consultants, Inc., Fort Wayne, Indiana

TIMOTHY A. WOODWARD, MD, Assistant Professor of Medicine, Division of Gastroenterology and Hepatology, Mayo Clinic, Jacksonville, Florida

RONALD W. YEH, MD, Fellow in Gastroenterology, Division of Gastroenterology and Hepatology, Stanford University School of Medicine, Stanford, California

YUKI YOUNG, MD, Gastroenterology Fellow, Division of Gastroenterology, Department of Medicine, University of California, San Francisco, California

CONTENTS

of the pancreatico-biliary system makes histologic diagnosis of malignancy at this region difficult. The ability to position the endoscopic ultrasound transducer at endoscopy in direct proximity to the pancreas and the bile duct, combined with the use of fine-needle aspiration, enables accurate preoperative staging of cancer, especially cancer too small to be characterized by CT or MRI. Endoscopic ultrasonography (EUS) identifies patients unlikely to be cured by surgery due to vascular invasion or regional nodal metastasis, thereby limiting procedure-related morbidity and mortality. This article focuses on the utility and recent advances of EUS in the evaluation of pancreatico-biliary cancer.

The palliation of pancreaticobiliary malignancies has changed over the last two decades. With the development of biliary stents, minimally invasive procedures have replaced surgical techniques. Endoscopically placed stents remain the mainstay for the palliative treatment of malignant biliary obstruction from unresectable pancreaticobiliary tumors. Further improvements in stent designs and advances in other endoscopic technologies are expected, and these should expand the role of minimally invasive palliation. This article reviews the current and anticipated roles of endoscopic techniques in the palliation of pancreaticobiliary malignancies.

Although colorectal cancer (CRC) is the second leading cause of cancer deaths in the United States, it is preventable. Screening modalities include fecal occult blood testing, flexible sigmoidoscopy, double-contrast barium enema, and colonoscopy. Colonoscopy allows effective detection and removal of precursor adenomatous polyps and is the dominant CRC screening modality. Emerging technologies include CT and MR colonography and fecal DNA tests. Effective and cost-effective surveillance after polypectomy and curative CRC resection requires balancing the protective effect of polypectomy while maximizing intervals between examinations; thus, estimation of the risk of recurrence determines the intensity of surveillance for individual patients.

Heredity plays an important causative role in a large percentage of colorectal cancers. Clinical recognition of the hereditary polyposis syndromes, hereditary nonpolyposis colorectal cancer, and common familial colorectal cancer is essential because screening, surveillance, and treatment among affected individuals and their family members differs from that recommended for the general population. More intensive cancer screening and surveillance is required if premature death is to be avoided. Genetic testing is commercially available for most of the hereditary colorectal cancer syndromes and can greatly facilitate the management of patients if properly undertaken.

Among the major innovations in radiology of the gastrointestinal (GI) system are the replacement of classic invasive diagnostic methods with noninvasive ones and the improvement in lesion characterization and staging of pancreatobiliary malignancies. Developments in imaging technology have led to many improvements in the field of diagnostic GI radiology. With its fast and thin-section scanning abilities, multidetector-row CT (MDCT) strengthens the place of CT as the most efficient tool to diagnose, characterize, and preoperatively stage pancreatic neoplasms. MR cholangiopancreatography has widely replaced endoscopic retrograde cholangiopancreatography in the diagnosis and staging of pancreatobiliary malignancies. MR imaging, using phased-array or endorectal coils, demonstrates local tumor invasion accurately in rectal cancers and thus allows an improved surgical planning. Virtual colonoscopy with MDCTs is an efficient screening method for colon cancer, and MDCT enterography is becoming the standard imaging technique for many small bowel disorders. The continuing developments in CT and MR technology will most probably further improve the accuracy of these and other imaging applications in the near future.

New techniques have expanded the role of endoscopy in the diagnosis, staging, therapy, and palliation of malignancies. Three major areas of emerging technologies—endoscopic ultrasound (EUS), luminal stent technology, and photodynamic therapy (PDT)—are discussed in this article. Although EUS and PDT have been used for more than two decades, they have only recently emerged as established integral methods in the armamentarium of the gastrointestinal endoscopist.

Gastrointestinal (GI) tract malignancies have a tremendous impact on society. Colorectal cancer is the second leading cause of cancer death in the United States and accounts for 10% of all cancer deaths. Significant research efforts are being directed toward using the interaction of light and tissue to detect pre-cancerous lesions of the GI tract. This article reviews the current status of various experimental optical technologies to detect pre-cancerous changes in the GI tract and focuses on the clinical applications of these technologies for the practicing gastroenterologist.

FORTHCOMING ISSUES

RECENT ISSUES

THE CLINICS ARE NOW AVAILABLE ONLINE!

Access your subscription at **www.theclinics.com**

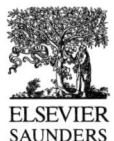
ELSEVIER
SAUNDERS

Gastrointest Endoscopy Clin N Am
15 (2005) xiii–xiv

GASTROINTESTINAL
ENDOSCOPY CLINICS
OF NORTH AMERICA

Foreword

Endoscopy and Oncology

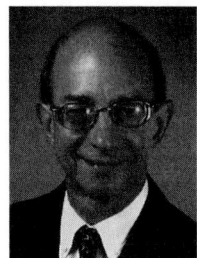

Charles J. Lightdale, MD
Consulting Editor

Gastrointestinal (GI) cancer has long been an important concern for the practicing gastroenterologist. Digestive cancer is a major worldwide health problem. It is estimated that 30% of all human cancers come from the digestive system, including the pancreas, biliary tree, and liver. These cancers, for the most part, have been highly lethal, with digestive cancers resulting in an estimated 36% of all cancer-related deaths.

The role of the gastroenterologist and GI endoscopist in the management of GI cancer has expanded in recent years. Diagnosis, which has generally been the main role for GI clinicians, continues to be a major focus, but there has been a shift in emphasis. The diagnosis of advanced cancer in symptomatic patients has yielded little gain, and there is a new approach using endoscopic inspection for screening and surveillance to detect the earliest stages of neoplasia with a greater likelihood of cure. New optical devices and new methods for analysis of biopsy material should facilitate improved diagnosis of early cancer and premalignant disease. Endoscopic therapy has emerged as a highly effective and minimally invasive way to control and cure early neoplasia of the digestive tract. Poly-pectomy has been a major advance, and most recently ablation and endoscopic mucosal resection seem to be highly successful in treating flat neoplastic areas involving the gut mucosa. Endoscopic ultrasonography (EUS) has resulted in improved accuracy for cancer staging, and EUS-guided fine-needle aspiration has been successful in obtaining tissue diagnosis outside the gut lumen. New EUS-

doi:10.1016/j.giec.2005.03.009
giendo.theclinics.com

guided therapies are being tested and have shown great potential. In advanced cancer, usually managed by multidisciplinary teams of oncologists, surgeons, and radiologists, the GI endoscopist has assumed a key role not only in diagnosis but in palliation with the use of stents and ablation and the placement of tubes for drainage and feeding.

When I first thought of an issue of the *Gastrointestinal Endoscopy Clinics of North America* devoted to Gastrointestinal Oncology, I simultaneously thought that Dr. Michael Kochman should be the Guest Editor. I am very pleased that he agreed to accept this task. Dr. Kochman has devoted much of his career to the diagnosis and treatment of digestive cancer, and he has a tremendous grasp of this field. He has edited an outstanding issue of the *Clinics* with a remarkable group of specialist authors to highlight the important and expanding role of endoscopy in GI oncology.

Charles J. Lightdale, MD
Department of Medicine
Columbia University Medical Center
161 Fort Washington Avenue, Room 812
New York, NY 10032, USA
E-mail address: CJL18@columbia.edu

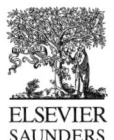

GASTROINTESTINAL
ENDOSCOPY CLINICS
OF NORTH AMERICA

ELSEVIER
SAUNDERS

Gastrointest Endoscopy Clin N Am
15 (2005) xv–xvi

Preface

Endoscopy and Oncology

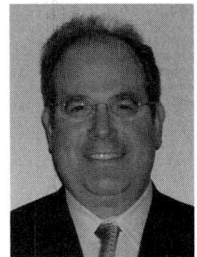
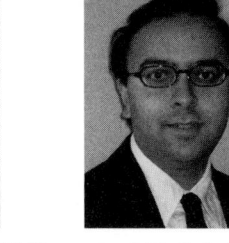

Michael L. Kochman, MD, FACP   Janak N. Shah, MD
Guest Editors

The area of Gastrointestinal Oncology is an active one; Clinical research and basic research have come together and changed the diagnostic and treatment protocols for a number of deadly malignancies. A multidisciplinary approach to the diagnosis and treatment seems to be the best paradigm because it allows for each individual medical specialty to apply its knowledge and expertise in an expeditious and effective manner.

Some of the cancers that we deal with are too often fatal. Our roles are changing: The boundaries between the medical subspecialties are blurring, and with progressive leadership we are better able to make the patients feel that their "team" is truly in sync and providing cutting-edge therapy. To this end, we gathered a nationally and internationally recognized group of clinical researchers and clinicians to provide a balanced approach to the endoscopic diagnosis and treatment of the most common of the gastrointestinal malignancies.

It is intended that this book will serve as a resource for trainees and clinicians in the medical and surgical fields. Those who infrequently diagnose or take care of patients with these neoplasms should be able to find enough easily accessible information to be able to converse with their patients and their families, and those who are routinely involved in the care of these patients will gain a better understanding of the capabilities and insight into the thought processes behind the often difficult diagnostic and treatment decisions that must be made.

1052-5157/05/$ – see front matter © 2005 Elsevier Inc. All rights reserved.
doi:10.1016/j.giec.2005.03.008   *giendo.theclinics.com*

We would like to thank the authors who did a phenomenal job conveying their expertise in their respective areas. It is difficult in these times to have genuine experts write articles due to the complex time demands placed upon them. They are to be congratulated. Charlie Lightdale, MD, who entrusted us with this project, deserves a special mention. His guidance and editorial skill over the years has been a tremendous boost, not only to us individually, but also to gastroenterology.

The staff at Elsevier was superb and demonstrated great professionalism. Their guidance and expertise shows in the polish of the final product. An individual thanks is due to Kerry Holland. Without her expertise the final product would not be as solid.

Michael L. Kochman, MD, FACP
Gastroenterology Division
Hospital of the University of Pennsylvania
3 Ravdin
3400 Spruce Street
Philadelphia, PA 19104, USA
E-mail address: Michael.kochman@uphs.upenn.edu

Janak N. Shah, MD
San Francisco VA Medical Center
4150 Clement Street
Building 203, Suite 2A79 GI Division (111B1)
San Francisco, CA 94121, USA
E-mail address: janak.shah@med.va.gov

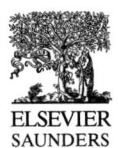

ELSEVIER
SAUNDERS

Gastrointest Endoscopy Clin N Am
15 (2005) 377–397

GASTROINTESTINAL
ENDOSCOPY CLINICS
OF NORTH AMERICA

Endoscopic Therapy for Barrett's Esophagus

Ronald W. Yeh, MD*, George Triadafilopoulos, MD

*Division of Gastroenterology and Hepatology, Stanford University School of Medicine,
Alway Building M-211, 300 Pasteur Drive, Stanford, CA 94305, USA*

Barrett's esophagus (BE) is a condition in which the normal esophageal squamous epithelium is replaced by specialized intestinal metaplasia. This condition is thought to develop when gastroesophageal reflux disease (GERD) damages the squamous epithelium. The injured esophagus heals through a metaplastic process whereby the squamous epithelium is replaced by intestine-like columnar and Alcian blue-positive goblet cells. BE increases the risk for developing esophageal adenocarcinoma [1,2].

The development of esophageal adenocarcinoma progresses from intestinal metaplasia with no dysplasia, to low-grade dysplasia (LGD), to high-grade dysplasia (HGD) (Fig. 1), and eventually to cancer [3]. It is unclear who is at risk and what the time course is for the progression to esophageal adenocarcinoma. Most patients with BE do not develop esophageal adenocarcinoma [4]. Furthermore, not all patients with BE and HGD develop adenocarcinoma. Levine et al [5] showed that during a 30-month follow-up, 26% of patients with HGD progressed to adenocarcinoma, 27% regressed to a less severe degree of dysplasia, and 47% remained stable. In another study with a mean 7.3-year surveillance for HGD, 16% of the patients developed cancer [4].

Once BE is diagnosed, the management involves controlling reflux symptoms, monitoring for the development of dysplasia and adenocarcinoma, and determining when and if therapeutic intervention is needed. Traditionally, esophagectomy has been recommended for patients who have HGD. This approach is advocated for several reasons: (1) Studies have shown that 33% to 50% of patients with HGD on biopsy have cancer present in the surgically resected esophagus [6–10]; (2) HGD is often multi-focal in nature; and (3) esophagectomy

---

* Corresponding author.
E-mail address: yehr@stanford.edu (R.W. Yeh).

1052-5157/05/$ – see front matter © 2005 Elsevier Inc. All rights reserved.
doi:10.1016/j.giec.2005.04.004

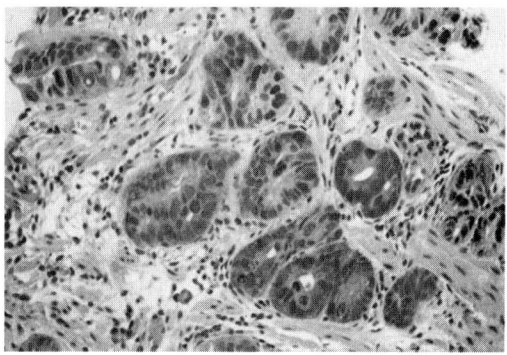

Fig. 1. Histologic appearance of BE with HGD.

removes all Barrett's mucosa, which prevents the development of new dysplastic lesions. Esophagectomy is not a benign procedure, especially in elderly and high-risk patients. Mortality rates have been reported to be in the range of 3% to 5%, and morbidity rates range from 18% to 48% [11,12].

It is believed that secondary prevention of Barrett's-related cancer can be achieved through the elimination of reflux combined with removal of the meta-plastic pre-malignant tissue. When the Barrett's epithelium is injured or removed and the gastroesophageal reflux is controlled, the reparative healing process can cause recolonization of the normal squamous mucosa. Endoscopic therapies using radiofrequency, suturing, and implantable biopolymers have been developed to control reflux, but none of them has been applied in patients with BE. The endo-scopic methods for removal of Barrett's metaplastic premalignant tissue can be classified as (1) thermal (argon-plasma coagulation [APC], electrocoagulation, laser irradiation, radiofrequency ablation), (2) photochemical (photodynamic therapy), or (3) mechanical (endoscopic mucosal resection). In this article, we review current published literature on endoscopic therapies for the management of BE.

Treatment of gastroesophageal reflux disease in the management of Barrett's esophagus

The importance of GERD control cannot be overemphasized. Control of heart-burn and regurgitation, healing of coexisting esophagitis, prevention of recurrent esophagitis, control of bile reflux, prevention of stricture formation, regression of Barrett's surface, and regression of dysplasia have been important endpoints for any patient with BE.

The intensity of anti-reflux therapy for patients with BE is highly con-troversial. Proponents of aggressive intra-esophageal acid control believe that acid and bile reflux is the main factor contributing to carcinogenesis. It is hy-pothesized that normalization or elimination of esophageal acid and bile exposure reduces the progression to HGD or adenocarcinoma by removal of such mucosal irritants. Several basic science studies have provided support for this hypothesis [13–16].

Proton-pump inhibitors (PPIs) and surgical antireflux therapies have been shown to be effective for improving or eliminating signs and symptoms of GERD in patients with BE [2]. Studies have reported regression of specialized intestinal metaplasia in a small number of patients who were treated with PPIs [17–21] and surgical anti-reflux therapies [22,23]. Furthermore, many uncontrolled studies have shown that endoscopic ablative therapy, combined with medical [24–28] or surgical reflux control [29,30], can result in squamous re-epithelialization of the Barrett's mucosa. Neither PPI therapy nor surgical anti-reflux therapy have been shown to eliminate or reduce cancer risk [31–35]. This may reflect the fact that neither of these approaches achieves complete control of acid or bile reflux in patients who have BE [36,37].

Recently, endoscopic treatments for GERD have been developed and have been approved by the FDA. The three major types of endoscopic therapy are (1) plication of gastric cardia folds using sutures, (2) thermal injury to the lower esophageal sphincter and cardia using radiofrequency, and (3) injection of ethylene vinyl alcohol polymer in the muscle of the gastroesophageal junction. All published data regarding safety and efficacy of these devices do not include patients who have BE. Thus, the use of such antireflux therapies to eliminate the risk of dysplasia and cancer in patients who have BE esophagus should be considered experimental.

Endoscopic therapies for Barrett's esophagus

Reversal of Barrett's epithelium with subsequent regrowth of squamous epithelium requires the control of gastroesophageal reflux and ablation of Barrett's epithelium. During the healing process, it is hypothesized that pluri-potent esophageal mucosal stem cells differentiate and expand, causing re-colonization of the treated esophagus by squamous mucosa instead of specialized intestinal metaplasia. The endoscopic methods for injuring and removing metaplastic premalignant tissue can be classified as thermal (APC, electrocoagulation, laser irradiation, radiofrequency ablation), photochemical (photodynamic therapy), or mechanical (endoscopic mucosal resection). We review the published literature on the safety and efficacy of each method.

Thermal ablation for the management of Barrett's esophagus

Argon-plasma coagulation

APC is a technique in which electrical energy is delivered through a jet of ionized argon gas flowing at 1 to 2 L/min from a probe to the tissue. This process allows the APC to cause noncontact injury to a large area of targeted tissue. The depth of injury is limited to 1 to 3 mm because current flow stops once charring of the surface mucosa has occurred [38]. The equipment needed for APC is inexpensive, easy to use, and available in most endoscopy units.

Many groups have evaluated the effectiveness of APC in ablating BE, and most of them involve the concurrent use of PPIs [27,30,38–48]. Five of the case series used antireflux surgery as a way to control reflux [30,46–48].

The success rate of complete endoscopic ablation of BE has ranged from 60% to 100% (Table 1) [49,50]. Buried glands and persistent intestinal metaplasia underneath the squamous re-epithelialization have been reported in 0% to 44% of cases. Long-term follow-up of successfully treated patients show recurrence of intestinal metaplasia ranging from 0% to 68%. In addition, adenocarcinoma arising under neo-squamous epithelium has been reported in patients achieving endoscopic and histologic clearance of BE [42,51–53]. Kahaleh and colleagues, using multivariate analysis, identified short-segment BE and normalization of acid exposure as the only independent predictive factors for sustained long-term re-epithelialization [42].

Experience with APC in the treatment of BE with HGD has been published by two groups. Van Laethem and colleagues [52] treated seven patients with HGD. Four patients had no evidence of intestinal metaplasia, one patient had persistent HGD, one patient had intestinal metaplasia, and one patient died of adenocarcinoma after a median follow-up of 24 months. Attwood and colleagues [54] treated 29 patients with HGD with 76% complete regression of dysplasia and conversion to neo-squamous esophageal mucosa. After a mean follow-up of 37 months, no patient died of esophageal adenocarcinoma. Four patients developed cancer, three of whom continued with ablation therapy, and one died of unrelated causes.

Frequently reported complications of APC therapy include chest discomfort and odynophagia. These symptoms can be managed by antacids and analgesia. Fever [44], bleeding [45], stricture formation [43–45], perforation, and death [38,41,44] have been reported.

Electrocoagulation

Multipolar electrocoagulation (MPEC) uses electrical energy to raise tissue temperature, which results in tissue desiccation and destruction. This technique requires a probe, passed through the channel of the endoscope, to be placed in contact with the target tissue. Power is applied until there is evidence of a white coagulum.

Sampliner and colleagues [55] initially reported squamous re-epithelialization of Barrett's mucosa with the use of MPEC and control of esophageal acid exposure with PPI therapy. Multiple case series have been published showing varying rates of residual BE (0% to 27%) (Table 2) [56–61]. Of the 296 patients who were treated with MPEC, all but four had nondysplastic BE. Acid suppression was achieved with PPIs, except in one trial in which patients underwent surgical anti-reflux therapy before MPEC ablation [5].

Table 1
Argon plasma coagulation for the treatment of Barrett's esophagus

Reference	n	Median APC sessions (range)	APC power setting (W)	Length of BE (cm) (range)	Endoscopic ablation (%)	Subsquamous intestinal metaplasia (%)	Median Follow-up (mo)	Intestinal metaplasia on follow-up (%)
Mork [27]	15	3 (1–8)	60	Median 4 (2–8)	86.7	0	6–13	7.7
Van Laethem [45]	31	2.4 (1–4)	60	Mean 4.5 (3–11)	81	24	12	47
Byrne [38]	30	4 (2–7)	60	Median 5 (3–17)	100	30	9	30
Grade[40]	9	Mean 1.7 (1–3)	60	Mean 3.5	100	22	NA	NA
Pereira-Lima [44]	33	Mean 1.96 (1–4)	65–70	Median 4 (0.5–7)	100	0	10.6	3
Schulz [43]	73	2 (1–5)	90	Median 4 (1–12)	99	0	12	0
Morris [44]	53	Mean 3	N/A	Mean 6 (3–15)	NA	30	38.5	NA
Tigges [30]	30	2 (1–7)	Up to 150	Mean 3 (1–10)	100	0	12	9
Basu [39]	50	4 (1–8)	30	Mean 5.9 (3–19)	68	44	12	68
Kahaleh [42]	39	3 (1–4)	60	Mean 4.7 (2–11)	70	44	36	62
Pagani [46]	94	Mean 3 (1–5)	60	NA	72	NA	Mean 12.5 and 26	12
Morino [47]	23	3.1 (2–6)	30–50	Mean 3.8 (2–8)	87	9	Mean 31.9	9
Ackroyd [48]	20	3 (2–4)	60	Mean 4 (2–13)	60	35	12	42
Pinotti [49]	19	2 (1–6)	50	NA	100	0	Mean 17	5
Hage [50]	14	NA	65	Mean 3 (3–4)	50	NA	18	33
Combined data	533				84	18		25

Abbreviations: APC, argon-plasma coagulation; BE, Barrett's esophagus; NA, not available.

Table 2
Multipolar electrocoagulation for the treatment of Barrett's esophagus

Reference	n	Anti-reflux	Length of BE	Follow-up (mo)	MPEC sessions	Residual (%)
Sharma [58]	11	Omeprazole 49 mg	4.4	24	9.5	27
Montes [57]	14	Anti-reflux surgery	4.8	21.6	3.7	0
Kovacs [56]	27	Lansoprazole 60 mg	3.4	4.5	NA	18.5
Sampliner [59]	58	Omeprazole 80 mg	3.4	6	3.5	22
Jackson [60]	8	Omeprazole 40 mg	4.3	12	NA	12.5
Guelrud [61]	178	Lansoprazole 60 mg	89% SSB	37	2.3–4.7	1.7
Combined data	296					14

Abbreviations: BE, Barrett's esophagus; MPEC, multipolar electrocoagulation; NA, not available; SSB, short segment BE.
From Sampliner RE. Multipolar electrocoagulation. Gastrointest Endosc Clin N Am 2003;13:449–55; with permission.

The reported complications of MPEC include transient odynophagia, dysphagia, chest pain, fever, bleeding, and stricture formation. No perforation has been reported.

Laser

Laser thermal ablation uses light energy to ablate the targeted tissue. Argon lasers, Nd:YAG lasers, and KTP:YAG lasers have been applied in the treatment of Barrett's mucosa. Nd:YAG lasers have a greater depth of penetration compared with KTP:YAG and argon lasers. The procedure is performed with the laser fiber placed through the biopsy channel of an endoscope. KTP:YAG and argon lasers produce visible light; Nd:YAG lasers produce infrared light and therefore require an aiming beam. The laser energy can be transferred to the targeted tissue through a contact or noncontact method.

Early studies by Berenson [25] and Sampliner [24] using argon and Nd:YAG laser showed that re-colonization of squamous mucosa was possible in an anacid environment. Luman and colleagues [62] were not successful in their treatment of four patients using Nd-YAG laser. Multiple groups have published case series with initial success ablation rate of 22% to 100% and a recurrence rate of 0% to 85% (Table 3). Complications related to laser ablation include retrosternal pain, dysphagia, odynophagia, nausea and vomiting, fever, epigastric pain, sore throat, headache [63], esophageal strictures, bleeding [63], and perforation [64].

Radiofrequency ablation

BaRRx's system consists of a custom radio frequency (RF) generator and a single-use treatment balloon catheter. The catheter is inserted endoscopically and positioned at the desired site of treatment. A short, controlled application of RF energy destroys the thin layer of Barrett's mucosa while preserving the muscular layer of the esophagus. Although recently the FDA granted a 510(k) clearance for the ablation of BE, there are no efficacy data available for this novel ablation method.

Table 3
Laser therapy for the treatment of Barrett's esophagus

Reference	n	Type of laser	Number of sessions (range)	Endoscopic ablation (%)	Subsquamous intestinal metaplasia (%)	Follow-up (mo)	Intestinal metaplasia on follow-up (%)
Barham [86]	16	KTP	Median 3 (1–6)	81	85	3–18	85
Salo [29]	11	Nd-YAG	Average 4 (1–8)	100	0	Average 26	0
Gossner [87]	8	KTP	Average 2.4	100	20	Average 10.6	20
Weston [63]	13	Nd-YAG	Average 2.7 (1–6)	77	0	Average 12.8	57
Fisher [64]	31	Nd-YAG	Average 6.5	83	0	Average 19.1	38
Bowers [88]	9	KTP	Median 2 (1–5)	22	NA	Average 6.8	11
Norberto [89]	15	Nd-YAG	Average 6.5 (3–17)	40	0	Average 28	NA
Combined data				71	17		35

Abbreviation: NA, not available.

In summary, APC, electrocoagulation, laser, and radiofrequency ablation of Barrett's mucosa have been studied. Most data pertain to patients with no dysplasia or LGD, but some studies have included patients with HGD. The results have shown variable rates of squamous re-epithelialization. There is high rate of subsquamous intestinal metaplasia, which can hinder future surveillance of Barrett's mucosa. Long-term follow-up shows a high rate of Barrett's mucosa recurrence. The combination of these factors, along with procedure-related complications, makes thermal ablation of Barrett's mucosa problematic for routine use in clinical practice.

Photodynamic therapy for the management of Barrett's esophagus

Photodynamic therapy (PDT) combines a photosensitizing drug, nonthermal light of a specific wavelength, and oxygen to cause tissue destruction. The photosensitizing drug is activated by a nonthermal light directed at the tissue, which causes the formation of singlet oxygen species that are highly reactive, unstable, and cause local tissue damage.

Hematoporphyrin derivative (HpD), porfimer sodium (Photofrin), 5-aminolaevulinic acid (5-ALA), and meta-tetrahydroxyphenyl chlorine (mTHPC) are the most frequently studied photosensitizing agents used in the treatment of BE. Photofrin, a purified form of HpD, is the only agent approved in the United States for use in the treatment of BE. Photofrin is usually administered intravenously at a dose of 2.0 mg/kg 48 hours before photoradiation at 630 nm of light. This agent localizes nonspecifically in tissue and can lead to full-thickness tissue necrosis of the esophagus and to stricture formation (Fig. 2). Photofrin can persist in body tissue for up to 3 months [65]; therefore, patients need to avoid sunlight and strong artificial light because ambient light may cause activation.

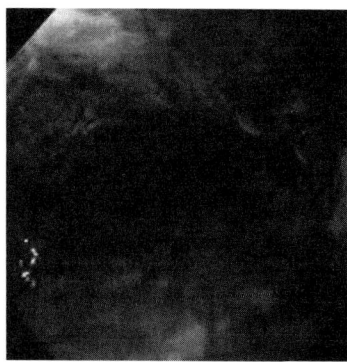

Fig. 2. Endoscopic appearance of the distal esophagus 24 hours after photodynamic therapy for HGD in a patient with BE. Such extensive changes early on were followed by complete re-epithelialization of BE by neo-squamous epithelium on follow-up endoscopy months later. (Courtesy of Herbert C. Wolfsen, MD, Jacksonville, Florida.)

5-ALA is an alternative agent available in Europe. 5-ALA is an orally administered pro-drug that has no photosensitizing properties. In body tissue, 5-ALA is converted into protoporphyrin IX, which is photosensitive. Protoporphyrin IX accumulates almost entirely in the mucosa, allowing for more superficial tissue injury and reducing the risk of stricture or perforation [66]. 5-ALA is given orally 4 to 6 hours before light treatment at 514 nm or 635 nm and has a reduced period of photosensitivity of 24 to 48 hours [67]. This drug is not available commercially for gastrointestinal (GI) use in the United States.

mTHPC is a second-generation photosensitizer that is injected intravenously and activated at a wavelength of 514 nm or 652 nm [68]. As compared with Photofrin, mTHPC has higher selectivity for neoplastic tissue and a decreased period of skin photosensitization (2 to 3 weeks) [69]. This agent has been used in Europe for treating early cancers of the head and neck and more recently for treating BE. This agent is not commercially available for GI use in the United States.

Major published data on PDT in patients with LGD and HGD are summarized in Tables 4 and 5, respectively. Most of the reports describe single-center, uncontrolled studies without standardized histologic analysis or treatment endpoints [70]. Photofrin is most frequently studied agent. In one study, over a mean series follow-up of 19 months, complete elimination of Barrett's mucosa was achieved in 44% and 50% of patients with HGD and LGD, respectively [70]. There was 34% rate of stricture formation, a 6% rate of subsquamous glandular mucosa detection, and early development of cancer after PDT [70]. In another study with a mean follow-up of 50.7 months, there was elimination of Barrett's mucosa in 54% and 71% of patients with HGD and LGD, respectively. There was a 30% rate of stricture formation, a 4.9% rate of subsquamous glandular mucosa detection, and 4.6% rate of subsquamous adenocarcinoma development.

Mayo Clinic investigators have reported similar experiences using Photofrin [71] and HpD [72], with complete elimination of BE with HGD in 56% and 35% of patients, respectively. Rates of stricture were 25% and 27%, respectively, and subsquamous glandular mucosa was found in 0% and 4% of patients, respectively.

Complete elimination of BE is possible in patients with BE with LGD or HGD. However, there is a 25% to 34% chance of esophageal stricture formation and continued risk of esophageal adenocarcinoma formation [70,73,74].

Several studies have been published on the safety and efficacy of 5-ALA in the treatment of BE. In a double-blind, randomized, placebo-controlled study of patients with BE with LGD, Ackroyd and colleagues [75] reported no evidence of dysplasia in patients treated with 5-ALA as compared with 33% in patients given placebo. There were no short- or long-term side effects, such as stricture formation, after 24 months of follow-up [75]. The same group published another study with a mean series follow-up of 53 months [76]. There was regression of LGD in 97% of patients, and 0% of patients developed strictures. Neither of these studies showed complete elimination of BE in any of the study patients.

Other researchers have reported similar results in patients with BE and HGD. Downgrading of HGD in all patients with no reported stricture forma-

Table 4
Photodynamic therapy for Barrett's esophagus with low-grade dysplasia

Reference	Method	Follow up (mo)	n	Subsquamous intestinal metaplasia (%)	Regression of LGD (%)	Elimination of intestinal metaplasia (%)	Stricture rate (%)[a]
Overholt [70]	PDT with photofrin with supplemental Nd:YAG	19 (4–48)	14	NA	93	50	34[a]
Overholt [74]	PDT with photofrin with supplemental Nd:YAG	50.7 (2–122)	14	NA	93	71	30[a]
Ackroyd [75]	5-ALA	24	18	0	100	0	0
Ackroyd [76]	5-ALA	53 (18–68)	40	3	97	0	0
Combined data					96	30	16

Abbreviations: 5-ALA, 5-aminolaevulinic acid; LGD, low-grade dysplasia; PDT, photodynamic therapy.

[a] Rates are reported for entire study population. Data were not subcategorized based on degree of dysplasia.

Table 5
Photodynamic therapy for Barrett's esophagus with high-grade dysplasia

Reference	Method	Follow up (mo) (range)	n	Subsquamous intestinal metaplasia (%)	Regression of HGD (%)	Elimination of intestinal metaplasia (%)	Stricture rate (%)
Overholt [70]	PDT with photofrin with supplemental Nd:YAG	19 (4–48)	73	NA	88	44	34[a]
Overholt [74]	PDT with photofrin with supplemental Nd:YAG	50.7 (2–122)	80	NA	78	54	30[a]
Wolfsen [71]	PDT with photofrin with supplemental APC	18.5 (1–56)	34	0	100	56	23[a]
Wang [72]	HpD	NA	26	NA	88	35	27[a]
Wolfsen [90]	PDT with photofrin	12	132	NA	72	41	36[a]
Etienne [68]	mTHPC	34 (12–68)	7	0	100	100	8[a]
Javaid [79]	mTHPC	27	6	NA	100	17	29[a]
Gossner [78]	5-ALA	9.9 (1–30)	10	6[a]	100	0	0[a]
Barr [77]	5-ALA	25–44	5	40	100	0	0[a]
Combined data					92	38.5	21

Abbreviations: 5-ALA, 5-aminolaevulinic acid; HGD, high-grade dysplasia; HpD, hematoporphyrin derivative; mTHPC, meta-tetrahydroxyphenyl chlorine; PDT, photodynamic therapy.

[a] Rates are reported for entire study population. Data were not subcategorized based on degree of dysplasia.

tion has been reported [77,78]. However, 5-ALA failed to eliminate BE in all patients studied.

There have been two small studies on the use of mTHPC with a total of 13 patients. These studies demonstrate the potential of this new agent in eliminating BE and in downgrading the histologic classification of dysplasia with decreased stricture rate [68,79].

In summary, PDT has been shown to eliminate BE and downgrade the histologic classification of dysplasia. However, no study has demonstrated that PDT can decrease the incidence and mortality of esophageal adenocarcinoma. The complication of stricture formation and the need to avoid sun light for up to 3 months after therapy may make this therapy unacceptable for many patients. Further research is needed to develop a new generation of photosensitizers with improved targeting of dysplastic and neoplastic tissue, rapid activation, and reduced cutaneous phototoxicity.

Endoscopic mucosal resection for the management of Barrett's esophagus

Endoscopic mucosal resection (EMR) allows the complete removal of mucosal lesions by resecting through the middle or deep layers of the submucosa. EMR can be used to cure early mucosal cancers in which there is little chance for lymph node metastasis and can provide tissue specimens for histopathologic staging and assessment of the adequacy of therapy. Four techniques (Fig. 3) are frequently used throughout the GI tract: (1) inject and cut; (2) inject, lift, and cut; (3) cap-assisted EMR; and (4) EMR with ligation.

The major published data on EMR for he treatment of BE are summarized in Table 6. Ell and colleagues [80] have reported on 64 patients with BE who underwent EMR for early carcinoma (61 patients) or HGD (three patients). Patients were separated into low- or high-risk groups based on size, macroscopic appearance, grade, and stage of lesion. Of the 35 low-risk patients who had lesions <20 mm, well or moderately differentiated adenocarcinoma or HGD, and depth limited to the mucosa, six patients (17%) had a local recurrence or metachronous carcinoma that required repeat EMR. Ninety-seven percent of the patients had complete local remission after an average of 12 months of therapy. There was bleeding in 20% of the low-risk patients [80]. In the high-risk group, defined as lesion diameter >20 mm and limited to mucosa based on staging procedure, macroscopically type III, poorly differentiated adenocarcinoma, or infiltration of the submucosa, 59% had complete remission after multiple resections. After an average follow-up of 10 months, local recurrence was observed in two patients, and metachronous cancer was observed in one patient.

The same group published their experience of 115 patients with BE and HGD or early adenocarcinoma treated with EMR ($n = 70$), PDT ($n = 32$), PDT + EMR ($n = 10$), and APC ($n = 3$) [81]. The complete remission rate was 98%. Metachronous cancer was found in 30% of patients after a mean follow-up of 34 months. EMR-related complications included five patients with bleeding episodes and three patients with stricture formation. Of the 19 patients who had

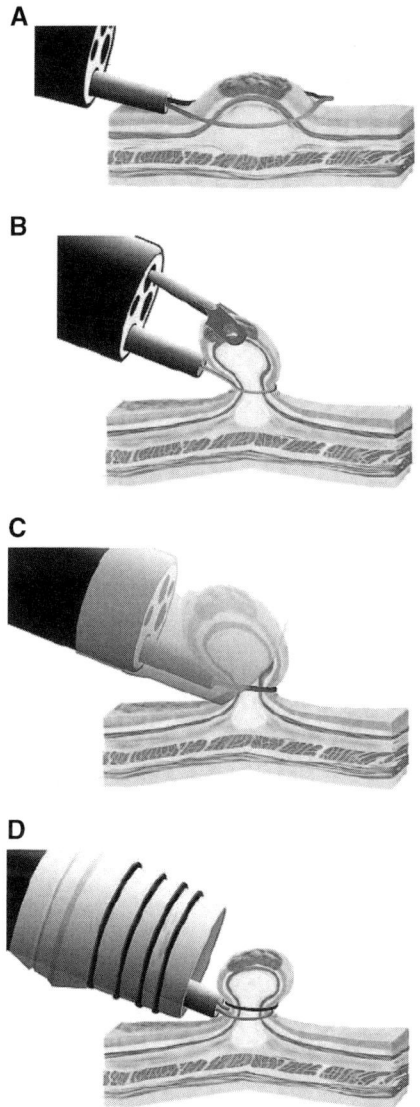

Fig. 3. Four types of commonly used EMR techniques. (*A*) Inject and cut technique. (*B*) Inject, lift, and cut technique. After submucosal injection, the mucosa is lifted with a pair of grasping forceps, which are passed through the second accessory channel of a double-channel endoscope. The forceps are retracted proximally while the snare is slightly advanced before it is closed at the base of the lesion. (*C*) EMR with cap. The cap has a gutter running circumferentially around its distal edge. This allows a specialized crescent-shaped snare to be preloaded inside the cap (not shown). After submucosal injection, the lesion is drawn into the cap by suction, and the snare is closed snugly. The snared lesion is released from the cap and resected. (*D*) EMR with ligation. This technique has been reported with or without prior submucosal injection. The lesion is snared by standard snare polypectomy after it has been ligated at its base with an endoscopic variceal ligation device. (*From* Soetikno RM, Gotoda T, Naka-nishi Y, et al. Endoscopic mucosal resection. Gastrointest Endosc 2003;57:567–79; with permission.)

Table 6
Endoscopic mucosal resection for Barrett's esophagus with high-grade dysplasia and adenocarcinoma

Reference	Method	Follow up in (mo) (range)	n	Complete remission	Recurrent or metachronous carcinoma (%)	Complication
Ell [80]	Inject-cut Ligate-cut	12	61 AC, 3 HGD	97% low risk group; 59% high risk group	14	Bleeding, 13%
May [81]	Inject-cut Ligate-cut	34 (24–60)	70 EMR	98%	30	Bleeding or stricture, 10%
Nijhawan [82]	Lift-cut Ligate-cut	14.6	25 (13 AC, 4 HGD, 8 other lesion)	NA	0	No complications
Seewald [83]	Cut without injection	9	12	100%	0	Bleeding, 13% Stricture, 17%
Giovannini [85]	Inject-cut Inject-lift-cut	18 (6–34)	9 AC, 12 HGD	85.7%	11	Bleeding, 19%
Combined data					11	12%

Abbreviations: AC, adenocarcinoma; EMR, endoscopic mucosal resection; HGD, high-grade dysplasia; NA, not available.

HGD, seven were treated with EMR, and 12 were treated with PDT. Complete remission was achieved in all patients, but after 9 months, 26% developed metachronous lesions requiring repeat local endoscopic therapy.

EMR has been used by other groups. Nijhawan and Wang [82] described 25 patients with BE with focal lesions who underwent EMR. On pathology, 13 patients had superficial adenocarcinoma, four patients had HGD, and eight patients had other low-risk lesions. EMR resulted in change of diagnosis in 44% of patients, with eight patients being reclassified from benign diagnoses to HGD or adenocarcinoma. Seven patients underwent additional PDT, and two patients received esophagectomy. There were no complications reported from the EMR. After 14.6 months of follow-up, no patient had cancer or HGD.

These studies suggest that EMR can be used to safely remove visible lesions from BE (Fig. 4). The tissue procurement through EMR can help in providing a more accurate diagnosis and aid in the further management of the patients. The high rate of metachronous or recurrent cancer suggests that the entire Barrett's mucosa needs to be ablated to prevent development of cancer.

Recently, Seewald and colleagues [83] reported the use of circumferential EMR in patients with BE containing multifocal high-grade intraepithelial neoplasia or intramucosal cancer and in patients with endoscopically nonidentifiable, early-stage, malignant mucosal change detected in random biopsy. In this study, 12 patients underwent circumferential EMR; five patients had multifocal lesions, and seven patients had no visible lesion. During a 9-month follow-up period, no recurrence of BE or malignancy was observed. Two of 12 patients (17%) developed strictures, and bleeding occurred in 4 of 31 (13%) EMR sessions. Additional studies on circumferential EMR suggest that the risk of developing esophageal stenosis can be minimized by creating a circumferential mucosal defect involving less than three fourths of the circumference of the esophagus [84].

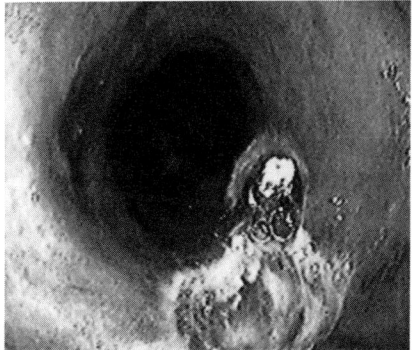

Fig. 4. Endoscopic appearance of the distal esophagus after endoscopic mucosal resection of nodular HGD in a patient who has BE. Complete mucosal healing with elimination of HGD was achieved, but intestinal metaplasia persisted, requiring endoscopic surveillance.

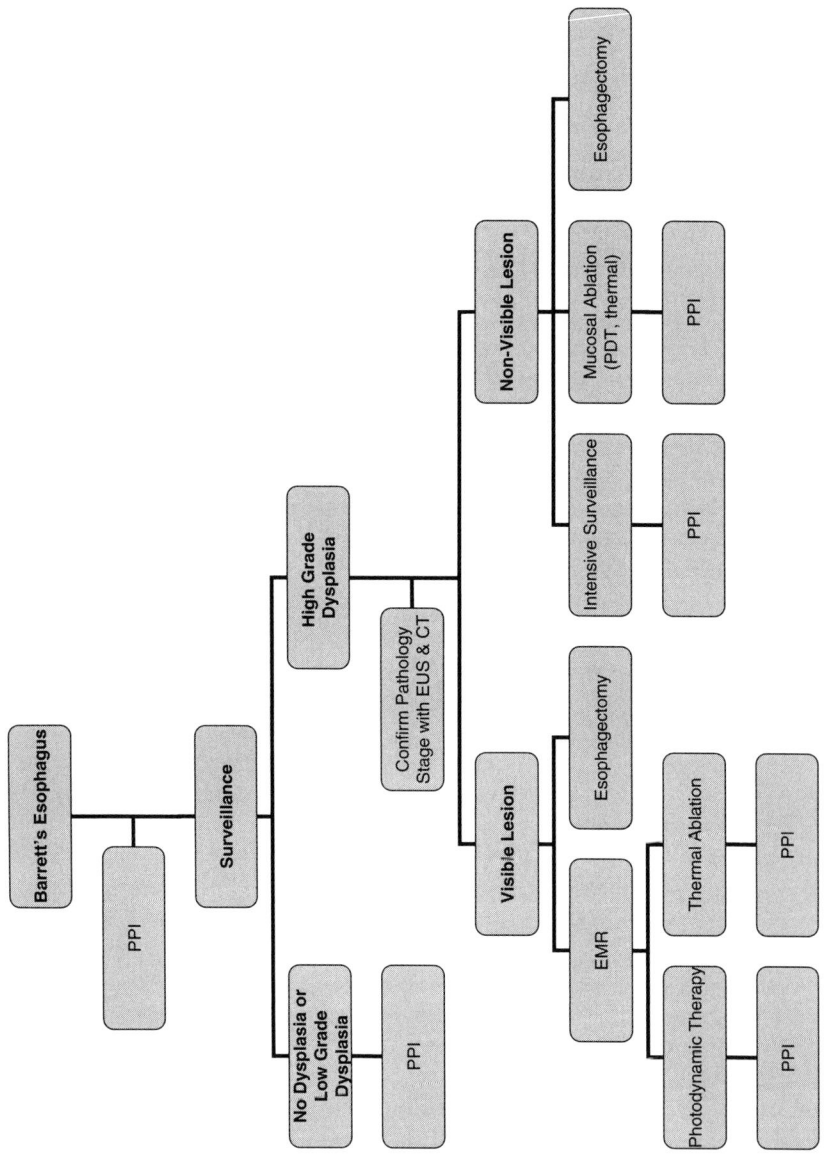

Another group in France reported their experience with 21 patients who underwent circumferential EMR spanning two separate sessions over 1 month to prevent esophageal stenosis. Twelve patients had high-grade intraepithelial neoplasia (HGIN), whereas nine patients had mucosal cancers. Eighteen patients had complete EMR resection. During mean follow-up of 18 months, two patients had local recurrence of HGIN and required repeat EMR. No patient reported dysphagia or had esophageal stenosis identified on endoscopy as a complication of EMR. Fifteen of 20 patients had squamous cells completely replacing the removed Barrett's mucosa [85].

In summary, current studies show that EMR can be used to remove dysplastic and early neoplastic Barrett's mucosa with minimal morbidity and mortality. However, with the high rate of metachronous lesions developing, EMR should be used to remove the entire Barrett's mucosa.

Summary

With the increase in the rate of esophageal adenocarcinoma in the United States and the Western world matched with the high morbidity and mortality of esophagectomy, there is an increasing need for new and effective techniques to treat and prevent esophageal adenocarcinoma. A wide variety of endoscopic mucosal ablative techniques have been developed for early esophageal neoplasia. However, long-term control of neoplastic risk has not been demonstrated. Most studies show that specialized intestinal metaplasia may persist underneath neosquamous mucosa, posing a risk for subsequent neoplastic progression.

Based on the data reviewed, we do not advise endoscopic mucosal ablation for patients with BE with no dysplasia or with LGD. Future studies need to show that this preventive interventional strategy can decrease cancer risk with minimal complications as compared with the current standard of care. We recommend endoscopic surveillance in addition to the use of PPIs for patients who have BE with no dysplasia or with LGD (Fig. 5). For patients with HGD, we recommend repeat endoscopy and biopsy along with pathologic confirmation of HGD by an expert pathologist. In cases of HGD, accurate staging work-up using endoscopic ultrasound and chest/upper abdomen CT should be performed to rule out extension into the submucosa or muscularis propria and metastasis to lymph node or distant structures. After thorough evaluation, if a patient is found to have HGD limited to the mucosa and if they decline surgical management, endoscopic ablation methods should be considered under a study protocol. Endoscopic mucosal resection should be offered to patients with visible lesions because this can be a potentially curative treatment and can offer histopathologic staging and assess-

Fig. 5. Algorithm for the management of BE with and without dysplasia. This algorithm represents the opinion of the authors based on current evidence and may vary depending on available local resources and expertise.

ment of the adequacy of therapy. Due to the concern for the development of metachronous lesions, complete Barrett's mucosal ablation should be considered using a combination of PDT, EMR, or thermal ablation. In patients who have HGD without visible lesions, complete Barrett's mucosal ablation should be considered using a combination of PDT, EMR, or thermal ablation (see Fig. 5).

References

[1] Cameron AJ, Ott BJ, Payne WS. The incidence of adenocarcinoma in columnar-lined (Barrett's) esophagus. N Engl J Med 1985;313:857–9.

[2] Spechler SJ. Clinical practice: Barrett's esophagus. N Engl J Med 2002;346:836–42.

[3] Hamilton S. Pathogenesis of columnar cell lined (Barrett's) esophagus. In: Spechler SJ, editor. Barrett's esophagus: pathophysiology, diagnosis, and management. New York: Elsevier; 1985. p. 29–37.

[4] Schnell TG, Sontag SJ, Chejfec G, et al. Long-term nonsurgical management of Barrett's esophagus with high-grade dysplasia. Gastroenterology 2001;120:1607–19.

[5] Levine DS. Management of dysplasia in the columnar-lined esophagus. Gastroenterol Clin North Am 1997;26:613–34.

[6] Pera M, Trastek VF, Carpenter HA, et al. Barrett's esophagus with high-grade dysplasia: an indication for esophagectomy? Ann Thorac Surg 1992;54:199–204.

[7] Edwards MJ, Gable DR, Lentsch AB, et al. The rationale for esophagectomy as the optimal therapy for Barrett's esophagus with high-grade dysplasia. Ann Surg 1996;223:585–9 [discussion: 589–91].

[8] Falk GW, Rice TW, Goldblum JR, et al. Jumbo biopsy forceps protocol still misses unsuspected cancer in Barrett's esophagus with high-grade dysplasia. Gastrointest Endosc 1999;49:170–6.

[9] Romagnoli R, Collard JM, Gutschow C, et al. Outcomes of dysplasia arising in Barrett's esophagus: a dynamic view. J Am Coll Surg 2003;197:365–71.

[10] Zaninotto G, Parenti AR, Ruol A, et al. Oesophageal resection for high-grade dysplasia in Barrett's oesophagus. Br J Surg 2000;87:1102–5.

[11] Heitmiller RF, Redmond M, Hamilton SR. Barrett's esophagus with high-grade dysplasia: an indication for prophylactic esophagectomy. Ann Surg 1996;224:66–71.

[12] Holscher AH, Bollschweiler E, Schroder W, et al. Prognostic differences between early squamous-cell and adenocarcinoma of the esophagus. Dis Esophagus 1997;10:179–84.

[13] Fitzgerald RC, Omary MB, Triadafilopoulos G. Dynamic effects of acid on Barrett's esophagus: an ex vivo proliferation and differentiation model. J Clin Invest 1996;98:2120–8.

[14] Shirvani VN, Ouatu-Lascar R, Kaur BS, et al. Cyclooxygenase 2 expression in Barrett's esophagus and adenocarcinoma: ex vivo induction by bile salts and acid exposure. Gastroenterology 2000;118:487–96.

[15] Souza RF, Shewmake K, Terada LS, et al. Acid exposure activates the mitogen-activated protein kinase pathways in Barrett's esophagus. Gastroenterology 2002;12:299–307.

[16] Ouatu-Lascar R, Fitzgerald RC, Triadafilopoulos G. Differentiation and proliferation in Barrett's esophagus and the effects of acid suppression. Gastroenterology 1999;117:327–35.

[17] Peters FT, Ganesh S, Kuipers EJ, et al. Endoscopic regression of Barrett's oesophagus during omeprazole treatment: a randomised double blind study. Gut 1999;45:489–94.

[18] Sharma P, Sampliner RE, Camargo E. Normalization of esophageal pH with high-dose proton pump inhibitor therapy does not result in regression of Barrett's esophagus. Am J Gastroenterol 1997;92:582–5.

[19] Gore S, Healey CJ, Sutton R, et al. Regression of columnar lined (Barrett's) oesophagus with continuous omeprazole therapy. Aliment Pharmacol Ther 1993;7:623–8.

[20] Sampliner RE. Effect of up to 3 years of high-dose lansoprazole on Barrett's esophagus. Am J Gastroenterol 1994;89:1844–8.

[21] Cooper BT, Neumann CS, Cox MA, et al. Continuous treatment with omeprazole 20 mg daily for up to 6 years in Barrett's oesophagus. Aliment Pharmacol Ther 1998;12:893–7.

[22] Sagar PM, Ackroyd R, Hosie KB, et al. Regression and progression of Barrett's oesophagus after antireflux surgery. Br J Surg 1995;82:806–10.

[23] Hofstetter WL, Peters JH, DeMeester TR, et al. Long-term outcome of antireflux surgery in patients with Barrett's esophagus. Ann Surg 2001;234:532–8 [discussion: 538–9].

[24] Sampliner RE, Hixson LJ, Fennerty MB, et al. Regression of Barrett's esophagus by laser ablation in an anacid environment. Dig Dis Sci 1993;38:365–8.

[25] Berenson MM, Johnson TD, Markowitz NR, et al. Restoration of squamous mucosa after ablation of Barrett's esophageal epithelium. Gastroenterology 1993;104:1686–91.

[26] Dumoulin FL, Terjung B, Neubrand M, et al. Treatment of Barrett's esophagus by endoscopic argon plasma coagulation. Endoscopy 1997;29:751–3.

[27] Mork H, Barth T, Kreipe HH, et al. Reconstitution of squamous epithelium in Barrett's oeso-phagus with endoscopic argon plasma coagulation: a prospective study. Scand J Gastroenterol 1998;33:1130–4.

[28] Overholt BF, Panjehpour M. Barrett's esophagus: photodynamic therapy for ablation of dys-plasia, reduction of specialized mucosa, and treatment of superficial esophageal cancer. Gastro-intest Endosc 1995;42:64–70.

[29] Salo JA, Salminen JT, Kiviluoto TA, et al. Treatment of Barrett's esophagus by endoscopic laser ablation and antireflux surgery. Ann Surg 1998;227:40–4.

[30] Tigges H, Fuchs KH, Maroske J, et al. Combination of endoscopic argon plasma coagulation and antireflux surgery for treatment of Barrett's esophagus. J Gastrointest Surg 2001;5:251–9.

[31] Abbas AE, Deschamps C, Cassivi SD, et al. Barrett's esophagus: the role of laparoscopic fundoplication. Ann Thorac Surg 2004;77:393–6.

[32] Oelschlager BK, Barreca M, Chang L, et al. Clinical and pathologic response of Barrett's esophagus to laparoscopic antireflux surgery. Ann Surg 2003;238:458–64 [discussion: 464–6].

[33] Csendes A. Surgical treatment of Barrett's esophagus: 1980–2003. World J Surg 2004;28: 225–31.

[34] Parrilla P, Martinez de Haro LF, Ortiz A, et al. Long-term results of a randomized prospective study comparing medical and surgical treatment of Barrett's esophagus. Ann Surg 2003;237: 291–8.

[35] Corey KE, Schmitz SM, Shaheen NJ. Does a surgical antireflux procedure decrease the incidence of esophageal adenocarcinoma in Barrett's esophagus? A meta-analysis. Am J Gastroenterol 2003;98:2390–4.

[36] Yeh RW, Gerson LB, Triadafilopoulos G. Efficacy of esomeprazole in controlling reflux symp-toms, intraesophageal, and intragastric pH in patients with Barrett's esophagus. Dis Esophagus 2003;16:193–8.

[37] Klaus A, Hinder RA. Medical therapy versus antireflux surgery in Barrett's esophagus: what is the best therapeutic approach? Dig Dis 2000;18:224–31.

[38] Byrne JP, Armstrong GR, Attwood SE. Restoration of the normal squamous lining in Barrett's esophagus by argon beam plasma coagulation. Am J Gastroenterol 1998;93:1810–5.

[39] Basu KK, Pick B, Bale R, et al. Efficacy and one year follow up of argon plasma coagulation therapy for ablation of Barrett's oesophagus: factors determining persistence and recurrence of Barrett's epithelium. Gut 2002;51:776–80.

[40] Grade AJ, Shah IA, Medlin SM, et al. The efficacy and safety of argon plasma coagulation therapy in Barrett's esophagus. Gastrointest Endosc 1999;50:18–22.

[41] Morris CD, Byrne JP, Armstrong GR, et al. Prevention of the neoplastic progression of Barrett's oesophagus by endoscopic argon beam plasma ablation. Br J Surg 2001;88:1357–62.

[42] Kahaleh M, Van Laethem JL, Nagy N, et al. Long-term follow-up and factors predictive of recurrence in Barrett's esophagus treated by argon plasma coagulation and acid suppression. Endoscopy 2002;34:950–5.

[43] Schulz H, Miehlke S, Antos D, et al. Ablation of Barrett's epithelium by endoscopic argon plasma coagulation in combination with high-dose omeprazole. Gastrointest Endosc 2000;51: 659–63.

[44] Pereira-Lima JC, Busnello JV, Saul C, et al. High power setting argon plasma coagulation for the eradication of Barrett's esophagus. Am J Gastroenterol 2000;95:1661–8.

[45] Van Laethem JL, Cremer M, Peny MO, et al. Eradication of Barrett's mucosa with argon plasma coagulation and acid suppression: immediate and mid term results. Gut 1998;43:747–51.

[46] Pagani M, Granelli P, Chella B, et al. Barrett's esophagus: combined treatment using argon plasma coagulation and laparoscopic antireflux surgery. Dis Esophagus 2003;16:279–83.

[47] Morino M, Rebecchi F, Giaccone C, et al. Endoscopic ablation of Barrett's esophagus using argon plasma coagulation (APC) following surgical laparoscopic fundoplication. Surg Endosc 2003;17:539–42.

[48] Ackroyd R, Tam W, Schoeman M, et al. Prospective randomized controlled trial of argon plasma coagulation ablation vs. endoscopic surveillance of patients with Barrett's esophagus after antireflux surgery. Gastrointest Endosc 2004;59:1–7.

[49] Pinotti AC, Cecconello I, Filho FM, et al. Endoscopic ablation of Barrett's esophagus using argon plasma coagulation: a prospective study after fundoplication. Dis Esophagus 2004;17: 243–6.

[50] Hage M, Siersema PD, van Dekken H, et al. 5-aminolevulinic acid photodynamic therapy versus argon plasma coagulation for ablation of Barrett's oesophagus: a randomised trial. Gut 2004;53: 785–90.

[51] Van Laethem JL, Peny MO, Salmon I, et al. Intramucosal adenocarcinoma arising under squamous re-epithelialisation of Barrett's oesophagus. Gut 2000;46:574–7.

[52] Van Laethem JL, Jagodzinski R, Peny MO, et al. Argon plasma coagulation in the treatment of Barrett's high-grade dysplasia and in situ adenocarcinoma. Endoscopy 2001;33:257–61.

[53] Shand A, Dallal H, Palmer K, et al. Adenocarcinoma arising in columnar lined oesophagus following treatment with argon plasma coagulation. Gut 2001;48:580–1.

[54] Attwood SE, Lewis CJ, Caplin S, et al. Argon beam plasma coagulation as therapy for high-grade dysplasia in Barrett's esophagus. Clin Gastroenterol Hepatol 2003;1:258–63.

[55] Sampliner RE, Fennerty B, Garewal HS. Reversal of Barrett's esophagus with acid suppression and multipolar electrocoagulation: preliminary results. Gastrointest Endosc 1996;44:532–5.

[56] Kovacs BJ, Chen YK, Lewis TD, et al. Successful reversal of Barrett's esophagus with multipolar electrocoagulation despite inadequate acid suppression. Gastrointest Endosc 1999;49:547–53.

[57] Montes CG, Brandalise NA, Deliza R, et al. Antireflux surgery followed by bipolar electrocoagulation in the treatment of Barrett's esophagus. Gastrointest Endosc 1999;50:173–7.

[58] Sharma P, Bhattacharyya A, Garewal HS, et al. Durability of new squamous epithelium after endoscopic reversal of Barrett's esophagus. Gastrointest Endosc 1999;50:159–64.

[59] Sampliner RE, Faigel D, Fennerty MB, et al. Effective and safe endoscopic reversal of nondysplastic Barrett's esophagus with thermal electrocoagulation combined with high-dose acid inhibition: a multicenter study. Gastrointest Endosc 2001;53:554–8.

[60] Jackson FW, Husson M, Wright S, et al. Eradication of Barrett's epithelium with multipolar electrocoagulation. Gastrointest Endosc 1997;45:AB71–187.

[61] Guelrud M, Herrera I. Multipolar electrocoagulation in the treatment of Barrett's esophagus. Gastrointest Endosc 1997;45:AB69.

[62] Luman W, Lessels AM, Palmer KR. Failure of Nd-YAG photocoagulation therapy as treatment for Barrett's oesophagus: a pilot study. Eur J Gastroenterol Hepatol 1996;8:627–30.

[63] Weston AP, Sharma P. Neodymium:yttrium-aluminum garnet contact laser ablation of Barrett's high grade dysplasia and early adenocarcinoma. Am J Gastroenterol 2002;97:2998–3006.

[64] Fisher RS, Bromer MQ, Thomas RM, et al. Predictors of recurrent specialized intestinal metaplasia after complete laser ablation. Am J Gastroenterol 2003;98:1945–51.

[65] Dougherty TJ, Gomer CJ, Henderson BW, et al. Photodynamic therapy. J Natl Cancer Inst 1998; 90:889–905.

[66] Claydon PE, Ackroyd R. 5-Aminolaevulinic acid-induced photodynamic therapy and photo-detection in Barrett's esophagus. Dis Esophagus 2004;17:205–12.

[67] Ackroyd R, Brown N, Vernon D, et al. 5-Aminolevulinic acid photosensitization of dysplastic Barrett's esophagus: a pharmacokinetic study. Photochem Photobiol 1999;70:656–62.

[68] Etienne J, Dorme N, Bourg-Heckly G, et al. Photodynamic therapy with green light and

m-tetrahydroxyphenyl chlorin for intramucosal adenocarcinoma and high-grade dysplasia in Barrett's esophagus. Gastrointest Endosc 2004;59:880–9.

[69] Prosst RL, Wolfsen HC, Gahlen J. Photodynamic therapy for esophageal diseases: a clinical update. Endoscopy 2003;35:1059–68.

[70] Overholt BF, Panjehpour M, Haydek JM. Photodynamic therapy for Barrett's esophagus: follow-up in 100 patients. Gastrointest Endosc 1999;49:1–7.

[71] Wolfsen HC, Woodward TA, Raimondo M. Photodynamic therapy for dysplastic Barrett esophagus and early esophageal adenocarcinoma. Mayo Clin Proc 2002;77:1176–81.

[72] Wang KK. Current status of photodynamic therapy of Barrett's esophagus. Gastrointest Endosc 1999;49:S20–3.

[73] van Hillegersberg R, Haringsma J, ten Kate FJ, et al. Invasive carcinoma after endoscopic ablative therapy for high-grade dysplasia in Barrett's oesophagus. Dig Surg 2003;20:440–4.

[74] Overholt BF, Panjehpour M, Halberg DL. Photodynamic therapy for Barrett's esophagus with dysplasia and/or early stage carcinoma: long-term results. Gastrointest Endosc 2003;58:183–8.

[75] Ackroyd R, Brown NJ, Davis MF, et al. Photodynamic therapy for dysplastic Barrett's oesophagus: a prospective, double blind, randomised, placebo controlled trial. Gut 2000;47:612–7.

[76] Ackroyd R, Kelty CJ, Brown NJ, et al. Eradication of dysplastic Barrett's oesophagus using photodynamic therapy: long-term follow-up. Endoscopy 2003;35:496–501.

[77] Barr H, Shepherd NA, Dix A, et al. Eradication of high-grade dysplasia in columnar-lined (Barrett's) oesophagus by photodynamic therapy with endogenously generated protoporphyrin IX. Lancet 1996;348:584–5.

[78] Gossner L, Stolte M, Sroka R, et al. Photodynamic ablation of high-grade dysplasia and early cancer in Barrett's esophagus by means of 5-aminolevulinic acid. Gastroenterology 1998;114:448–55.

[79] Javaid B, Watt P, Krasner N. Photodynamic therapy (PDT) for oesophageal dysplasia and early carcinoma with mTHPC (m-tetrahydroxyphenyl chlorin): a preliminary study. Lasers Med Sci 2002;17:51–6.

[80] Ell C, May A, Gossner L, et al. Endoscopic mucosal resection of early cancer and high-grade dysplasia in Barrett's esophagus. Gastroenterology 2000;118:670–7.

[81] May A, Gossner L, Pech O, et al. Local endoscopic therapy for intraepithelial high-grade neoplasia and early adenocarcinoma in Barrett's oesophagus: acute-phase and intermediate results of a new treatment approach. Eur J Gastroenterol Hepatol 2002;14:1085–91.

[82] Nijhawan PK, Wang KK. Endoscopic mucosal resection for lesions with endoscopic features suggestive of malignancy and high-grade dysplasia within Barrett's esophagus. Gastrointest Endosc 2000;52:328–32.

[83] Seewald S, Akaraviputh T, Seitz U, et al. Circumferential EMR and complete removal of Barrett's epithelium: a new approach to management of Barrett's esophagus containing high-grade intraepithelial neoplasia and intramucosal carcinoma. Gastrointest Endosc 2003;57:854–9.

[84] Katada C, Muto M, Manabe T, et al. Esophageal stenosis after endoscopic mucosal resection of superficial esophageal lesions. Gastrointest Endosc 2003;57:165–9.

[85] Giovannini M, Bories E, Pesenti C, et al. Circumferential endoscopic mucosal resection in Barrett's esophagus with high-grade intraepithelial neoplasia or mucosal cancer: preliminary results in 21 patients. Endoscopy 2004;36:782–7.

[86] Barham CP, Jones RL, Biddlestone LR, et al. Photothermal laser ablation of Barrett's oesophagus: endoscopic and histological evidence of squamous re-epithelialisation. Gut 1997;41:281–4.

[87] Gossner L, May A, Stolte M, et al. KTP laser destruction of dysplasia and early cancer in columnar-lined Barrett's esophagus. Gastrointest Endosc 1999;49:8–12.

[88] Bowers SP, Mattar SG, Waring PJ, et al. KTP laser ablation of Barrett's esophagus after anti-reflux surgery results in long-term loss of intestinal metaplasia: potassium-titanyl-phosphate. Surg Endosc 2003;17:49–54.

[89] Norberto L, Polese L, Angriman I, et al. High-energy laser therapy of Barrett's esophagus: preliminary results. World J Surg 2004;28:350–4.

[90] Wolfsen HC. Photodynamic therapy for mucosal esophageal adenocarcinoma and dysplastic Barrett's esophagus. Dig Dis 2002;20:5–17.

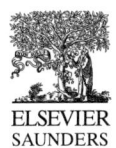

ELSEVIER
SAUNDERS

Gastrointest Endoscopy Clin N Am
15 (2005) 399–429

GASTROINTESTINAL
ENDOSCOPY CLINICS
OF NORTH AMERICA

Endoscopic Ultrasound for Luminal Malignancies

Raghuram P. Reddy, MD[a], Michael J. Levy, MD[a],*, Maurits J. Wiersema, MD[b]

[a]Developmental Endoscopy Unit, Division of Gastroenterology and Hepatology, Mayo Clinic,
200 First Street SW, Rochester, MN 55905, USA
[b]GI Consultants, Inc., 1900 Carew Street, Suite 1, Fort Wayne, IN 46805, USA

Luminal gastrointestinal (GI) tract cancers are responsible for substantial morbidity and mortality. In the United States, an estimated 187,000 new esophageal, gastric, and colorectal cancers will be diagnosed this year, resulting in more than 82,000 cancer-related deaths [1]. Accurate staging is required to determine the prognosis, to guide management, and to improve patient outcomes. Since the first pairing of ultrasonography with endoscopy in 1980 [2], technologic advances and the increased availability of trained endosonographers have propelled endoscopic ultrasonography (EUS) to the forefront of luminal GI cancer staging. EUS produces high-resolution images of the GI tract wall and adjacent structures, which are necessary to optimize locoregional staging [3,4]. The development of linear EUS allows fine needle aspiration (FNA) of lesions within and outside the GI tract wall, which further enhances staging accuracy. EUS is regarded as an essential component of initial staging for luminal GI cancers and is increasingly used for restaging after chemoradiation and for postresection surveillance. In this article we discuss the role of EUS for evaluating luminal GI cancers.

Luminal cancer staging

Initial evaluation of patients with luminal GI cancers centers on the assessment of operative risk and tumor stage. Comorbid conditions may preclude a

---

* Corresponding author.
E-mail address: levy.michael@mayo.edu (M.J. Levy).

1052-5157/05/$ – see front matter © 2005 Elsevier Inc. All rights reserved.
doi:10.1016/j.giec.2005.03.004

Box 1. Esophageal cancer staging

Primary tumor (T)

- TX: Primary tumor cannot be assessed
- T0: No evidence of primary tumor
- Tis: Carcinoma in situ
- T1: Tumor invades lamina propria or submucosa
- T2: Tumor invades muscularis propria
- T3: Tumor invades adventitia
- T4: Tumor invades adjacent structures

Regional lymph nodes (N)

- NX: Regional lymph nodes cannot be assessed
- N0: No regional lymph node metastasis
- N1: Regional lymph node metastasis

Distant metastasis (M)

- MX: Distant metastasis cannot be assessed
- M0: No distant metastasis
- M1: Distant metastasis
- Tumors of the lower thoracic esophagus:
    M1a: Metastasis in celiac lymph nodes
    M1b: Other distant metastasis
- Tumors of the midthoracic esophagus:
    M1a: Not applicable
    M1b: Nonregional lymph nodes or other distant metastasis
- Tumors of the upper thoracic esophagus:
    M1a: Metastasis in cervical nodes
    M1b: Other distant metastasis

AJCC stage groupings

- Stage 0
    Tis, N0, M0
- Stage I
    T1, N0, M0
- Stage IIA
    T2, N0, M0
    T3, N0, M0

- Stage IIB
    - T1, N1, M0
    - T2, N1, M0
- Stage III
    - T3, N1, M0
    - T4, any N, M0
- Stage IV
    - Any T, any N, M1
- Stage IVA
    - Any T, any N, M1a
- Stage IVB
    - Any T, any N, M1b

From American Joint Committee on Cancer. Esophagus. In: AJCC cancer staging manual. 6th edition. New York: Springer; 2002. p. 91–8.

---

patient with a potentially resectable tumor from undergoing surgery. Accurate luminal cancer staging is necessary to determine the prognosis, to guide administration of chemoradiation, to distinguish patients with potentially resectable localized cancers, and to select the ideal means and extent of resection. Early detection is crucial for improving prognosis, and the determination of resectability is required to avoid unnecessary surgical intervention in favor of less morbid interventions. Accurate staging helps standardize study protocols and facilitates data exchange, which enhances our research efforts and improves patient care.

Halsted [5] and others in the early 20th century observed that solid tumors progress through a series of stages, starting at the primary tumor site and spreading to lymphatics and distant organs. Pierre Denoix developed the Tumor (T), Node (N), Metastasis (M) classification system for cancer staging in the 1940s, which was adopted by the International Union Against Cancer (UICC) in 1953 [6]. The American Joint Committee on Cancer (AJCC) was organized in 1959 to develop a system of clinical staging for cancer. Since its inception, the AJCC has followed the TNM system. In 1987 the AJCC and UICC TNM systems were unified, leading to greater worldwide acceptance (Boxes 1–3). Cancers are further grouped as stage I through IV based on homogeneity with respect to survival. Staging as defined by TNM classification depends on characteristics of the primary tumor, namely, depth of tumor infiltration into the lumen wall and adjacent structures (T stage), regional lymph node involvement (N stage), and the presence or absence of distant metastasis (M stage). Advanced tumor depth and lymph node metastases have been shown to be poor prognostic indicators [7–16]. Some data suggest that nodal metastasis may have the greatest impact on survival [17–21]. Staging usually begins with noninvasive

Box 2. Gastric cancer staging

Primary tumor (T)

- TX: Primary tumor cannot be assessed
- T0: No evidence of primary tumor
- Tis: Carcinoma in situ: intraepithelial tumor without invasion of the lamina propria
- T1: Tumor invades lamina propria or submucosa
- T2: Tumor invades the muscularis propria or the subserosa
    T2a: Tumor invades muscularis propria
    T2b: Tumor invades subserosa
- T3: Tumor penetrates the serosa (visceral peritoneum) without invading adjacent structures
- T4: Tumor invades adjacent structures

Regional lymph nodes (N)

- NX: Regional lymph node(s) cannot be assessed
- N0: No regional lymph node metastasis
- N1: Metastasis in 1 to 6 regional lymph nodes
- N2: Metastasis in 7 to 15 regional lymph nodes
- N3: Metastasis in more than 15 regional lymph nodes

Distant metastasis (M)

- MX: Distant metastasis cannot be assessed
- M0: No distant metastasis
- M1: Distant metastasis

AJCC stage groupings

- Stage 0
    Tis, N0, M0
- Stage IA
    T1, N0, M0
- Stage IB
    T1, N1, M0
    T2a, N0, M0
    T2b, N0, M0
- Stage II
    T1, N2, M0
    T2a, N1, M0

```
            T2b, N1, M0
            T3, N0, M0
          • Stage IIIA
            T2a, N2, M0
            T2b, N2, M0
            T3, N1, M0
            T4, N0, M0
          • Stage IIIB
            T3, N2, M0
          • Stage IV
            T4, N1, M0
            T4, N2, M0
            T4, N3, M0
            T1, N3, M0
            T2, N3, M0
            T3, N3, M0
            Any T, any N, M1
```

From American Joint Committee on Cancer. Stomach. In: AJCC Cancer Staging Manual. 6th edition. New York: Springer; 2002. p. 99–112.

imaging, such as CT, MRI, or PET, which are generally superior to EUS for excluding distant metastatic disease. EUS is subsequently performed and offers a clear advantage over noninvasive imaging modalities with regard to locoregional staging accuracy for GI luminal cancers [22–36].

Endoscopic ultrasonography appearance

Primary tumor

EUS imaging of the GI wall lumen identifies five distinct layers that appear as hyperechoic (bright or echorich) layers alternating with hypoechoic (dark or echo-poor) layers (Fig. 1 and Table 1) [37]. These layers are numbered from one to five, with the first layer located closest to the transducer (luminal side) and the fifth layer located in the outermost (adventitial or serosal) layer. The first layer is hyperechoic and represents the interface between the balloon and superficial mucosa. The deep mucosa appears as a hypoechoic (or black) layer. The central hyperechoic layer accounts for the submucosa and an interface echo. The muscularis propria appears as a hypoechoic fourth layer in which one can often visualize a thin hyperechoic line representing an interface echo between the inner circular and outer longitudinal muscle layers. The outermost hyperechoic layer corresponds to the adventitia that surrounds the esophagus and dis-

Box 3. Rectal cancer staging

Primary tumor (T)

- TX: Primary tumor cannot be assessed
- T0: No evidence of primary tumor
- Tis: Carcinoma in situ: intraepithelial or invasion of the lamina propria
- T1: Tumor invades submucosa
- T2: Tumor invades muscularis propria
- T3: Tumor invades through the muscularis propria into the subserosa, or into nonperitonealized pericolic or perirectal tissues
- T4: Tumor directly invades other organs or structures or perforates visceral peritoneum

Regional lymph nodes (N)

- NX: Regional nodes cannot be assessed
- N0: No regional lymph node metastasis
- N1: Metastasis in one to three regional lymph nodes
- N2: Metastasis in four or more regional lymph nodes

Distant metastasis (M)

- MX: Distant metastasis cannot be assessed
- M0: No distant metastasis
- M1: Distant metastasis

AJCC stage groupings

- Stage 0
    Tis, N0, M0
- Stage I
    T1, N0, M0
    T2, N0, M0
- Stage IIA
    T3, N0, M0
- Stage IIB
    T4, N0, M0
- Stage IIIA
    T1, N1, M0
    T2, N1, M0

- Stage IIIB
    T3, N1, M0
    T4, N1, M0
- Stage IIIC
    Any T, N2, M0
- Stage IV
    Any T, Any N, M1

From American Joint Committee on Cancer. Colon and rectum. In: AJCC Cancer Staging Manual. 6th edition. New York: Springer; 2002. p. 111–23.

tal two thirds of the rectum or serosa that overlies the stomach, small intestine, and proximal one third of the rectum.

Unlike standard dedicated echoendoscopes, ultrasound miniprobes operate at substantially higher frequencies (up to 30 MHz), providing higher-resolution imaging and allowing delineation of nine wall layers [23,38]. The first and second layers represent the superficial mucosa (hyper- and hypoechoic, respectively). The third layer is hyperechoic and represents the lamina propria. The fourth layer, which is hypoechoic, signifies the muscularis mucosa. The fifth layer

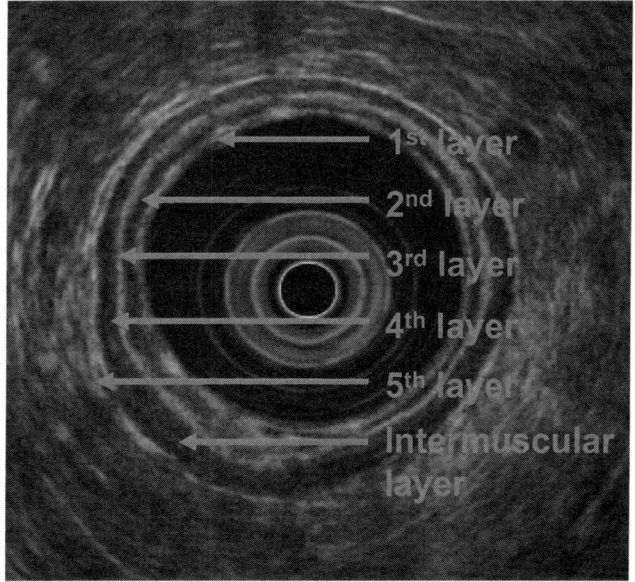

Fig. 1. Gastrointestinal wall layers as demonstrated by EUS. Five distinct layers are present that appear as hyperechoic (bright or echorich) layers alternating with hypoechoic (dark or echopoor) layers.

Table 1
Gastrointestinal wall layers as detected by standard endoscopic ultrasound

Layer	Sonographic appearance	Histologic correlation
First[a]	Hyperechoic	Interface between superficial mucosa and water-filled balloon or water-filled lumen
Second	Hypoechoic	Deep mucosa
Third	Hyperechoic	Submucosa
Fourth	Hypoechoic	Muscularis propria
Fifth[b]	Hyperechoic	Adventitia or serosa

[a] The first layer is positioned closest to the transducer (luminal side).
[b] The fifth layer is the outermost (adventitial or serosal) layer.

or submucosa is hyperechoic. The sixth, seventh, and eighth layers (appearing hypo-, hyper-, and hypoechoic, respectively) indicate the inner circular muscle, intervening interface echo, and outer longitudinal muscle fibers of the muscularis propria. The ninth layer accounts for the adventitia and appears hyperechoic. The greater resolution of these miniprobes may have particular value for superficial esophageal cancers for which nonsurgical therapies, such as endoscopic mucosal resection and photodynamic therapy, may be appropriate [38,39].

Luminal GI cancers ultrasonographically appear as hypoechoic areas that infiltrate in a centripetal fashion from the mucosa to deeper tissues, resulting in disruption of normal wall layers (Table 2). T1 tumors infiltrate the mucosa (layer 1 with or without layer 2) and may extend to the submucosa (layer 3), but no deeper (Fig. 2). T2 tumors infiltrate as deep as the muscularis propria (layer 4) (Fig. 3), whereas T3 tumors infiltrate into the adventitia or serosa (layer 5) (Fig. 4). T4 tumors directly infiltrate adjacent major structures, such as the heart or diaphragm for esophageal cancers and prostate or vagina for rectal cancers (Fig. 5). These T-staging criteria hold true for all GI luminal cancers except gastric cancer, which may penetrate the muscularis propria and infiltrate the gastrocolic or gastrohepatic ligaments or into the greater or lesser omentum

Table 2
T staging according to depth of primary tumor infiltration[a]

Tumor stage	EUS appearance
T1	Tumor infiltrates the mucosa with or without submucosa (layers 1–3)
T2	Tumor infiltrates the muscularis propria (layer 4)
T3	Tumor infiltrates the adventitia or serosa (layer 5)
T4	Tumor infiltrates adjacent major structures

Abbreviation: EUS, endoscopic ultrasonography.
[a] These T-staging criteria hold true for all GI luminal cancers except gastric cancer, which may penetrate the muscularis propria and infiltrate the gastrocolic or gastrohepatic ligaments or into the greater or lesser omentum without perforating the overlying visceral peritoneum. If perforation occurs of the overlying visceral peritoneum, the tumor should be classified as T3.

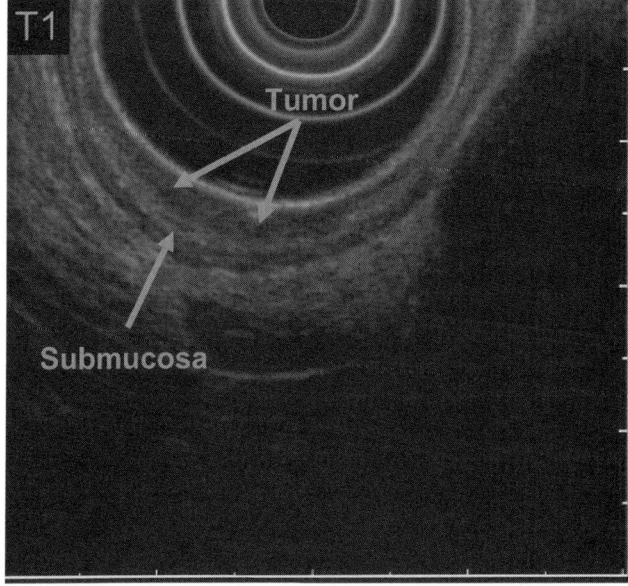

Fig. 2. The esophageal cancer involves the first and second wall layers. Just deep to the tumor, the submucosa is intact, and there is no evidence of tumor infiltration into the muscularis propria (T1).

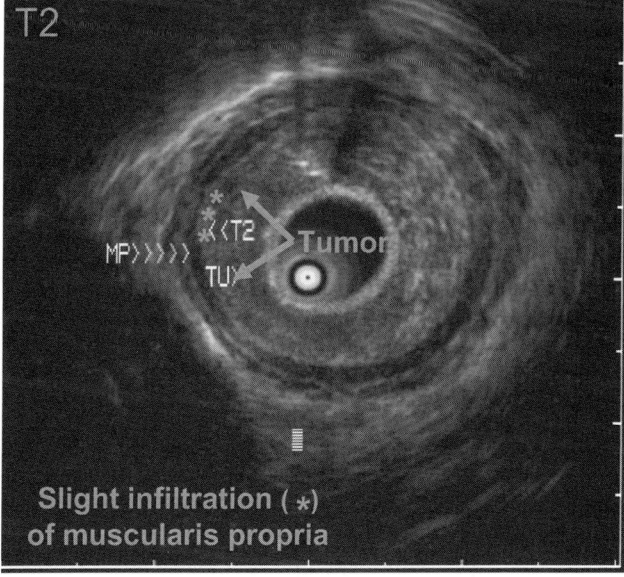

Fig. 3. The esophageal cancer involves the first, second, and third wall layers, corresponding to the superficial mucosa, deep mucosa, and submucosa, respectively. Irregularity of the interface between the third and fourth wall layers results from focal tumor infiltration into the muscularis propria (T2).

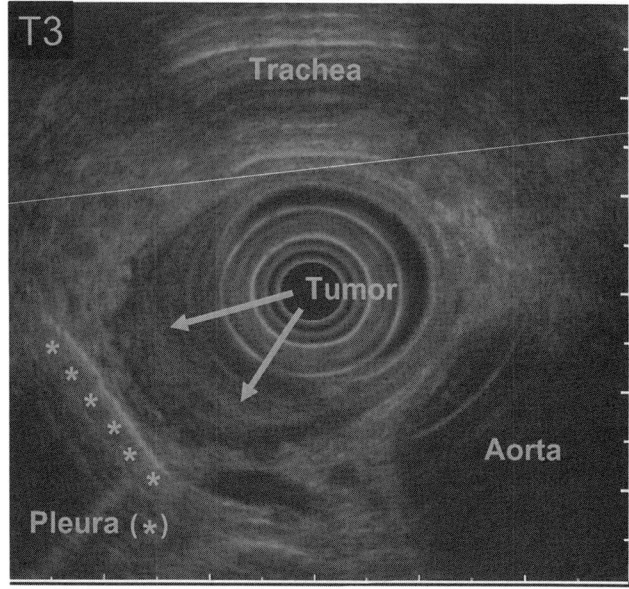

Fig. 4. The esophageal cancer extends through all wall layers. Surrounding structures, such as the right pleura, are not involved, and the tumor is stage T3.

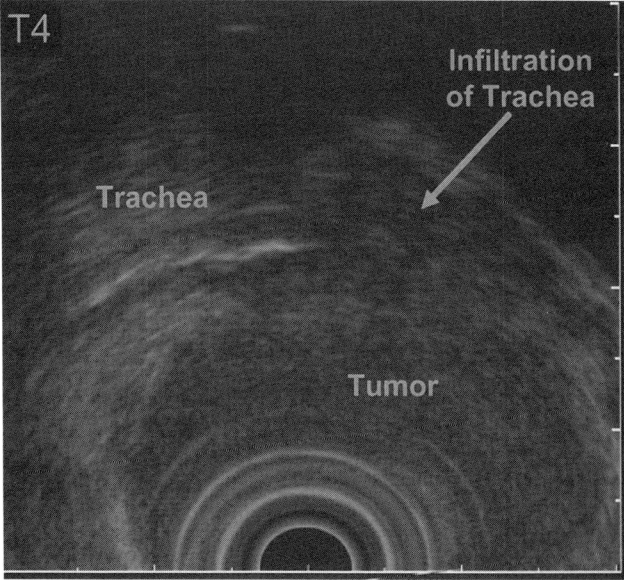

Fig. 5. The esophageal cancer extends through all wall layers and is thereby at least T3. Further tumor extension into the tracheas designates this tumor as T4.

Table 3
Endoscopic ultrasonography criteria for assessment of lymph nodes

Lymph node features	Benign	Malignant
Size (width)	<10 mm	>10 mm
Shape	Elongated/oblong	Round
Border	Irregular	Smooth
Echogenicity	Echorich	Echopoor

without perforating the overlying visceral peritoneum. If perforation occurs of the overlying visceral peritoneum, the tumor should be classified as T3.

Malignant tissue cannot be accurately distinguished from inflammation and fibrosis with EUS. The latter occurs with ulcerated masses and occurs after chemoradiation. Fibrosis and inflammation may lead to overstaging, particularly in patients with T2 tumors [40–48]. Although overstaging is of concern and may lead to inappropriate administration of chemoradiation, some researchers have found this to be an uncommon occurrence [49–51]. Overstaging may also result from tangential imaging resulting in overestimation of tumor depth. Conversely, microscopic tumor invasion cannot be detected by EUS and is associated with understaging [30,52]. Understaging may also occur with tumor stenosis, which limits the extent of the evaluation [53].

Lymph nodes

The typical EUS characteristics of malignant lymph nodes are echopoor appearance, round shape, a smooth border, and size > 1 cm in the shortest axis. (Table 3 and Fig. 6A, B) [54–56]. When lymph nodes meet all four criteria, there is an 80% to 100% chance of metastatic involvement [54–56]. However, only 25% of malignant lymph nodes have all of these features. Additionally, overlap in appearance between benign and malignant lymph nodes makes EUS N staging problematic. For instance, malignant perirectal lymph nodes secondary to rectal cancer are often "benign-appearing" according to the aforementioned criteria (Fig. 6C). Overstaging occurs with enlarged reactive lymph nodes that mimic malignant lymphadenopathy.

Technique

EUS staging of luminal GI tract cancers is typically performed in an ambulatory setting. EUS for esophageal or gastric cancer staging requires an overnight fast. When incomplete gastric emptying is suspected, a 1- to 2-day diet of clear liquids is helpful to avoid retained food. Although some clinicians perform rectal EUS after administering enemas alone, we prefer a full colon prep to optimize acoustic coupling, minimize image artifacts from intraluminal contents, and reduce luminal fecal material when EUS-FNA is done. Conscious sedation is routinely given for upper GI EUS, but it is optional for rectal EUS. Patients are examined in the left lateral position. Repositioning is occasionally needed to improve imaging, in particular for superficial tumors in the stomach or rectum. Routine administration of prophylactic antibiotics is unnecessary for EUS-FNA of solid upper GI lesions [57–59]. Although some clinicians advocate the routine use of prophylactic antibiotics for perirectal EUS-FNA [60], there are emerging data suggesting this practice may be unnecessary [61].

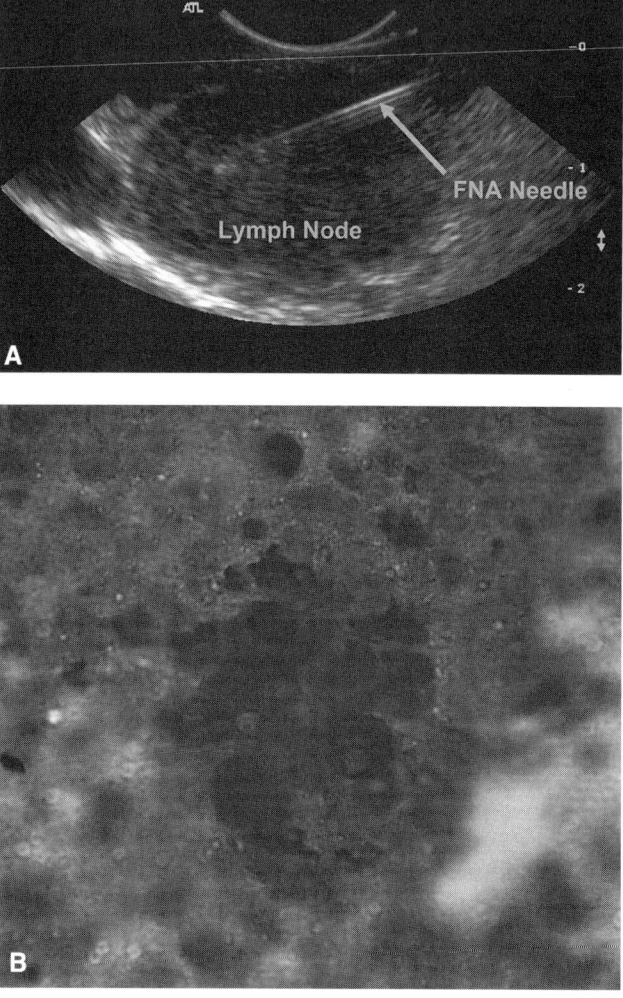

Fig. 6. (*A*) The lymph node has typical malignant characteristics of echopoor, round with a smooth border, and is > 1 cm in width. (*B*) Cytology collected during EUS-FNA of the lymph node confirms metastatic adenocarcinoma. (*C*) A benign-appearing subcarinal lymph node. Other than a width of > 1 cm, this lymph node meets no criteria to suggest malignant infiltration.

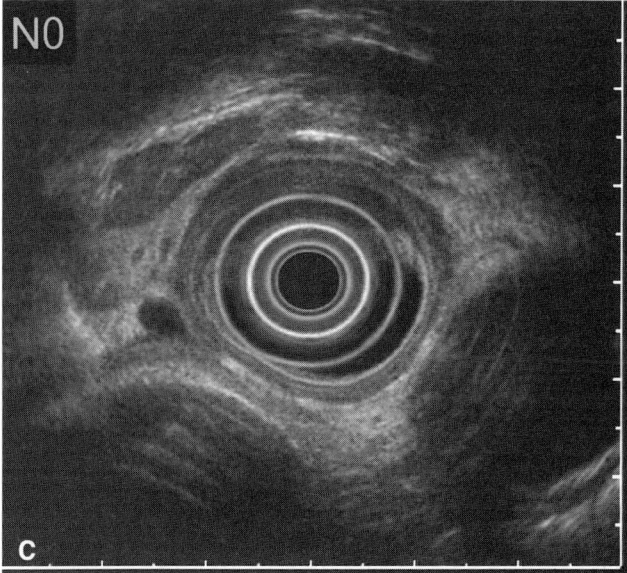

Fig. 6 (*continued*).

EUS is preceded by esophagogastroduodenoscopy or flexible sigmoidoscopy, as appropriate, to document the proximal and distal tumor extent, circumferential extent, and relation to other structures to facilitate the EUS examination and to aid resection. Mucosal biopsies are taken if they had not been done previously. For rectal cancers, a manual examination is performed to assess the tumor, the findings of which have been shown to correlate with tumor stage and resectability.

Although some clinicians perform only a linear examination, we feel that initial radial EUS is mandatory for optimal luminal cancer staging and examination efficiency. We focus the initial one to two pull-throughs on a lymph node survey and search for metastatic disease (Fig. 7). We begin the LN survey from the third portion of the duodenum for upper GI EUS and proximal to the iliac vessels (about 30 cm) for lower GI EUS. T staging is performed through a focused examination overlying the primary tumor, keeping in mind the need to examine the tumor in a perpendicular axis, ideally at a scanning distance approximating the focal zone. The use of variable frequencies and insufflation of nonaerated water into the lumen can improve T-stage accuracy, as does avoidance of balloon overinflation and compression of the primary tumor. Balloon overinflation often leads to rapid slippage of the echoendoscope through a stenotic tumor and limited examination quality. Linear EUS is performed to sample periluminal lymph nodes identified by radial EUS. During EUS-FNA, one should avoid traversing the primary tumor with the needle to minimize false-positive cytology and tumor seeding.

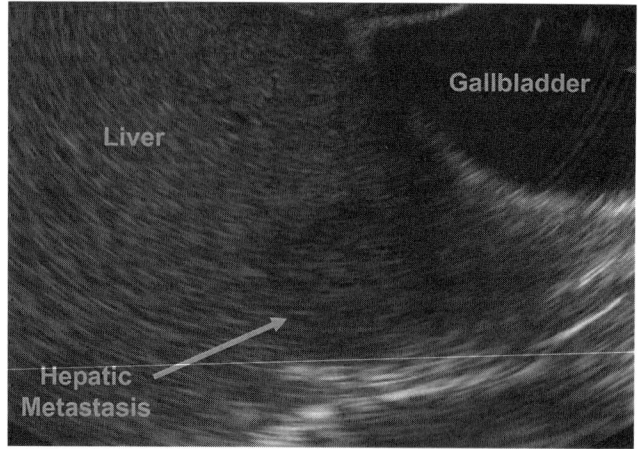

Fig. 7. Hypoechoic appearance of a hepatic metastasis in a patient with an esophageal cancer. Metastases to the liver can also be hyperechoic or mixed in appearance.

Small-caliber (~2–3 mm diameter) flexible miniprobes may be used for patients with stenotic lesions precluding the use of a dedicated echoendoscope. These probes are passed through standard endoscopes. They operate at higher frequencies (up to 30 MHz) than standard EUS and produce a greater resolution image but at a corresponding loss in penetration. Rectal EUS can be performed with rigid instruments that have a lower cost. Most clinicians favor flexible echoendoscopes to facilitate traversal of stenotic tumors and to allow assessment and biopsy of lymph nodes in the left iliac region.

Esophageal cancer

Although esophageal cancer is relatively uncommon, there has been a recent marked increased incidence of adenocarcinomas arising in the distal esophagus [62–64]. Esophageal cancer is associated with a high mortality, as demonstrated by the expected number of new cases this year in the United States (14,250) being nearly matched by the expected number of deaths (13,300) [1]. As these data suggest, most patients with esophageal cancer already have locally advanced disease at initial presentation. The overall 5-year survival rate is < 10% [65].

The practice of surveillance endoscopy in patients with Barrett's esophagus has increased the detection of early malignant lesions that are amenable to endoscopic mucosal resection (EMR) or photodynamic therapy [66–72]. Lymph node metastasis is unlikely in early cancers, and EMR may be curative if the esophageal tumor does not invade the muscularis mucosa [73]. Nodal metastasis is present in up to 10% of patients with a tumor invading only the muscularis mucosa, and for such patients EMR and PDT should not be offered [73,74].

Approximately 50% to 75% of all other patients with esophageal cancer have more advanced disease. For locally advanced cancers (greater than stage IIB-III), standard surgical techniques and wide resections provide unsatisfactory survival benefit [20,21,75]. Multimodality treatment protocols target this group, attempting to downstage the primary tumor, thereby increasing resectability rates, eliminating or delaying micrometastases, and potentially prolonging survival [76]. Patients with a complete pathologic response to neoadjuvant therapy have a demonstrable advantage, with 5-year survival rates of 60% to 100% [77]. A meta-analysis of six randomized controlled trials (RCTs) found that patients receiving chemoradiation before surgical resection had downstaging of their tumors and decreased 3-year mortality rates compared with patients undergoing surgery alone [78]. However, preoperative administration of radiotherapy and chemotherapy for patients with early-stage disease (stage IIA or lower) is associated with increased postoperative mortality and no survival advantage. Surgical resection is standard for early-stage disease, whereas most advanced cancers are managed with palliative therapy alone [9]. The influence of staging on clinical management highlights the need for accurate staging to improve patient outcomes.

Numerous studies have found EUS superior to CT for tumor (T) (85% versus 55%) and lymph node (N) (81% versus 56%) staging of esophageal cancer [22–24,26,28–30,35,37,55,79–88]. These preliminary results were supported by the findings of a recent meta-analysis of 13 studies [89]. Despite the advantage of EUS, identification of malignant lymph nodes remains problematic, with reported accuracy rates of 50% to 90% [22–24,26,28–30,35,37,55,79–88]. In most trials, EUS-FNA improves sensitivity by an additional 10% over EUS alone. A recent prospective, blinded study by Vazquez-Sequeiros et al [90] found the N-stage accuracy for EUS-FNA (87%) to be greater than EUS (74%) and CT (51%) in esophageal carcinoma. The presence of malignant celiac and cervical nodes must be carefully examined given the impact on stage, prognosis, and management [91]. As many as 30% of patients with advanced esophageal cancer have celiac lymph node metastasis [92], and EUS-FNA has a sensitivity of 88% to 100% for their detection [93–95], often after a negative radial EUS examination [93].

Obstructing esophageal cancers

Approximately 13% to 40% of the patients undergoing EUS have a non-traversable obstructing esophageal tumor [26,28,30,88,90]. Some clinicians advocate dilatation, given the greater accuracy of EUS for T and N staging for traversable versus nontraversable tumors (81% versus 28% and 86% versus 72%, respectively) [96]. Others caution against routine dilatation given the associated risk and tendency for advanced disease in the majority of these patients. Although initial studies reported perforation rates as high as 24% [97–99], more recent studies find this practice to be safe (Fig. 8) [100–102].

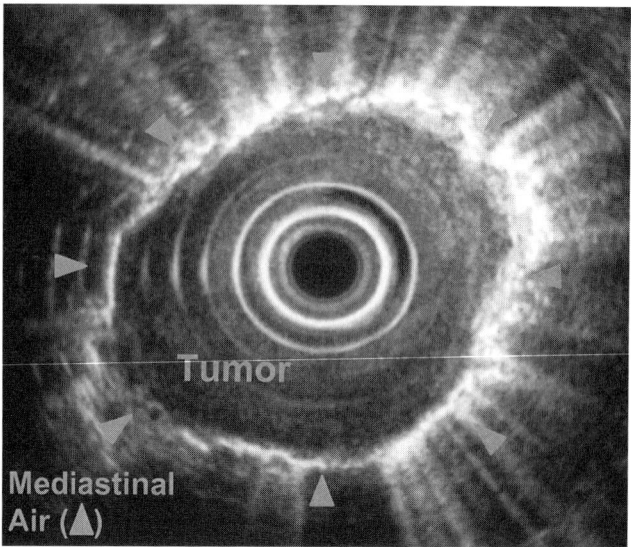

Fig. 8. Pneumomediastinum in a patient secondary to esophageal perforation developing while attempting to traverse a stenotic esophageal tumor with the echoendoscope.

Miniprobes may improve T- and N-stage accuracy, but the limited depth of penetration impairs complete assessment of locoregional spread [103]. A small-caliber (7 mm) wire-guided echoendoscope without fiberoptic capability is available for staging stenotic tumors (Olympus MH-908). The use of this instrument in 130 patients allowed complete endoscopic staging in 90% (27/30) cases, compared with 60% (60/100) in whom it was not used [104].

In our practice, if the initial standard gastroscope cannot traverse the stenosis, we do not dilate because we are infrequently able to pass the echoendoscope even with this intervention. For patients with circumferential stenosis permitting passage of a gastroscope but not the echoendoscope, judicious dilation is undertaken using stepwise balloon dilatation to a maximum of 15 mm. We are cautious when semi-circumferential involvement is present because the normal (and hence thinner) esophageal wall may be at increased risk of tearing in this setting, particularly if the proximal esophagus is dilated.

Restaging after chemoradiation

Esophageal carcinomas are often restaged after neoadjuvant chemoradiation therapy to identify patients most likely to benefit from surgical resection. In this setting, EUS has a T-stage accuracy of about 30% and an N-stage accuracy (without FNA) of < 60% [105–109]. Overstaging is common because EUS cannot reliably distinguish tumor from inflammation and fibrosis. The addition of FNA may allow distinction. Some clinicians advocate determination of tumor cross-sectional area, with a 50% or greater reduction indicating a therapeutic response [108]. Chak et al [110] reported a survival benefit for patients who achieved this degree of response.

Detection of locoregional recurrence

Most esophageal cancer recurrences are locoregional irrespective of the therapy administered [111,112]. EUS is ideal for detecting intra- and extra-luminal recurrence offering a sensitivity of >92% and specificity of >96%, which are superior to standard endoscopy and CT [113–115].

Impact of endoscopic ultrasonography on management

In a study by Vazquez-Sequeiros et al [90], treatment decisions were altered in 77% of patients based on EUS-FNA findings. Mortensen et al [116] performed EUS-FNA in 14 patients; the management strategy was altered in 13 patients with nodal metastasis. To evaluate the impact of EUS and EUS-FNA on tumor recurrence and survival, the outcomes between two cohorts of patients with esophageal cancer with no discernible difference in stage-based management strategy were compared [117]. Patients were staged preoperatively by CT alone or by CT and EUS/EUS-FNA. The two groups were well matched with respect to age, gender, and tumor location and stage. The group undergoing combined CT and EUS/EUS-FNA had a significantly lower recurrence rate and a survival advantage. The improved outcomes theoretically resulted from superior staging with EUS, which may have optimized clinical decision-making.

EUS also has an economic impact. Shumaker et al [118] estimated that for every 100 patients with esophageal cancer, preoperative EUS would obviate the need for neoadjuvant care in 14 patients with stage I disease and would avoid surgery in 12 patients with stage IV disease, resulting in an average cost savings of $3443 per patient. In their opinion, initial EUS allows a significant proportion of patients (26% in their series) to avoid multimodal therapy with a reduction in medical expenses. These conclusions must be carefully considered given the authors' assumption that all patients with esophageal cancer not undergoing EUS staging would have routinely been managed with multimo-dality therapy including surgery. In a decision analysis model comparing EUS-guided FNA to CT-guided FNA and surgery, Harewood and Wiersema [119] concluded that EUS-guided FNA was less costly than the other strategies for staging esophageal cancer. This was particularly true in patients with a high prevalence (>16%) of metastatic celiac lymph nodes and when the sensitivity of EUS-FNA was >66% [119]. Wallace et al [120] used the decision-analysis model as well and compared the cost and effectiveness of different strategies for esophageal cancer staging. Under baseline assumptions, CT + EUS-FNA was the least expensive strategy and offered more quality-adjusted life-years than all other strategies with the exception of PET + EUS-FNA. The authors concluded that the combination of PET + EUS-FNA is preferred for staging patients with esophageal cancer despite the higher cost of PET.

Gastric cancer

The term "gastric cancer" generally refers to adenocarcinoma, which accounts for 90% to 95% of all gastric malignancies, whereas mucosa-associated lymphoid tissue (MALT) lymphoma accounts for 4% to 8% of gastric cancers. Gastric cancer remains the second-most common cause of cancer-related deaths worldwide, accounting for 10% of cases despite an overall decreasing incidence in industrialized countries [121]. Cancer of the distal half of the stomach has been decreasing in the United States, whereas the incidence of cancer of the cardia and gastroesophageal junction has been rapidly rising [62,122,123].

Gastric cancer prognosis strongly correlates with tumor stage and grade [14–16]. Surgery may be curative in localized distal gastric cancer. Most patients (80% to 90%) have advanced disease at presentation and a 5-year prognosis of only 3% to 13% [124]. Radical surgery with curative intent is the cornerstone of therapy for advanced gastric cancer [125], but locoregional and peritoneal recurrence are common [126]. Survival is not improved with chemotherapy or radiotherapy alone [127–129]. A large phase III multicenter RCT including 556 patients with 5-year median follow-up reported improved survival with postoperative chemoradiation therapy for completely resected stage IB to stage IV M0 gastric adenocarcinoma compared with surgery alone [130]. These findings highlight the need for accurate preoperative staging, particularly when multimodal therapy is planned [131,132].

EUS is the most sensitive modality for locoregional staging of gastric cancer, with a T-stage accuracy of 60% to 90% and an N-stage accuracy of 50% to 80% [29,30,132–140]. A meta-analysis of 13 studies found EUS to be superior to CT for staging accuracy [89]. Willis et al [139] reported that curative resection can be accurately predicted by preoperative EUS. EUS differentiation of T2 and T3 gastric cancers is difficult. The serosa covering the gastric wall is thin and represented on EUS as an interface echo only. Subserosal fat located between the serosa and muscularis propria appears as a bright layer with EUS, and tumor extension into the subserosal layer (T2) is often misclassified as T3. Areas of the stomach, notably the lesser curve and the posterior wall of the fundus, contain no serosal cover because of the peritoneal reflection, which often leads to overstaging of T2 tumors. Carcinomas in these areas are classified as T2 tumors histopathologically even when they show transmural tumor growth [80].

Adenocarcinoma of the gastric cardia, gastroesophageal junction (GEJ), and lower esophageal cancers have similar characteristics, risk factors, and prognoses. Differentiation may be difficult due to longitudinal extension. Multimodal therapy is favored except for early-stage or widely metastatic disease. The overall T-stage accuracy of EUS for cardia and GEJ cancers (70% to 85%) is superior to CT (15% to 50%) [141–147]. EUS is the most accurate modality for nodal staging of cardia and GEJ cancers (60% to 80%). A meta-analysis of four studies confirmed the superior locoregional staging accuracy of EUS compared with CT for adenocarcinoma of the gastric cardia [89].

Gastric mucosa-associated lymphoid tissue lymphoma

Gastric MALT lymphoma is a low-grade lymphoma that is usually associated with *Helicobacter pylori* infection [148–150]. Since the identification of *H. Pylori* as a causal agent, surgical resection has largely been replaced by antibiotic therapy for *H. Pylori* eradication or chemotherapy and radiotherapy with no apparent decrease in survival [151–156]. Complete remission follows *H. Pylori* eradication in 50% to 80% of the patients in a stage-dependent manner [152,154, 157–159]. Relapse is more likely when EUS demonstrates tumor infiltration beyond the submucosa [154,158] or nodal spread [158]. There are no clear guidelines for managing patients that fail *H. Pylori* eradication therapy. Chemotherapy, radiotherapy, surgery, or any combination of these therapies may be attempted when *H. Pylori* eradication fails.

For MALT lymphoma, EUS has a T-stage accuracy of 80% to 97% [53,158, 160,161] and an N-stage accuracy of 77% to 90%. The addition of cytology, flow cytometry, or immunocytochemistry of aspirates from the tumor or lymph nodes may affect staging [162].

Surveillance with routine endoscopy and mucosal biopsy is favored at frequent intervals until *H. Pylori* eradication and histologic remission is documented [163,164]. Thereafter, endoscopic and histologic surveillance is often repeated at 3- to 6-month intervals [163,164]. Evidence supporting surveillance by EUS after *H. Pylori* eradication is insufficient [165–167]. EUS documentation of normalization of wall thickness lags behind histologic remission but has been suggested as a useful marker [165,166]. The utility of EUS for detecting MALT recurrence may be limited by the tendency to underestimate surface extension [160]. There are no reports of EUS surveillance after chemotherapy or radiotherapy.

Rectal cancer staging

The management of rectal cancer has changed considerably over the last several decades. Rectal cancer prognosis strongly correlates with locoregional disease extent, and treatment strategies depend on tumor stage. For advanced locoregional disease, postoperative chemoradiotherapy improves local control and survival [168,169]. These findings led the National Institutes of Health Consensus Conference in 1990 to recommend postoperative chemoradiotherapy for all patients with stage II-III rectal cancer (tumor extension into perirectal fat or mesorectal or pelvic lymph nodes) [170]. Subsequently, several RCTs have reported that preoperative adjuvant therapy decreases the local relapse rate compared with surgery alone [171–173] or postoperative adjuvant therapy [174–176]. In addition, the Swedish Rectal Cancer Trial reported that preoperative adjuvant therapy is beneficial only to patients with advanced locoregional disease and is associated with a survival advantage [170,177–179].

These findings were later supported by the results of a meta-analysis of 14 RCTs [180]. In addition to improved local control and long-term survival, pre-operative adjuvant therapy increases the chance for sphincter-sparing surgery in patients who may otherwise require abdominoperineal resection. Accurate rectal cancer staging is therefore essential to identify patients most likely to benefit from neoadjuvant therapy while avoiding unnecessary administration to patients with early-stage disease.

Although CT and MRI are sensitive for the detection of metastatic disease from rectal cancer, they are less useful for locoregional staging. EUS has become the preferred modality for locoregional staging due to its high-resolution imaging of the lumen wall and surrounding structures. EUS offers greater accuracy (80% to 95%) than CT (65% to 75%) or conventional MRI (75% to 85%) for T staging of rectal cancer [50,51,181–185]. Endorectal coil MRI is nearly as accurate as EUS but is more expensive [50,186]. A decision-analysis suggests that the most cost-effective strategy for evaluating nonmetastatic proximal rectal cancer is combined CT and EUS [49]. The main benefit of EUS is to improve T-stage accuracy.

Although EUS lymph node staging accuracy for rectal cancer is low (70% to 75%), it compares favorably with CT (accuracy 55% to 65%) and MRI (accuracy 60% to 65%). Nearly 50% of malignant perirectal lymph nodes are smaller than 5 mm, and only about 20% are detected by EUS [187]. Although the addition of FNA may improve N-stage accuracy, the data are limited. We previously reported similar N-stage accuracy (80%) for CT, EUS, and EUS-FNA. In this setting, FNA is most likely to affect the care of patients with early T-stage disease, and many clinicians restrict the use of FNA to this subgroup of patients. EUS-FNA should also be performed in patients with suspected peri-iliac lymphadenopathy because this represents distant metastases (M1). The limitations of EUS in rectal cancer are highlighted in a recent abstract describing 51 patients with rectal cancer undergoing EUS, of whom 15 patients underwent EUS-FNA of perirectal nodes [188]. EUS identified only 4 of 12 patients (33%) with pathologically positive lymph nodes (pN+) at resection. The overall N-stage accuracy was 70%. In contrast, EUS-FNA correctly identified positive lymph nodes in all six patients with pN+ disease. EUS-FNA correctly predicted lymph node status in 13 of 15 patients (87%). Further study is needed to clarify the utility of EUS-FNA in this setting.

Obstructing rectal cancers

Up to 17% of rectal cancers are nontraversable, which leads to impaired staging. Echoendoscopes are more likely than rigid instruments to traverse the tumor because they are flexible, smaller in diameter, and can be advanced under endoscopic guidance [189]. Obstructing tumors are typically advanced stage, and the echoendoscope may be wedged into the tumor to provide limited staging information.

Impact of endoscopic ultrasonography on management

In a study from our center, we performed CT and EUS in a cohort of 80 patients with nonmetastatic rectal cancer [49]. Using surgical pathology as the gold standard, preoperative CT and EUS led to understaging in 39% and 15% of patients, respectively. The addition of EUS to CT altered the management of nearly one third of patients, identifying those likely to benefit from preoperative chemoradiation. We also compared two cohorts of patients, one staged by CT imaging alone versus one staged by EUS and EUS-FNA. Even though there was no difference in the stage-based multimodal therapy between the two groups, there was a statistically significant reduction in tumor recurrence risk (hazard ratio 0.72, 95% confidence interval 0.52–0.97) for those undergoing EUS and EUS-FNA. Survival was similar in the two groups when adjusted for age, gender, and timing of therapy. EUS-FNA more appropriately guided stage-dependent management and improved outcomes, likely because of superior staging accuracy.

Restaging after neoadjuvant therapy

Preoperative neoadjuvant chemoradiotherapy is routinely administered for advanced locoregional disease to downstage rectal cancers. The resulting necro-inflammatory and fibrotic changes are sonographically indistinguishable from malignant tissue. As a result, EUS restaging has a T-stage accuracy of only 50%, and overstaging occurs in 40% of patients [190,191].

Recurrent rectal cancer

Local rectal cancer recurrence develops in 30% to 50% of patients after surgical resection with curative intent and is influenced by tumor stage and use of adjuvant therapy (Fig. 9) [192–194]. Curative resection of recurrent disease requires early detection, which is difficult to accomplish with standard endoscopy because recurrence tends to be extraluminal within regions of inflammation and fibrosis [195,196]. This pattern of recurrence hampers detection with CT [195,196]. CT is further impaired due to metal surgical clips and poor resolution for lesions <2 cm in diameter [196].

EUS sensitivity (100%) for detecting recurrent rectal cancer is superior to CT (82% to 85%) [197,198]. The major limitation of EUS in this setting is poor specificity for distinguishing carcinoma from inflammation and fibrosis. Unlike initial rectal cancer staging, FNA improves accuracy, as demonstrated in a study by Hunerbein et al [199] and confirmed by Lohnert et al [200]. Specificity improved from 57% to 93%, and accuracy improved from 75% to 79% to 92% to 100%. In the study by Lohnert et al [200], 31 of 116 patients with recurrent rectal cancer had lesions amenable to reoperation, the smallest of which was only 3 mm. These findings confirm the utility of EUS for detecting early recurrence and improving survival. The optimal timing for postopera-

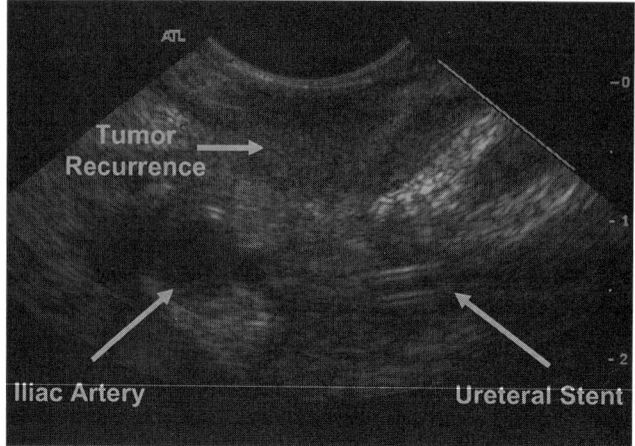

Fig. 9. Recurrent rectal cancer in a patient in whom endoscopic surveillance was normal.

tive EUS surveillance is unclear. Lohnert et al performed EUS surveillance at 3-month intervals for the first 2 years and then at 6-month intervals for an additional year. An aggressive approach to surveillance is warranted in patients with the greatest likelihood of recurrence (eg, advanced cancers before resection or cancers undergoing transanal excision).

Summary

EUS is the most accurate method for locoregional staging of luminal GI cancers. EUS should be performed in patients being considered for surgery once distant metastases have been excluded by noninvasive imaging modalities. The addition of EUS-FNA has further improved lymph node staging accuracy. Although EUS has a limited role in restaging patients after chemotherapy or radiation therapy, it is the most sensitive technique for detecting locoregional tumor recurrence. The findings of EUS and EUS-FNA in these varied settings serve to determine prognosis, guide management, and improve patient outcomes.

References

[1] Jemal A, Tiwari RC, Murray T, et al. Cancer statistics, 2004. CA Cancer J Clin 2004;54:8–29.
[2] DiMagno EP, Buxton JL, Regan PT, et al. Ultrasonic endoscope. Lancet 1980;1:629–31.
[3] Rifkin MD, Gordon SJ, Goldberg BB. Sonographic examination of the mediastinum and up-
      per abdomen by fiberoptic gastroscope. Radiology 1984;151:175–80.
[4] Nickl NJ, Cotton PB. Clinical application of endoscopic ultrasonography. Am J Gastroenterol
      1990;85:675–82.
[5] Harvey AM. Early contributions to the surgery of cancer: William S. Halsted, Hugh H. Young
      and John G. Clark. Johns Hopkins Med J 1974;135:399–417.
[6] Denoix PF. TNM classification. Bull Inst Nat Hyg (Paris) 1944;1:52–82.

[7] Berdejo L. Transhiatal versus transthoracic esophagectomy for clinical stage I esophageal carcinoma. Hepatogastroenterology 1995;42:789–91.

[8] DeMeester TR. Esophageal carcinoma: current controversies. Semin Surg Oncol 1997;13: 217–33.

[9] Fockens P, Kisman K, Merkus MP, et al. The prognosis of esophageal carcinoma staged irresectable (T4) by endosonography. J Am Coll Surg 1998;186:17–23.

[10] Korst RJ, Rusch VW, Venkatraman E, et al. Proposed revision of the staging classification for esophageal cancer. J Thorac Cardiovasc Surg 1998;115:660–9 [discussion 69–70].

[11] Seitz JF, Perrier H, Monges G, et al. Analyse multifactorielle des facteurs pronostiques et predictifs de reponse a la radiochimiotherapie concomitante dans les cancers epidermoides de l'oesophage: interet de l'immunodetection de la proteine p53. Gastroenterol Clin Biol 1995;19:465–74.

[12] Stark SP, Romberg MS, Pierce GE, et al. Transhiatal versus transthoracic esophagectomy for adenocarcinoma of the distal esophagus and cardia. Am J Surg 1996;172:478–81 [discussion 81–2].

[13] Pommier RF, Vetto JT, Ferris BL, et al. Relationships between operative approaches and outcomes in esophageal cancer. Am J Surg 1998;175:422–5.

[14] Adachi Y, Yasuda K, Inomata M, et al. Pathology and prognosis of gastric carcinoma: well versus poorly differentiated type. Cancer 2000;89:1418–24.

[15] Nakamura K, Ueyama T, Yao T, et al. Pathology and prognosis of gastric carcinoma: findings in 10,000 patients who underwent primary gastrectomy. Cancer 1992;70:1030–7.

[16] Siewert JR, Bottcher K, Stein HJ, et al. Relevant prognostic factors in gastric cancer: ten-year results of the German Gastric Cancer Study. Ann Surg 1998;228:449–61.

[17] Siewert JR, Fink U, Beckurts KT, et al. Surgery of squamous cell carcinoma of the esophagus. Ann Oncol 1994;5(Suppl 3):1–7.

[18] Roder JD, Busch R, Stein HJ, et al. Ratio of invaded to removed lymph nodes as a predictor of survival in squamous cell carcinoma of the oesophagus. Br J Surg 1994;81:410–3.

[19] Edwards JM, Hillier VF, Lawson RA, et al. Squamous carcinoma of the oesophagus: histological criteria and their prognostic significance. Br J Cancer 1989;59:429–33.

[20] Hagen JA, Peters JH, DeMeester TR. Superiority of extended en bloc esophagogastrectomy for carcinoma of the lower esophagus and cardia. J Thorac Cardiovasc Surg 1993;106:850–8 [discussion 58–9].

[21] DeMeester TR, Zaninotto G, Johansson KE. Selective therapeutic approach to cancer of the lower esophagus and cardia. J Thorac Cardiovasc Surg 1988;95:42–54.

[22] Flamen P, Lerut A, Van Cutsem E, et al. The utility of positron emission tomography for the diagnosis and staging of recurrent esophageal cancer. J Thorac Cardiovasc Surg 2000;120: 1085–92.

[23] Murata Y, Suzuki S, Hashimoto H. Endoscopic ultrasonography of the upper gastrointestinal tract. Surg Endosc 1988;2:180–3.

[24] Tio TL, Coene PP, den Hartog Jager FC, et al. Preoperative TNM classification of esophageal carcinoma by endosonography. Hepatogastroenterology 1990;37:376–81.

[25] Dittler HJ, Bollschweiler E, Siewert JR. Was leistet die Endosonographie im praoperativen Staging des Osophaguskarzinoms? Dtsch Med Wochenschr 1991;116:561–6.

[26] Vilgrain V, Mompoint D, Palazzo L, et al. Staging of esophageal carcinoma: comparison of results with endoscopic sonography and CT. AJR Am J Roentgenol 1990;155:277–81.

[27] Botet JF, Lightdale CJ, Zauber AG, et al. Preoperative staging of gastric cancer: comparison of endoscopic US and dynamic CT. Radiology 1991;181:426–32.

[28] Botet JF, Lightdale CJ, Zauber AG, et al. Preoperative staging of esophageal cancer: comparison of endoscopic US and dynamic CT. Radiology 1991;181:419–25.

[29] Grimm H, Binmoeller KF, Hamper K, et al. Endosonography for preoperative locoregional staging of esophageal and gastric cancer. Endoscopy 1993;25:224–30.

[30] Rosch T, Lorenz R, Zenker K, et al. Local staging and assessment of resectability in carcinoma of the esophagus, stomach, and duodenum by endoscopic ultrasonography. Gastrointest Endosc 1992;38:460–7.

[31] Quint LE, Glazer GM, Orringer MB. Esophageal imaging by MR and CT: study of normal anatomy and neoplasms. Radiology 1985;156:727–31.

[32] Petrillo R, Balzarini L, Bidoli P, et al. Esophageal squamous cell carcinoma: MRI evaluation of mediastinum. Gastrointest Radiol 1990;15:275–8.

[33] Takashima S, Takeuchi N, Shiozaki H, et al. Carcinoma of the esophagus: CT vs MR imaging in determining resectability. AJR Am J Roentgenol 1991;156:297–302.

[34] Lehr L, Rupp N, Siewert JR. Assessment of resectability of esophageal cancer by computed tomography and magnetic resonance imaging. Surgery 1988;103:344–50.

[35] Koch J, Halvorsen Jr RA. Staging of esophageal cancer: computed tomography, magnetic resonance imaging, and endoscopic ultrasound. Semin Roentgenol 1994;29:364–72.

[36] Rosch T. Endosonographic staging of esophageal cancer: a review of literature results. Gastrointest Endosc Clin North Am 1995;5:537–47.

[37] Kimmey MB, Martin RW, Haggitt RC, et al. Histologic correlates of gastrointestinal ultrasound images. Gastroenterology 1989;96:433–41.

[38] Hasegawa N, Niwa Y, Arisawa T, et al. Preoperative staging of superficial esophageal carcinoma: comparison of an ultrasound probe and standard endoscopic ultrasonography. Gastrointest Endosc 1996;44:388–93.

[39] Murata Y, Suzuki S, Ohta M, et al. Small ultrasonic probes for determination of the depth of superficial esophageal cancer. Gastrointest Endosc 1996;44:23–8.

[40] Souquet JC, Napoleon B, Pujol B, et al. Endosonography-guided treatment of esophageal carcinoma. Endoscopy 1992;24(Suppl 1):324–8.

[41] Garcia-Aguilar J, Pollack J, Lee SH, et al. Accuracy of endorectal ultrasonography in preoperative staging of rectal tumors. Dis Colon Rectum 2002;45:10–5.

[42] Beynon J. An evaluation of the role of rectal endosonography in rectal cancer. Ann R Coll Surg Engl 1989;71:131–9.

[43] Feifel G, Hildebrandt U, Dhom G. Assessment of depth of invasion in rectal cancer by endosonography. Endoscopy 1987;19:64–7.

[44] Yamashita Y, Machi J, Shirouzu K, et al. Evaluation of endorectal ultrasound for the assessment of wall invasion of rectal cancer: report of a case. Dis Colon Rectum 1988;31:617–23.

[45] Boyce GA, Sivak Jr MV, Lavery IC, et al. Endoscopic ultrasound in the pre-operative staging of rectal carcinoma. Gastrointest Endosc 1992;38:468–71.

[46] Cho E, Nakajima M, Yasuda K, et al. Endoscopic ultrasonography in the diagnosis of colorectal cancer invasion. Gastrointest Endosc 1993;39:521–7.

[47] Herzog U, von Flue M, Tondelli P, et al. How accurate is endorectal ultrasound in the preoperative staging of rectal cancer? Dis Colon Rectum 1993;36:127–34.

[48] Glaser F, Schlag P, Herfarth C. Endorectal ultrasonography for the assessment of invasion of rectal tumours and lymph node involvement. Br J Surg 1990;77:883–7.

[49] Harewood GC, Wiersema MJ. Cost-effectiveness of endoscopic ultrasonography in the evaluation of proximal rectal cancer. Am J Gastroenterol 2002;97:874–82.

[50] Meyenberger C, Huch Boni RA, Bertschinger P, et al. Endoscopic ultrasound and endorectal magnetic resonance imaging: a prospective, comparative study for preoperative staging and follow-up of rectal cancer. Endoscopy 1995;27:469–79.

[51] Thaler W, Watzka S, Martin F, et al. Preoperative staging of rectal cancer by endoluminal ultrasound vs. magnetic resonance imaging: preliminary results of a prospective, comparative study. Dis Colon Rectum 1994;37:1189–93.

[52] Fockens P, Van den Brande JH, van Dullemen HM, et al. Endosonographic T-staging of esophageal carcinoma: a learning curve. Gastrointest Endosc 1996;44:58–62.

[53] Caletti G, Fusaroli P, Bocus P. Endoscopic ultrasonography. Endoscopy 1998;30:198–221.

[54] Bhutani MS, Hawes RH, Hoffman BJ. A comparison of the accuracy of echo features during endoscopic ultrasound (EUS) and EUS-guided fine-needle aspiration for diagnosis of malignant lymph node invasion. Gastrointest Endosc 1997;45:474–9.

[55] Catalano MF, Sivak Jr MV, Rice T, et al. Endosonographic features predictive of lymph node metastasis. Gastrointest Endosc 1994;40:442–6.

[56] Grimm H, Hamper K, Binmoeller KF, et al. Enlarged lymph nodes: malignant or not? Endoscopy 1992;24(Suppl 1):320–3.

[57] Barawi M, Gottlieb K, Cunha B, et al. A prospective evaluation of the incidence of bacteremia associated with EUS-guided fine-needle aspiration. Gastrointest Endosc 2001;53:189–92.

[58] Levy MJ, Norton ID, Wiersema MJ, et al. Prospective risk assessment of bacteremia and other infectious complications in patients undergoing EUS-guided FNA. Gastrointest Endosc 2003; 57:672–8.

[59] Janssen J, Konig K, Knop-Hammad V, et al. Frequency of bacteremia after linear EUS of the upper GI tract with and without FNA. Gastrointest Endosc 2004;59:339–44.

[60] Wiersema MJ, Harewood GC. Endoscopic ultrasound for rectal cancer. Gastroenterol Clin North Am 2002;31:1093–105.

[61] Levy MJ, Kumar S, Norton ID, et al. Prospective risk assessment of bacteremia in patients undergoing endoscopic ultrasound-guided fine needle aspiration (EUS-FNA) of rectal and perirectal lesions [abstract]. Gastrointest Endosc 2004;59:AB108.

[62] Blot WJ, Devesa SS, Kneller RW, et al. Rising incidence of adenocarcinoma of the esophagus and gastric cardia. JAMA 1991;265:1287–9.

[63] Devesa SS, Blot WJ, Fraumeni Jr JF. Changing patterns in the incidence of esophageal and gastric carcinoma in the United States. Cancer 1998;83:2049–53.

[64] Pera M, Cameron AJ, Trastek VF, et al. Increasing incidence of adenocarcinoma of the esophagus and esophagogastric junction. Gastroenterology 1993;104:510–3.

[65] DeCamp Jr MM, Swanson SJ, Jaklitsch MT. Esophagectomy after induction chemoradiation. Chest 1999;116(Suppl):466S–9S.

[66] Overholt BF, Panjehpour M, Haydek JM. Photodynamic therapy for Barrett's esophagus: follow-up in 100 patients. Gastrointest Endosc 1999;49:1–7.

[67] May A, Gossner L, Pech O, et al. Local endoscopic therapy for intraepithelial high-grade neoplasia and early adenocarcinoma in Barrett's oesophagus: acute-phase and intermediate results of a new treatment approach. Eur J Gastroenterol Hepatol 2002;14:1085–91.

[68] May A, Gossner L, Pech O, et al. Intraepithelial high-grade neoplasia and early adenocarcinoma in short-segment Barrett's esophagus (SSBE): curative treatment using local endoscopic treatment techniques. Endoscopy 2002;34:604–10.

[69] Gossner L, May A, Sroka R, et al. Photodynamic destruction of high grade dysplasia and early carcinoma of the esophagus after the oral administration of 5-aminolevulinic acid. Cancer 1999; 86:1921–8.

[70] Gossner L, Stolte M, Sroka R, et al. Photodynamic ablation of high-grade dysplasia and early cancer in Barrett's esophagus by means of 5-aminolevulinic acid. Gastroenterology 1998;114: 448–55.

[71] Takeshita K, Tani M, Inoue H, et al. Endoscopic treatment of early oesophageal or gastric cancer. Gut 1997;40:123–7.

[72] Ell C, May A, Gossner L, et al. Endoscopic mucosal resection of early cancer and high-grade dysplasia in Barrett's esophagus. Gastroenterology 2000;118:670–7.

[73] Tajima Y, Nakanishi Y, Ochiai A, et al. Histopathologic findings predicting lymph node metastasis and prognosis of patients with superficial esophageal carcinoma: analysis of 240 surgically resected tumors. Cancer 2000;88:1285–93.

[74] Tio TL. Diagnosis and staging of esophageal carcinoma by endoscopic ultrasonography. Endoscopy 1998;30(Suppl 1):A33–40.

[75] Hulscher JB, van Sandick JW, de Boer AG, et al. Extended transthoracic resection compared with limited transhiatal resection for adenocarcinoma of the esophagus. N Engl J Med 2002; 347:1662–9.

[76] Rice TW, Blackstone EH, Adelstein DJ, et al. Role of clinically determined depth of tumor invasion in the treatment of esophageal carcinoma. J Thorac Cardiovasc Surg 2003;125: 1091–102.

[77] Refaely Y, Krasna MJ. Multimodality therapy for esophageal cancer. Surg Clin North Am 2002;82:729–46.

[78] Fiorica F, Di Bona D, Schepis F, et al. Preoperative chemoradiotherapy for oesophageal cancer: a systematic review and meta-analysis. Gut 2004;53:925–30.

[79] Binmoeller KF, Seifert H, Seitz U, et al. Ultrasonic esophagoprobe for TNM staging of highly stenosing esophageal carcinoma. Gastrointest Endosc 1995;41:547–52.

[80] Dittler IIJ, Siewert JR. Role of endoscopic ultrasonography in esophageal carcinoma. Endoscopy 1993;25:156–61.

[81] Heintz A, Hohne U, Schweden F, et al. Preoperative detection of intrathoracic tumor spread of esophageal cancer: endosonography versus computed tomography. Surg Endosc 1991;5: 75–8.

[82] Peters JH, Hoeft SF, Heimbucher J, et al. Selection of patients for curative or palliative resection of esophageal cancer based on preoperative endoscopic ultrasonography. Arch Surg 1994; 129:534–9.

[83] Ziegler K, Sanft C, Zeitz M, et al. Evaluation of endosonography in TN staging of oesophageal cancer. Gut 1991;32:16–20.

[84] Takemoto T, Ito T, Aibe T, et al. Endoscopic ultrasonography in the diagnosis of esophageal carcinoma, with particular regard to staging it for operability. Endoscopy 1986;18(Suppl 3): 22–5.

[85] Romagnuolo J, Scott J, Hawes RH, et al. Helical CT versus EUS with fine needle aspiration for celiac nodal assessment in patients with esophageal cancer. Gastrointest Endosc 2002;55: 648–54.

[86] Rice TW. Clinical staging of esophageal carcinoma. CT, EUS, and PET. Chest Surg Clin N Am 2000;10:471–85.

[87] Suntharalingam M, Haas ML, Sonett JR, et al. Accurate lymph node assessment prior to trimodality therapy for esophageal cancer. Cancer J 2001;7:509–15.

[88] Tio TL, Cohen P, Coene PP, et al. Endosonography and computed tomography of esophageal carcinoma: preoperative classification compared to the new (1987) TNM system. Gastroenterology 1989;96:1478–86.

[89] Kelly S, Harris KM, Berry E, et al. A systematic review of the staging performance of endoscopic ultrasound in gastro-oesophageal carcinoma. Gut 2001;49:534–9.

[90] Vazquez-Sequeiros E, Norton ID, Clain JE, et al. Impact of EUS-guided fine-needle aspiration on lymph node staging in patients with esophageal carcinoma. Gastrointest Endosc 2001; 53:751–7.

[91] Parmar KS, Zwischenberger JB, Reeves AL, et al. Clinical impact of endoscopic ultrasound-guided fine needle aspiration of celiac axis lymph nodes (M1a disease) in esophageal cancer. Ann Thorac Surg 2002;73:916–20 [discussion 20–1].

[92] Earlam R, Cunha-Melo JR. Oesophageal squamous cell carcinoma: I. A critical review of surgery. Br J Surg 1980;67:381–90.

[93] Reed CE, Mishra G, Sahai AV, et al. Esophageal cancer staging: improved accuracy by endoscopic ultrasound of celiac lymph nodes. Ann Thorac Surg 1999;67:319–21 [discussion 22].

[94] Giovannini M, Monges G, Seitz JF, et al. Distant lymph node metastases in esophageal cancer: impact of endoscopic ultrasound-guided biopsy. Endoscopy 1999;31:536–40.

[95] Catalano MF, Alcocer E, Chak A, et al. Evaluation of metastatic celiac axis lymph nodes in patients with esophageal carcinoma: accuracy of EUS. Gastrointest Endosc 1999;50:352–6.

[96] Catalano MF, Van Dam J, Sivak Jr MV. Malignant esophageal strictures: staging accuracy of endoscopic ultrasonography. Gastrointest Endosc 1995;41:535–9.

[97] Van Dam J, Rice TW, Catalano MF, et al. High-grade malignant stricture is predictive of esophageal tumor stage: risks of endosonographic evaluation. Cancer 1993;71:2910–7.

[98] Heit HA, Johnson LF, Siegel SR, et al. Palliative dilation for dysphagia in esophageal carcinoma. Ann Intern Med 1978;89:629–31.

[99] Tulman AB, Boyce Jr HW. Complications of esophageal dilation and guidelines for their prevention. Gastrointest Endosc 1981;27:229–34.

[100] Pfau PR, Ginsberg GG, Lew RJ, et al. Esophageal dilation for endosonographic evaluation of malignant esophageal strictures is safe and effective. Am J Gastroenterol 2000;95:2813–5.

[101] Kallimanis GE, Gupta PK, al-Kawas FH, et al. Endoscopic ultrasound for staging esophageal cancer, with or without dilation, is clinically important and safe. Gastrointest Endosc 1995; 41:540–6.

[102] Wallace MB, Hawes RH, Sahai AV, et al. Dilation of malignant esophageal stenosis to allow EUS guided fine-needle aspiration: safety and effect on patient management. Gastrointest Endosc 2000;51:309–13.

[103] Menzel J, Hoepffner N, Nottberg H, et al. Preoperative staging of esophageal carcinoma: miniprobe sonography versus conventional endoscopic ultrasound in a prospective histopathologically verified study. Endoscopy 1999;31:291–7.

[104] Mallery S, Van Dam J. Increased rate of complete EUS staging of patients with esophageal cancer using the nonoptical, wire-guided echoendoscope. Gastrointest Endosc 1999;50:53–7.

[105] Zuccaro Jr G, Rice TW, Goldblum J, et al. Endoscopic ultrasound cannot determine suitability for esophagectomy after aggressive chemoradiotherapy for esophageal cancer. Am J Gastroenterol 1999;94:906–12.

[106] Mallery S, DeCamp M, Bueno R, et al. Pretreatment staging by endoscopic ultrasonography does not predict complete response to neoadjuvant chemoradiation in patients with esophageal carcinoma. Cancer 1999;86:764–9.

[107] Kalha I, Kaw M, Fukami N, et al. The accuracy of endoscopic ultrasound for restaging esophageal carcinoma after chemoradiation therapy. Cancer 2004;101:940–7.

[108] Isenberg G, Chak A, Canto MI, et al. Endoscopic ultrasound in restaging of esophageal cancer after neoadjuvant chemoradiation. Gastrointest Endosc 1998;48:158–63.

[109] Beseth BD, Bedford R, Isacoff WH, et al. Endoscopic ultrasound does not accurately assess pathologic stage of esophageal cancer after neoadjuvant chemoradiotherapy. Am Surg 2000; 66:827–31.

[110] Chak A, Canto MI, Cooper GS, et al. Endosonographic assessment of multimodality therapy predicts survival of esophageal carcinoma patients. Cancer 2000;88:1788–95.

[111] Denham JW, Steigler A, Kilmurray J, et al. Relapse patterns after chemo-radiation for carcinoma of the oesophagus. Clin Oncol (R Coll Radiol) 2003;15:98–108.

[112] Nakagawa S, Kanda T, Kosugi S, et al. Recurrence pattern of squamous cell carcinoma of the thoracic esophagus after extended radical esophagectomy with three-field lymphadenectomy. J Am Coll Surg 2004;198:205–11.

[113] Muller C, Kahler G, Schoele J. Endosonographic examination of gastrointestinal anastomoses with suspected locoregional tumor recurrence. Surg Endosc 2000;14:45–50.

[114] Fockens P, Manshanden CG, van Lanschot JJ, et al. Prospective study on the value of endosonographic follow-up after surgery for esophageal carcinoma. Gastrointest Endosc 1997;46: 487–91.

[115] Catalano MF, Sivak Jr MV, Rice TW, et al. Postoperative screening for anastomotic recurrence of esophageal carcinoma by endoscopic ultrasonography. Gastrointest Endosc 1995;42: 540–4.

[116] Mortensen MB, Pless T, Durup J, et al. Clinical impact of endoscopic ultrasound-guided fine needle aspiration biopsy in patients with upper gastrointestinal tract malignancies: a prospective study. Endoscopy 2001;33:478–83.

[117] Harewood GC, Kumar KS. Assessment of clinical impact of endoscopic ultrasound on esophageal cancer. J Gastroenterol Hepatol 2004;19:433–9.

[118] Shumaker DA, de Garmo P, Faigel DO. Potential impact of preoperative EUS on esophageal cancer management and cost. Gastrointest Endosc 2002;56:391–6.

[119] Harewood GC, Wiersema MJ. A cost analysis of endoscopic ultrasound in the evaluation of esophageal cancer. Am J Gastroenterol 2002;97:452–8.

[120] Wallace MB, Nietert PJ, Earle C, et al. An analysis of multiple staging management strategies for carcinoma of the esophagus: computed tomography, endoscopic ultrasound, positron emission tomography, and thoracoscopy/laparoscopy. Ann Thorac Surg 2002;74:1026–32.

[121] Parkin DM. Global cancer statistics in the year 2000. Lancet Oncol 2001;2:533–43 [erratum appears in Lancet Oncol 2001;2:596].

[122] Fuchs CS, Mayer RJ. Gastric carcinoma. N Engl J Med 1995;333:32–41.

[123] Craanen ME, Dekker W, Blok P, et al. Time trends in gastric carcinoma: changing patterns of type and location. Am J Gastroenterol 1992;87:572-9.

[124] Wanebo HJ, Kennedy BJ, Chmiel J, et al. Cancer of the stomach: a patient care study by the American College of Surgeons. Ann Surg 1993;218:583-92.

[125] Roukos DH. Current status and future perspectives in gastric cancer management. Cancer Treat Rev 2000;26:243-55.

[126] Gunderson LL, Sosin H. Areas of failure found at reoperation (second or symptomatic look) following "curative surgery" for adenocarcinoma of the rectum: clinicopathologic correlation and implications for adjuvant therapy. Cancer 1974;34:1278-92.

[127] Chang HM, Jung KH, Kim TY, et al. A phase III randomized trial of 5-fluorouracil, doxorubicin, and mitomycin C versus 5-fluorouracil and mitomycin C versus 5-fluorouracil alone in curatively resected gastric cancer. Ann Oncol 2002;13:1779-85.

[128] Fenoglio-Preiser CM, Noffsinger AE, Belli J, et al. Pathologic and phenotypic features of gastric cancer. Semin Oncol 1996;23:292-306.

[129] Scheiman JM, Cutler AF. Helicobacter pylori and gastric cancer. Am J Med 1999;106:222-6.

[130] Macdonald JS, Smalley SR, Benedetti J, et al. Chemoradiotherapy after surgery compared with surgery alone for adenocarcinoma of the stomach or gastroesophageal junction. N Engl J Med 2001;345:725-30.

[131] Takemoto T, Tada M, Dittler HJ, et al. Impact of staging on treatment of gastric carcinoma. Endoscopy 1993;25:46-50.

[132] Dittler HJ, Siewert JR. Role of endoscopic ultrasonography in gastric carcinoma. Endoscopy 1993;25:162-6.

[133] Akahoshi K, Misawa T, Fujishima H, et al. Preoperative evaluation of gastric cancer by endoscopic ultrasound. Gut 1991;32:479-82.

[134] Akahoshi K, Misawa T, Fujishima H, et al. Regional lymph node metastasis in gastric cancer: evaluation with endoscopic US. Radiology 1992;182:559-64.

[135] Caletti G, Ferrari A, Brocchi E, et al. Accuracy of endoscopic ultrasonography in the diagnosis and staging of gastric cancer and lymphoma. Surgery 1993;113:14-27.

[136] Hunerbein M, Dohmoto M, Rau B, et al. Endosonography and endosonography-guided biopsy of upper-GI-tract tumors using a curved-array echoendoscope. Surg Endosc 1996;10:1205-9.

[137] Lightdale CJ. Endoscopic ultrasonography in the diagnosis, staging and follow-up of esophageal and gastric cancer. Endoscopy 1992;24(Suppl 1):297-303.

[138] Tio TL, Schouwink MH, Cikot RJ, et al. Preoperative TNM classification of gastric carcinoma by endosonography in comparison with the pathological TNM system: a prospective study of 72 cases. Hepatogastroenterology 1989;36:51-6.

[139] Willis S, Truong S, Gribnitz S, et al. Endoscopic ultrasonography in the preoperative staging of gastric cancer: accuracy and impact on surgical therapy. Surg Endosc 2000;14:951-4.

[140] Ziegler K, Sanft C, Zimmer T, et al. Comparison of computed tomography, endosonography, and intraoperative assessment in TN staging of gastric carcinoma. Gut 1993;34:604-10.

[141] Andriulli A, Recchia S, De Angelis C, et al. Endoscopic ultrasonographic evaluation of patients with biopsy negative gastric linitis plastica. Gastrointest Endosc 1990;36:611-5.

[142] Singh S, Macleod G, Walker T, et al. Endoscopic fine-needle aspiration cytology in the diagnosis of linitis plastica. Br J Surg 1994;81:1010.

[143] de Manzoni G, Pedrazzani C, Di Leo A, et al. Experience of endoscopic ultrasound in staging adenocarcinoma of the cardia. Eur J Surg Oncol 1999;25:595-8.

[144] Francois E, Peroux J, Mouroux J, et al. Preoperative endosonographic staging of cancer of the cardia. Abdom Imaging 1996;21:483-7.

[145] Greenberg J, Durkin M, Van Drunen M, et al. Computed tomography or endoscopic ultrasonography in preoperative staging of gastric and esophageal tumors. Surgery 1994;116: 696-701 [discussion 701-2].

[146] Hordijk ML, Zander H, van Blankenstein M, et al. Influence of tumor stenosis on the accuracy of endosonography in preoperative T staging of esophageal cancer. Endoscopy 1993;25: 171-5.

[147] Kienle P, Buhl K, Kuntz C, et al. Prospective comparison of endoscopy, endosonography and computed tomography for staging of tumours of the oesophagus and gastric cardia. Digestion 2002;66:230–6.

[148] Nakamura S, Yao T, Aoyagi K, et al. Helicobacter pylori and primary gastric lymphoma: a histopathologic and immunohistochemical analysis of 237 patients. Cancer 1997;79:3–11.

[149] Parsonnet J, Hansen S, Rodriguez L, et al. Helicobacter pylori infection and gastric lymphoma. N Engl J Med 1994;330:1267–71.

[150] Wotherspoon AC, Ortiz-Hidalgo C, Falzon MR, et al. Helicobacter pylori-associated gastritis and primary B-cell gastric lymphoma. Lancet 1991;338:1175–6.

[151] Cogliatti SB, Schmid U, Schumacher U, et al. Primary B-cell gastric lymphoma: a clinico-pathological study of 145 patients. Gastroenterology 1991;101:1159–70.

[152] Nobre-Leitao C, Lage P, Cravo M, et al. Treatment of gastric MALT lymphoma by Helicobacter pylori eradication: a study controlled by endoscopic ultrasonography. Am J Gastroenterol 1998; 93:732–6.

[153] Pinotti G, Zucca E, Roggero E, et al. Clinical features, treatment and outcome in a series of 93 patients with low-grade gastric MALT lymphoma. Leuk Lymphoma 1997;26:527–37.

[154] Sackmann M, Morgner A, Rudolph B, et al. Regression of gastric MALT lymphoma after eradication of Helicobacter pylori is predicted by endosonographic staging. MALT Lymphoma Study Group. Gastroenterology 1997;113:1087–90.

[155] Schechter NR, Portlock CS, Yahalom J. Treatment of mucosa-associated lymphoid tissue lymphoma of the stomach with radiation alone. J Clin Oncol 1998;16:1916–21.

[156] Weston AP, Banerjee SK, Horvat RT, et al. Prospective long-term endoscopic and histologic follow-up of gastric lymphoproliferative disease of early stage IE low-grade B-cell mucosa-associated lymphoid tissue type following Helicobacter pylori eradication treatment. Int J Oncol 1999;15:899–907.

[157] Roggero E, Zucca E, Pinotti G, et al. Eradication of Helicobacter pylori infection in primary low-grade gastric lymphoma of mucosa-associated lymphoid tissue. Ann Intern Med 1995;122: 767–9.

[158] Ruskone-Fourmestraux A, Lavergne A, Aegerter PH, et al. Predictive factors for regression of gastric MALT lymphoma after anti-Helicobacter pylori treatment. Gut 2001;48:297–303.

[159] Wotherspoon AC, Doglioni C, Diss TC, et al. Regression of primary low-grade B-cell gastric lymphoma of mucosa-associated lymphoid tissue type after eradication of Helicobacter pylori. Lancet 1993;342:575–7.

[160] Palazzo L, Roseau G, Ruskone-Fourmestraux A, et al. Endoscopic ultrasonography in the local staging of primary gastric lymphoma. Endoscopy 1993;25:502–8.

[161] Schuder G, Hildebrandt U, Kreissler-Haag D, et al. Role of endosonography in the surgical management of non-Hodgkin's lymphoma of the stomach. Endoscopy 1993;25:509–12.

[162] Ribeiro A, Vazquez-Sequeiros E, Wiersema LM, et al. EUS-guided fine-needle aspiration combined with flow cytometry and immunocytochemistry in the diagnosis of lymphoma. Gastrointest Endosc 2001;53:485–91.

[163] Savio A, Franzin G, Wotherspoon AC, et al. Diagnosis and posttreatment follow-up of Helicobacter pylori-positive gastric lymphoma of mucosa-associated lymphoid tissue: histology, polymerase chain reaction, or both? Blood 1996;87:1255–60.

[164] Savio A, Zamboni G, Capelli P, et al. Relapse of low-grade gastric MALT lymphoma after Helicobacter pylori eradication: true relapse or persistence? Long-term post-treatment follow-up of a multicenter trial in the north-east of Italy and evaluation of the diagnostic protocol's adequacy. Recent Results Cancer Res 2000;156:116–24.

[165] Levy M, Hammel P, Lamarque D, et al. Endoscopic ultrasonography for the initial staging and follow-up in patients with low-grade gastric lymphoma of mucosa-associated lymphoid tissue treated medically. Gastrointest Endosc 1997;46:328–33.

[166] Lugering N, Menzel J, Kucharzik T, et al. Impact of miniprobes compared to conventional endosonography in the staging of low-grade gastric malt lymphoma. Endoscopy 2001;33: 832–7.

[167] Puspok A, Raderer M, Chott A, et al. Endoscopic ultrasound in the follow up and response assessment of patients with primary gastric lymphoma. Gut 2002;51:691–4.

[168] Krook JE, Moertel CG, Gunderson LL, et al. Effective surgical adjuvant therapy for high-risk rectal carcinoma. N Engl J Med 1991;324:709–15.

[169] Anonymous. Prolongation of the disease-free interval in surgically treated rectal carcinoma. Gastrointestinal Tumor Study Group. N Engl J Med 1985;312:1465–72.

[170] Anonymous. NIH consensus conference. Adjuvant therapy for patients with colon and rectal cancer. JAMA 1990;264:1444–50.

[171] Anonymous. Improved survival with preoperative radiotherapy in resectable rectal cancer. Swedish Rectal Cancer Trial. N Engl J Med 1997;336:980–7 [erratum appears in N Engl J Med 1997;336:1539].

[172] Anonymous. Randomised trial of surgery alone versus radiotherapy followed by surgery for potentially operable locally advanced rectal cancer. Medical Research Council Rectal Cancer Working Party. Lancet 1996;348:1605–10.

[173] Minsky BD. Adjuvant therapy for rectal cancer: a good first step. N Engl J Med 1997;336:1016–7.

[174] Hyams DM, Mamounas EP, Petrelli N, et al. A clinical trial to evaluate the worth of preoperative multimodality therapy in patients with operable carcinoma of the rectum: a progress report of National Surgical Breast and Bowel Project Protocol R-03. Dis Colon Rectum 1997;40:131–9.

[175] Grann A, Feng C, Wong D, et al. Preoperative combined modality therapy for clinically resectable uT3 rectal adenocarcinoma. Int J Radiat Oncol Biol Phys 2001;49:987–95.

[176] Sauer R, Becker H, Hohenberger W, et al. Preoperative versus postoperative chemoradiotherapy for rectal cancer. N Engl J Med 2004;351:1731–40.

[177] Pahlman L, Glimelius B. Pre- or postoperative radiotherapy in rectal and rectosigmoid carcinoma: report from a randomized multicenter trial. Ann Surg 1990;211:187–95.

[178] Kapiteijn E, Marijnen CA, Nagtegaal ID, et al. Preoperative radiotherapy combined with total mesorectal excision for resectable rectal cancer. N Engl J Med 2001;345:638–46.

[179] Frykholm GJ, Glimelius B, Pahlman L. Preoperative or postoperative irradiation in adeno-carcinoma of the rectum: final treatment results of a randomized trial and an evaluation of late secondary effects. Dis Colon Rectum 1993;36:564–72.

[180] Camma C, Giunta M, Fiorica F, et al. Preoperative radiotherapy for resectable rectal cancer: a meta-analysis. JAMA 2000;284:1008–15.

[181] Kwok H, Bissett IP, Hill GL. Preoperative staging of rectal cancer. Int J Colorectal Dis 2000;15:9–20.

[182] Hildebrandt U, Klein T, Feifel G, et al. Endosonography of pararectal lymph nodes: in vitro and in vivo evaluation. Dis Colon Rectum 1990;33:863–8.

[183] Tio TL, Coene PP, van Delden OM, et al. Colorectal carcinoma: preoperative TNM classification with endosonography. Radiology 1991;179:165–70.

[184] Guinet C, Buy JN, Ghossain MA, et al. Comparison of magnetic resonance imaging and computed tomography in the preoperative staging of rectal cancer. Arch Surg 1990;125:385–8.

[185] Rifkin MD, Ehrlich SM, Marks G. Staging of rectal carcinoma: prospective comparison of endorectal US and CT. Radiology 1989;170:319–22.

[186] Gualdi GF, Casciani E, Guadalaxara A, et al. Local staging of rectal cancer with transrectal ultrasound and endorectal magnetic resonance imaging: comparison with histologic findings. Dis Colon Rectum 2000;43:338–45.

[187] Spinelli P, Schiavo M, Meroni E, et al. Results of EUS in detecting perirectal lymph node metastases of rectal cancer: the pathologist makes the difference. Gastrointest Endosc 1999;49:754–8.

[188] Park HH, Nguyen PT, Tran Q, et al. Endoscopic ultrasound-guided fine needle aspiration in the staging of rectal cancer. Gastrointest Endosc 2000;51:AB171.

[189] Hawes RH. New staging techniques: endoscopic ultrasound. Cancer 1993;71(Suppl):4207–13.

[190] Rau B, Hunerbein M, Barth C, et al. Accuracy of endorectal ultrasound after preoperative radiochemotherapy in locally advanced rectal cancer. Surg Endosc 1999;13:980–4.

[191] Napoleon B, Pujol B, Berger F, et al. Accuracy of endosonography in the staging of rectal cancer treated by radiotherapy. Br J Surg 1991;78:785–8.

[192] Pahlman L, Glimelius B. Local recurrences after surgical treatment for rectal carcinoma. Acta Chir Scand 1984;150:331–5.

[193] Phillips RK, Hittinger R, Blesovsky L, et al. Local recurrence following 'curative' surgery for large bowel cancer: I. The overall picture. Br J Surg 1984;71:12–6.

[194] Heald RJ, Ryall RD. Recurrence and survival after total mesorectal excision for rectal cancer. Lancet 1986;1:1479–82.

[195] Mascagni D, Corbellini L, Urciuoli P, et al. Endoluminal ultrasound for early detection of local recurrence of rectal cancer. Br J Surg 1989;76:1176–80.

[196] Ramirez JM, Mortensen NJ, Takeuchi N, et al. Endoluminal ultrasonography in the follow-up of patients with rectal cancer. Br J Surg 1994;81:692–4.

[197] Novell F, Pascual S, Viella P, et al. Endorectal ultrasonography in the follow-up of rectal cancer: is it a better way to detect early local recurrence? Int J Colorectal Dis 1997;12:78–81.

[198] Rotondano G, Esposito P, Pellecchia L, et al. Early detection of locally recurrent rectal cancer by endosonography. Br J Radiol 1997;70:567–71.

[199] Hunerbein M, Totkas S, Moesta KT, et al. The role of transrectal ultrasound-guided biopsy in the postoperative follow-up of patients with rectal cancer. Surgery 2001;129:164–9.

[200] Lohnert MS, Doniec JM, Henne-Bruns D. Effectiveness of endoluminal sonography in the identification of occult local rectal cancer recurrences. Dis Colon Rectum 2000;43:483–91.

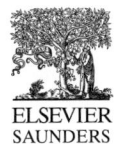
ELSEVIER
SAUNDERS

Gastrointest Endoscopy Clin N Am
15 (2005) 431–454

GASTROINTESTINAL
ENDOSCOPY CLINICS
OF NORTH AMERICA

Endoscopic Mucosal Resection: Treatment of Neoplasia

Alberto Larghi, MD, PhD, Irving Waxman, MD*

Department of Endoscopy and Therapeutics, Section of Gastroenterology, The University of Chicago, 5758 S. Maryland Avenue, MC 9028, Chicago, Illinois 60637, USA

Endoscopic mucosal resection (EMR), or mucosectomy, represents a major therapeutic advance in the management of gastrointestinal (GI) malignancy. First introduced in Japan under the name "strip-off biopsy" as an endoscopic diagnostic technique for gastric cancer [1], EMR has rapidly become a therapeutic modality that provides a valid alternative to surgical resection for the treatment of early cancers of the GI tract. By excision through the middle or deeper part of the submucosa, EMR allows complete and curative removal of areas of affected mucosa. This is accomplished with minimal cost, morbidity, and mortality and with little or no impact on the long-term quality of life of patients. Several EMR techniques have been described that are alternatively used dependent upon the anatomic conditions, the macroscopic appearance of the lesion to be resected, and the endoscopist's personal experience. This article discusses the techniques, indications, and outcomes of EMR in the management of GI neoplasia.

Early cancer: definition, diagnosis, and evaluation

The term "early cancer" refers to a localized tumor potentially curable after complete resection because of the absence or low risk of lymph node metastasis. In the GI tract, this term corresponds to lesions confined within the submucosa layer. Most of the early cancers are identified during screening of high-risk

---

* Corresponding author.

E-mail address: iwaxman@medicine.bsd.uchicago.edu (I. Waxman).

1052-5157/05/$ – see front matter © 2005 Elsevier Inc. All rights reserved.
doi:10.1016/j.giec.2005.04.003

conditions or incidentally during endoscopic procedures performed in the search for other lesions. The endoscopic appearance of early cancers may be subtle and difficult to recognize unless rigorous endoscopic examinations are performed. Learning to identify these lesions represents the first step in the process of early endoscopic detection [2,3]. To facilitate this process, additional techniques have been developed, such as chromoendoscopy and magnification, increasing potential for detection of lesions at an early stage [4,5].

Endoscopic appearance

Lesions that have the potential at endoscopy to be early cancers are called "superficial." The endoscopic appearance of superficial lesions was first described in Japan for gastric cancer. The Japanese Gastric Cancer Association recognizes three main types of superficial lesions: type I polypoid, type II nonpolypoid and non-excavated, and type III nonpolypoid with an ulcer (Fig. 1). Type I is further divided as Ip for pedunculated lesions and Is for sessile lesions; type II is further divided as IIa for slightly elevated lesions, IIb for completely flat lesions, IIc for slightly depressed lesions [6]. This classification has been applied to describe superficial lesions at other sites [7–10].

The depth of invasion, in particular the presence of tumor penetration into the submucosa, can be predicted by the morphology of a superficial lesion, providing an endoscopic staging. For a type I lesion, the risk of submucosal invasion increases with the diameter. For type II lesion, invasion of the submucosa is more frequent in depressed lesions (IIc) than in other subtypes [11].

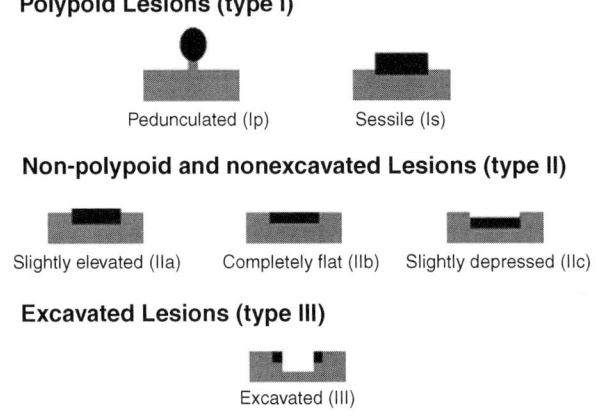

Polypoid Lesions (type I)

Pedunculated (Ip)   Sessile (Is)

Non-polypoid and nonexcavated Lesions (type II)

Slightly elevated (IIa)   Completely flat (IIb)   Slightly depressed (IIc)

Excavated Lesions (type III)

Excavated (III)

Fig. 1. The endoscopic appearance of superficial lesions as classified by the Japanese Gastric Cancer Association. (*From* Participants in the Paris Workshop. The Paris endoscopic classification of superficial neoplastic lesions: esophagus, stomach, and colon: November 30 to December 1, 2002. Gastrointest Endosc 2003;58(Suppl):S3–43; with permission.)

Chromoendoscopy and magnification

Any abnormal area of mucosa identified during the endoscopic examination may need evaluation with chromoendoscopy. Chromoendoscopy provides a detailed macroscopic analysis of the lesion and a precise delineation of its margins, and thus of its extension, with the potential of improving the curative effects of EMR [5]. A variety of stains have been realized. Lugol's iodine (1.5% to 2.0%) has been used for the evaluation of squamous cell esophageal cancer with a sensitivity and specificity of 96% and 63%, respectively [12]. Indigo carmine (0.5% to 1.0%) is the most frequent dye used on abnormal areas of the stomach and the colon [11,13]. Methylene blue (0.5% to 1.0%) has been evaluated to enhance the detection of endoscopically unapparent high-grade dysplasia (HGD) and early-stage cancer in Barrett's esophagus (BE) with conflicting results [14]. Better results have been obtained with methylene blue combined with acetic acid [15]. Chromoendoscopy with high magnification videoendoscopes may further improve visualization of mucosal detail, increasing the possibility of predicting completeness of EMR and identifying lesions unsuitable for EMR [16,17]. Tissue spectroscopy and optical coherence tomography are promising techniques that may improve the endoscopist's ability to detect subtle neoplastic changes of the GI mucosa, although they are unlikely to become part of the routine diagnostic armamentarium [18,19].

Estimation of the depth of tumor penetration

The less-than-perfect reliability of endoscopic staging with the adjunct of chromoendoscopy and magnification endoscopy for the estimation of cancer depth before EMR can be improved by the use of endoscopic ultrasonography (EUS), in particular high-frequency US probe sonography (HFUPS). HFUPS may distinguish nine layers within the wall of GI organs, in contrast to a five-layered structure seen with conventional EUS, thus providing better images that are useful in the evaluation of transmural penetration and in differentiating cancers limited to the mucosa from those with submucosal penetration. The main limitation of HFUPS is its tendency to overstage early lesions. The diagnostic accuracy of HFUPS in assessing depth of tumor invasion in the esophagus, stomach, and colon ranges from 67% to 94% among the published studies [20–25]. This high variability in HFUPS accuracy may reflect the use of probes with different penetration (15 MHz versus 20 MHz) and differences in the patient populations studied. The accuracy of HFUPS is significantly better for elevated type lesions than for depressed ones [23].

When different techniques are used in combination to select lesions suitable for EMR, the overall accuracy is high [26]. Because of the limitations of these staging techniques, it has been suggested that when a lesion meeting the generally accepted criteria of size and appearance is encountered, EMR can be performed without prior HFUPS as long as the lesion can safely be removed in its entirety [27,28]. Submucosal injection used to facilitate EMR can also help in the decision of whether or not to continue with the procedure [29]. The observation of a bleb formation with elevation of the overlying mucosa indicates the absence of deep submucosal involvement and the feasibility of EMR [30]. On the other hand, the dense fibrosis associated with deep submucosal invasion prevents fluid infiltration through the submucosal connective tissue, decreasing bleb formation and elevation of the lesion [30]. This so-called "nonlifting sign" has been found to have 100% sensitivity, 99% specificity, and 83% positive predictive value for invasive carcinoma in patients with early cancer of the colon [31]. Depth of tumor invasion can be precisely established by histologic analysis of EMR specimens, which is part of the diagnostic algorithm for the evaluation of early gastric cancer [32] and, as recently suggested, for HGD and early adenocarcinoma arising in BE [33].

Endoscopic mucosal resection

Techniques

The EMR techniques can be separated into two major groups: nonsuction ("lift-and-cut") and suction ("suck-and-cut") (Fig. 2).

"Lift-and-cut" methods

The simplest method in this group is the inject-and-cut technique, which represents an evolution of the of strip-off biopsy technique described by Tada in 1984 [1]. Lifting of the mucosal lesion is obtained by submucosal injection of a solution with the creation of a submucosal bleb that is strangulated by a snare and resected using electric cutting current. To maintain the fluid injection at the site of resection and render the procedure even safer than when saline alone is injected, the addition of epinephrine to decrease bleeding and the use of hypertonic saline, a 50% dextrose solution, or sodium hyaluronate to enhance formation of a good bulge have been described [34–37]. Indigo carmine is often added to the injectant to provide blue-green color to the expanded submucosa to help in the assessment of depth during and after resection. Different types of snares have been described, but there is no randomized study defining the ideal solution. Large lesions typically require piecemeal resection [38]. Whenever possible, inject-and-cut endoscopic piecemeal resections should be completed during a single session.

A double-channel endoscope facilitates the inject-lift-cut technique. After performing submucosal injection in standard fashion, a grasping forceps is used to pull the target lesion into an opened diathermy loop that has been introduced through the second working channel. The snare is then closed, and the lesion is resected [39].

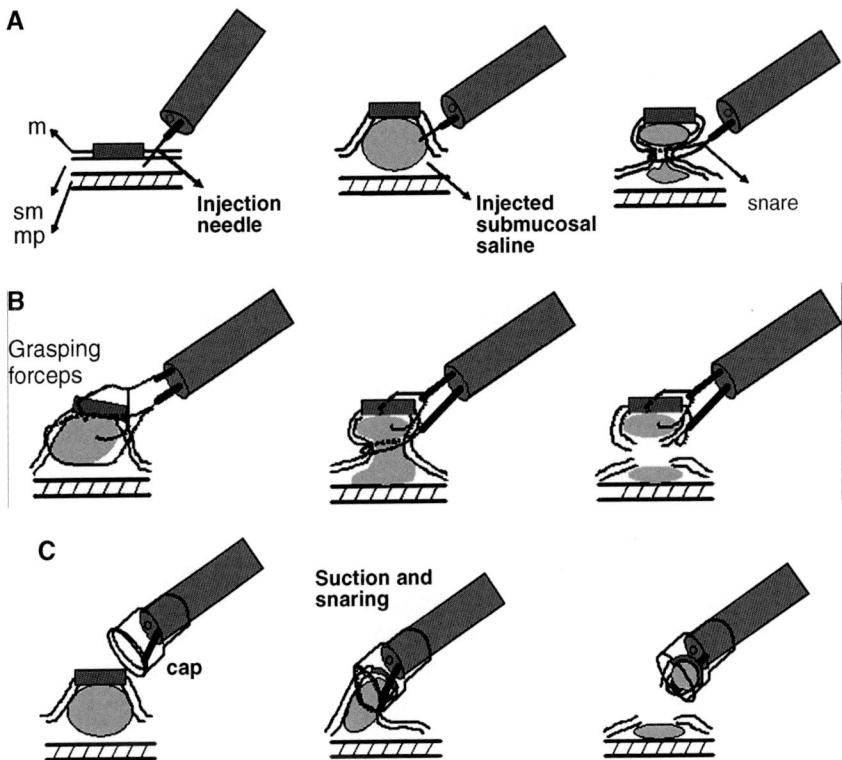

Fig. 2. Diagrams illustrating endoscopic mucosal resection techniques. (*A*) Strip biopsy technique. The lesion is injected at its base with sterile saline solution to raise the submucosa. A snare is placed at the base of the lesion, and the lesion is resected using the standard technique. (*B*) Lift-and-cut technique. The lesion is adequately raised, and the lesion is grasped with a rat tooth forceps advanced through an open snare using a double-channel endoscope. It is lifted with the forceps, the snare is placed at the base of the lesion, and resection ensues. (*C*) Cap technique. After saline solution injection, the lesion is suctioned into a pre-fitted cap placed at the tip of the endoscope and resected with a pre-looped snare in the tip of the cap. (*From* Raju GS, Waxman I. High-frequency US probe sonography-assisted endoscopic mucosal resection. Gastrointest Endosc 2000;52(Suppl):S39–49; with permission.)

"Suck-and-cut" methods

The lesion is aspirated and separated from the muscular coat and is resected by (1) simple suction with a monofilament snare, (2) endoscopic aspiration mucosectomy [40], (3) endoscopic mucosal resection using a cap-fitted panendoscope (EMRC) [41], (4) endoscopic mucosal resection tube (EMRT) [42–44], and (5) endoscopic mucosal resection using a ligating device (EMRL) [45–47].

Soehendra's technique [48] is a simple EMR technique that does not require accessory devices except for a specially designed snare made of monofilament stainless steel wire of 0.4 mm diameter. A large-channel endoscope is essential to provide enough suction alongside an inserted snare. The size of a resected specimen is smaller with this method than with other techniques. The EMRC is a simpler and easier refinement of EMR methods and can be used in any part of the GI tract, with the exception of the small intestine [49]. The technique requires a specialized transparent plastic cap that is fitted to the tip of a standard diagnostic or therapeutic endoscope. Typically, after marking the periphery of the lesion, diluted epinephrine (1:100,000) or saline solution is injected into the submucosa. A special crescent-shaped snare is pre-looped into the groove of the rim of the cap, and the injected area is suctioned into the cap. The snare is tightened around the created pseudopolyp, the entrapped tissue is pushed outside the cap with the snare, and blended current cautery is applied. Different-sized caps are available, according to the diameter of the endoscope. The largest of these caps has a diameter of 18 mm and has been designed to perform en bloc resection. The EMRL technique is similar to EMRC and uses a standard endoscopic variceal ligation device that is fitted on a single-channel endoscope. The lesion to be resected is sucked and ligated with [50] or without [9] prior submucosal injection before standard polypectomy is performed. In the EMRT technique, a specially designed transparent silicon-rubbed made tube, 65 cm in length and 18 mm in external diameter, is used. After submucosal injection, a crescent snare is inserted through a side channel of the tube and opened to enclose the target lesion. Finally, the lesion is drawn up into the tube using the suction of an endoscope that has been inserted in the tube and is resected by applying high-frequency current. Large segments of mucosa can be resected with this technique [44].

The observation of an increased rate of local recurrence when piecemeal resection is performed has stimulated Japanese investigators to develop new EMR techniques able to obtain large en bloc resection. A promising technique using a modified needle-knife with a ceramic ball at its top, also called insulation-tipped electrosurgical knife (IT knife), has been described in early gastric cancer EGC [51,52]. The ceramic ball at the tip of needle-knife prevents electrosurgical current from flowing toward the deeper layer of the gastric wall during resection. A circumferential cut around the lesion is initially made, and, after submucosal injection of a mixture of hyaluronic acid, epinephrine, and indigo carmine, the lesion is exfoliated en bloc using the IT knife. This new technique has been termed "endoscopic submucosal dissection."

Endoscopic mucosal resection complications

The most frequent complication of EMR is bleeding, which, according to the definition and the type of lesion resected, has been reported to occur in 1.5% [27,53] to 24% [54] of cases. Bleeding usually occurs during the procedure or within the first 24 hours after the procedure. Endoscopic hemostasis can be achieved in the vast majority of patients. Different hemostatic techniques can be used, although endoscopic clipping carries the advantage of a significantly lower risk of perforation as compared with other therapies [55]. Most of the data of endoscopic clipping in the western literature are from patients who experienced post-polypectomy bleeding [56,57]. Although the use of endoclips has been shown to be effective in the control of active bleeding after polypectomy, prophylactic clip placement to close the defects after EMR does not prevent delayed bleeding [58].

The most worrisome complication, perforation, is uncommon with EMR techniques. Perforation occurs by including the muscle layer in the snare resection. Inoue et al [59] reviewed the recorded videotapes of EMRC (two perforations in 380 cases of GI lesions; esophagus $n = 1$, colon $n = 1$) to determine the cause of perforation. Lack of submucosal saline solution injection was the major cause of perforation. Large-volume injection, which creates a large bleb and potentially reduces the risk of perforation, was recommended. Furthermore, strangulation of the target mucosa at the middle part of the created bleb (not at the base) decreases the risk of perforation [59]. Endosonographic assessment of submucosal dissection may be useful to evaluate whether the mucosal lesion is lifted up sufficiently from the proper muscle layer after local saline solution injection and to confirm that the muscle layer is kept outside the strangulating snare, which is useful in averting the risk of perforation [60]. Immediately recognized perforation has been successfully sealed with endoclips [61–63], whereas large perforations require immediate surgery.

Although the development of stenosis is limited to the esophagus, it is an important complication of EMR that seems to be associated, at least in animal models, with deep thermal injury of the esophageal wall [64]. Katada et al [65] analyzed their experience with EMR treatment of 216 superficial esophageal lesions in 137 patients and found that esophageal stenosis developed after EMR of 13 lesions (6%). All of these cases occurred in the 49 patients (27%) who underwent more than 75% circumferential EMR and may be avoided by two-stage resections at approximately 8-week intervals [66]. The same rate of esophageal stenosis occurring 4 weeks after circumferential EMR for the treatment of HGD and intramucosal carcinoma in BE have been reported by Seewald et al [67]. These early strictures were successfully dilated without evidence of recurrence after a mean follow-up of 1 year [67].

Esophagus

The presence of lymphatic vessels in the esophageal mucosa makes it unique among GI hollow viscus organs. Mucosal and submucosal lymphatics form a complex interconnecting network of vessels that intermittently pierce the muscularis propria, draining into regional lymph nodes and, in some patients, directly into the thoracic duct. This lymphatic anatomy allows early and widespread dissemination of esophageal carcinoma. In squamous cell carcinoma (SCC), the risk of lymph node metastasis for intraepithelial lesions (m1) and cancers invading the lamina propria (m2) is low, whereas cancers invading the muscularis mucosa (m3) and the upper third of the submucosal layer (sm1) are associated with a 10% to 19% incidence of lymph node metastasis, which increases to more than 40% with deeper extension into the middle and lower two thirds of the submucosal layer (sm2 and sm3) [53,68]. Moreover, in m1 and m2 cancers, vascular invasion does not usually occur, as opposed to m3 lesions, which carry a 25% risk of vascular invasion in the absence of lymph node metastasis [69]. Although almost all the data on EMR treatment of SCC are reported dividing mucosa and submucosa in the above-mentioned six layers, EMR specimens do not contain the entire submucosa, and this precise histopathologic subclassification cannot always be performed. Invasion in the submucosa should be measured with a micrometric scale from of the muscularis mucosae. Cancer invasion within 200 μm of the submucosa has been found to be associated with a small risk of lymph node metastasis [70].

In BE, the available surgical experience suggests that the risk of lymph node metastasis increases with depth of invasion. Lymph node metastases have been reported to occur in 0% to 33% of patients with adenocarcinoma limited to the mucosa [71–74]. This risk increases to up to 50% when submucosal invasion occurs. The wide range of lymph node metastasis reported in mucosal cancer arising in BE reflects the small number of patients included in each single study. A more realistic estimation of 1% to 3% risk of lymph node metastasis is obtained when the data from all studies are pooled. All the studies have distinguished mucosal from submucosal invasion, whereas whether different levels of mucosal invasion (m1, m2, m3) as described in SCC are associated with different potential for metastatic disease has not been investigated. It is possible to grade tumor penetration in BE according to various depths of mucosal invasion, although its clinical significance remains to be established [33]. Based on the available evidence, in patients with BE and HGD or adenocarcinoma, EMR should be performed for lesions proved to be confined to the mucosa by other staging means. Representative cases of EMR in SCC and BE are shown in Figs. 3 and 4.

Indications for endoscopic mucosal resection

Absolute indications for EMR in esophageal SCC include superficial (m1 to m2 lesions), limited (3.0 cm; <3/4 circumferential involvement), and few (1 to 4) lesions [75]. Relative indications include deep (m3 to sm1), extensive (>3.0 cm; >3/4 circumferential involvement), and multiple (>5) lesions (Table 1) [43]. In a nationwide questionnaire to the members of the Japanese Society for Esophageal Diseases, based on 2418 patients with superficial esophageal cancers from 143 institutions, the indication for EMR was limited to m1 and m2 superficial cancer in 76% of the institutions surveyed, whereas the remaining 24% represented selected cases with m3 and sm disease [53]. Moreover, in the large majority of the cases lesion size was restricted to a maximum diameter of 2 cm.

Lesions in the middle and lower thoracic esophagus and those affecting the posterolateral wall are easily amenable for EMR, whereas lesions in the cervical

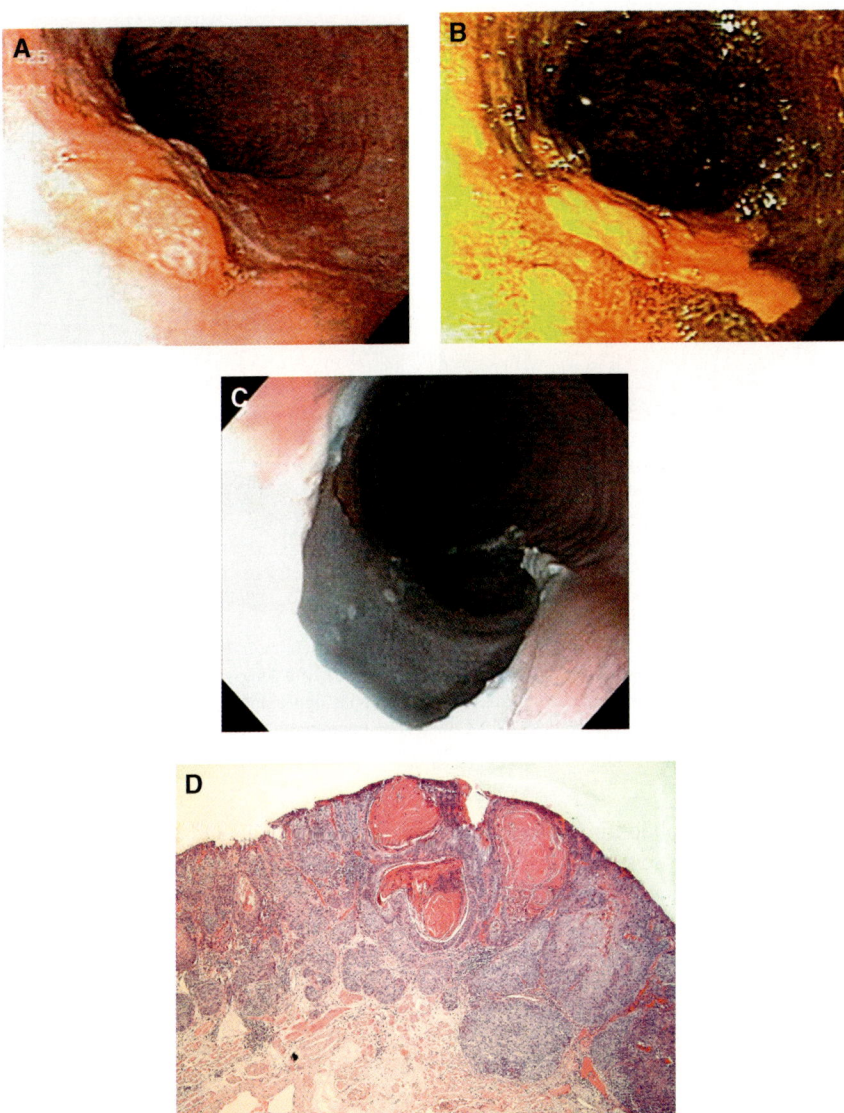

Fig. 3. Superficial esophageal squamous cell carcinoma. (*A*) Endoscopic image showing an elevated area (IIa) in the mid-esophagus; the biopsy was consistent with squamous cell carcinoma. (*B*) Chromoendoscopy with Lugol's iodine (1.5%) stain. (*C*) Mucosal defect after endoscopic mucosectomy performed in a piecemeal fashion using the endoscopic mucosal resection cap technique. (*D*) Low-power photomicrograph of part of one of the resected specimens revealing a well-differentiated squamous cell carcinoma focally extending into the inner circular layer of the muscularis mucosa (m3 disease).

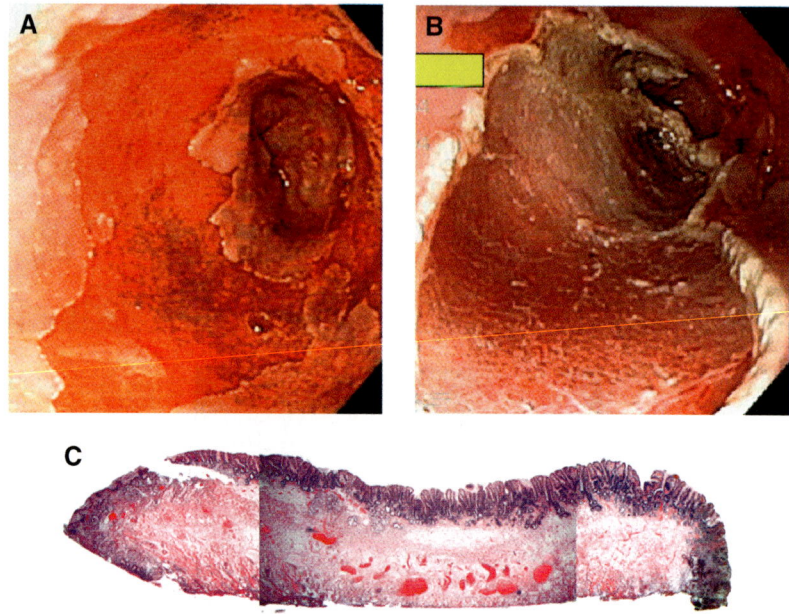

Fig. 4. Barrett's esophagus (BE). (*A*) Endoscopic appearance of a long-segment of BE in a patient with biopsy proven high-grade dysplasia. (*B*) Endoscopic appearance of the mucosectomy site with exposure of the deep submucosa. (*C*) Low-power micrograph (H&E) of an entire endoscopic mucosal resection specimen.

esophagus and abdominal esophagus and those affecting the anterior wall are more difficult to resect.

The indications for EMR in the treatment of BE are not well established. The Wiesbaden group, which has the largest experience reported to date, has performed EMR preferably in the presence of endoscopically visible lesions

Table 1
Indications for endoscopic mucosal resection in early cancers of the GI tract [75,108]

	Esophagus	Stomach	Colon
Surface morphology	I, IIa, IIb, IIc, IIc + IIa	I, IIa, IIb, IIc + IIa	I, IIa, IIb, IIc + IIa, LST
Dimension	2 cm	I, IIa, IIb: 2cm	I, IIa, LST: <3 cm
		IIc: 1 cm	IIc + IIa: <1 cm
			IIa + IIc: <1 cm
Transverse extension	30%		
Depth of invasion	m1, m2, m3 ??	m1, m2, m3, sm1 ??	m1, m2, m3 sm1a, sm1b
Histology	Squamous/glandular high-grade dysplasia/cancer	Glandular high-grade dysplasia/cancer	
Safety margin of resection	2 mm	2 mm	

Abbreviation: LST, lateral spreading tumor.

proven to be HGD or adenocarcinoma confined to the mucus [9,76,77]. This approach carries the risk of leaving in place metachronous lesions and Barrett's epithelium with the potential for recurrent disease. The possibility that circumferential EMR would be equally safe or provide better results broadening the indications for EMR to include patients with invisible flat lesions has been preliminarily evaluated [78,79], but additional data in larger cohorts of patients are needed. No information on maximum lesion size or grade of tumor differentiation for performing EMR is available.

Long-term outcome

An important source of information regarding patients with esophageal SCC treated with EMR is the registry periodically published by the Japanese Society for Esophageal Diseases (www.jsed.umin.ac.jp). The results are not stratified according to the histologic type, subclassification of invasion depth, or lymphatic or vascular involvement and cannot be used to determine the exact outcomes of patients who had EMR. Nevertheless, a low disease-specific mortality is reported.

In the study based on a nationwide questionnaire to the members of the Japanese Society for Esophageal Diseases, the outcome of 396 patients with esophageal cancer who were treated with EMR is reported, stratified according to the depth of invasion [53]. There was no significant difference in prognosis between m3 and m1 or m2 cancers. Only 1 of 46 patients with invasion of the muscularis mucosae died from tumor recurrence. In the 915 patients with mucosal disease who were analyzed in this study, vascular invasion and lymph node metastasis were higher in patients with m3 disease than in those with tumors limited to the epithelial layer and the lamina propria. This result may be due to the smaller number of patients with m3 lesions ($n = 46$) who underwent EMR versus surgery and suggests a selection bias, although a detailed explanation of the staging procedures was not provided. This study also demonstrated the observation of similar survival rates of patients with mucosal and sm1 disease treated with EMR as compared with those treated with surgery. This result parallels a more recent study by Shimizu et al [80] suggesting that EMR may be safe and effective for the long-term management of patients with SCC invading the muscularis mucosae and the upper third of the submucosa.

The largest published single-author experience for the treatment of esophageal SCC with EMR is the one from Makuuchi [44]. Using the EMR-tube method, the authors removed 540 lesions from 351 patients with SCC. Most of the patients ($n = 249$) had m1 or m2 disease, 87 patients had m3 or sm1 invasion, and the remaining 15 had sm2 or sm3 lesions. Local recurrence occurred after a mean follow-up of 9 months in four patients in the m1/m2 group, in six patients in the m3/sm1 group, and in one patient with sm2 disease. All recurrences were successfully treated with endoscopic therapy, except in one patient with a concomitant lower pharyngeal cancer, where surgical resection was performed. Twenty-six patients (7.4%) developed a second lesion at a mean follow-up of 26 months. Lymph node metastasis and death from cancer were observed only in patients with sm1 and sm2 disease. The overall 5-year disease-specific survival was 97.9%; similar results were reported by Inoue [59].

Outcome data in BE are limited. In 2000, Ell et al [9] reported the first prospective series of 64 patients with early cancer or HGD in BE treated with EMR. Complete remission was achieved in 82.5% of the cases (97% in the low-risk group and 59 in the high-risk group). During a mean follow-up of 1 year, 14% of the patients developed recurrent or metachronous lesions that were successfully treated with a combination of different endoscopic therapies, including repeat EMR. The effectiveness of EMR has been subsequently confirmed by the same group in two other reports [76,77], one involving patients with short-segment BE only [76] and by an American group [81–84]. The follow-up of all these studies was not long enough to draw definite conclusions. The publication by the Ell et al [85] reported no difference in the 5-year survival between patients who had undergone endoscopic treatment for early cancer in BE, and the average German population of the same age and sex may provide an answer to this important question.

Stomach

The risk of lymph node metastasis in gastric adenocarcinoma increases with the depth of tumor penetration. Lesions confined to the mucosa are associated with a lower risk of lymph node involvement (0% to 3%), which increases to 20% for tumors extending deep in the submucosa [86,87]. In Japan, where the incidence of gastric cancer is high, the observation of a 5-year survival >90% in patients with EGC after gastrectomy with complete removal of primary and secondary lymph nodes has stimulated the search for an alternative and less invasive treatment [88,89]. Through retrospective analysis of surgically resected specimens, Japanese investigators have determined that the diameter of the tumor, lymphatic involvement, depth of submucosal invasion, and extent of horizontal cancerous submucosal involvement significantly correlated with nodal involvement [90]. These observations have been translated into clinical practice with the development of criteria to select cancers associated with a low probability of lymph node metastasis that may be amenable to endoscopic treatment. Regarding submucosal invasion, a subdivision to stratify depth of tumor penetration by using a micrometric scale as in SCC has been proposed, with a proposed cutoff value for invasion in the submucosa of 500 μm [91]. In a review of 245 cases of EGC, the incidence of lymph node metastasis in lesions with submucosal invasion above the cutoff value (sm1) was 2% compared with 20% in those with deeper penetration (sm2) [92]. Some authors have suggested a more strict value of 300 μm [93].

Indications for endoscopic mucosal resection

The indications to perform EMR therapy in EGC are constantly revised and updated based on the results of new published studies, and after 20 years from the introduction of EMR in Japan they are a matter of profound debate among Japanese institutions. Absolute indications for gastric EMR include well- or moderately differentiated type IIa adenocarcinoma (the slightly elevated type) smaller than 2 cm or type IIc (slightly depressed type) without ulcer formation smaller than 1 cm (Table 1) [75]. Lymph node metastasis is found in only 0.01% of such cases, and prognosis after this treatment is comparable to that of surgical resection for EGC in completely resected cases [94]. For type IIc undifferentiated EGC, a consensus has not been reached.

Relative indications include (1) well-differentiated mucosal cancer <30 mm in size without ulcer or ulcer scar, (2) well-differentiated mucosal cancer <20 mm in size with ulcer or ulcer scar, (3) poorly differentiated cancer <10 mm in size, and (4) sm1 cancer <20 mm in size without ulcer or ulcer scars [95–97]. Nevertheless, the results of a recent study from Gotoda et al [98] may expand the role of EMR in EGC if confirmed by long-term prospective studies. By comparing 3016 intramucosal EGC with those of 2249 submucosal tumors, the authors found that lesions invading the submucosa could not be distinguished from those confined to the mucosa by comparing size, appearance, location, or histologic information obtained from conventional biopsies. The best predictor of lymph node metastasis was the presence or absence of lymphatic or vascular involvement, information that is available only after histologic analysis of the resected specimen [98].

Long-term outcome

The large majority of data on the outcome of EMR for the treatment of EGC have been published in the Japanese literature. In most cases, long-term follow-up results were not clearly stated. To clarify the effectiveness of EMR as curative treatment of EGC, Kojima et al [99] performed a review of a total of 1832 cases from 12 major Japanese institutions. In 10 series, the indications mentioned above were used for patient selection. In the remaining two institutions, a combination of elevated lesions <30 mm, depressed lesions <20 mm, and ulcerated lesions <10 mm were included. Using different EMR techniques, en bloc resection was performed in 76% of the 641 cases. The follow-up ranged from 4 months to 11 years. Complete resection was achieved in 1353 cases (76%). In incompletely resected cases, residual cancer was successfully treated with endoscopic retreatment or surgery. Recurrence after histopathologically documented eradication was observed in 1.9% of the patients; these data were derived mostly from a series with expanded indications. Only one patient died of metastatic gastric cancer, accounting for a disease-specific survival rate of 99%.

Ono et al [100] reported on a large, single-center experience describing 445 patients with ECG treated with EMR over an 11-year period. Patient selection was based on the generally accepted criteria, although the maximum diameter of the treated lesions was extended to 30 mm instead of 20 mm. In 74 patients (15%), histopathologic evaluation of the resected specimens showed submucosal invasion illustrating the difficulty in obtaining a correct pre-EMR diagnosis. Among 405 intramucosal cancers, complete resection was achieved in 278 cases (69%); in 43 patients (11%), lateral margins were involved, whereas in the remaining 84 patients (20%), diathermic burn, mechanical damage, or failure to retrieve specimens prevented evaluation of the completeness of the resection. Local recurrences occurred in five cases (2%) of complete resection versus 17 cases (18%) of the 95 patients with confirmed incomplete or non-evaluable resection. All of these patients underwent surgery and remain disease free. No deaths related to EGC were observed. The authors attributed the cause of the high local recurrence rate to the use of a piecemeal resection technique and the inappropriate assessment of the multiple fragments of resected specimens. In addition, the authors found that the IT knife allowed safe resection of larger lesions in a single piece, increasing the average rate of complete resection to more than 90% and facilitating histologic evaluation [100]. This observation needs confirmation in a larger cohort of patients.

Colon

In the colon, lymph node metastasis occurs only after penetration of the submucosa and is directly correlated to the depth of submucosal penetration by the tumor. Some investigators use a semiquantitative evaluation of invasion depth in the colonic submucosa in three sectors (1, 2, and 3) of equivalent thickness. The submucosal lesions involving the upper third (sm1) are further subclassified into a, b, and c according to the horizontal extension from less than a quarter to more than half [101]. In cancers with discrete submucosal invasion (sm1a and sm1b), lymph node metastasis are found rarely, as compared with more advanced stages (sm1c and beyond) where nodal metastasis are frequent [102,103]. The cutoff value at which an EMR can be considered safe has been estimated to be at 500 μm by some authors [27,104] and at 1000 μm by others [105]. Lesions invading superficially into the submucosa (≤500 μm) have been found to be associated with a 2% risk of nodal involvement as compared with 11% to 15% beyond this value [27,104]. As for esophageal SSC and EGC, involvement of colonic lymphatics and venules has been found to be a better predictor of lymph node metastasis than depth of invasion [106].

From a morphologic point of view, depressed lesions (IIc) have significantly higher incidence of submucosal invasion as compared with protruded (IIa) and elevated lesions (IIb) [107]. Generally, the larger the diameter of each, the higher the ratio of submucosal invasion, although IIc lesions are likely to be

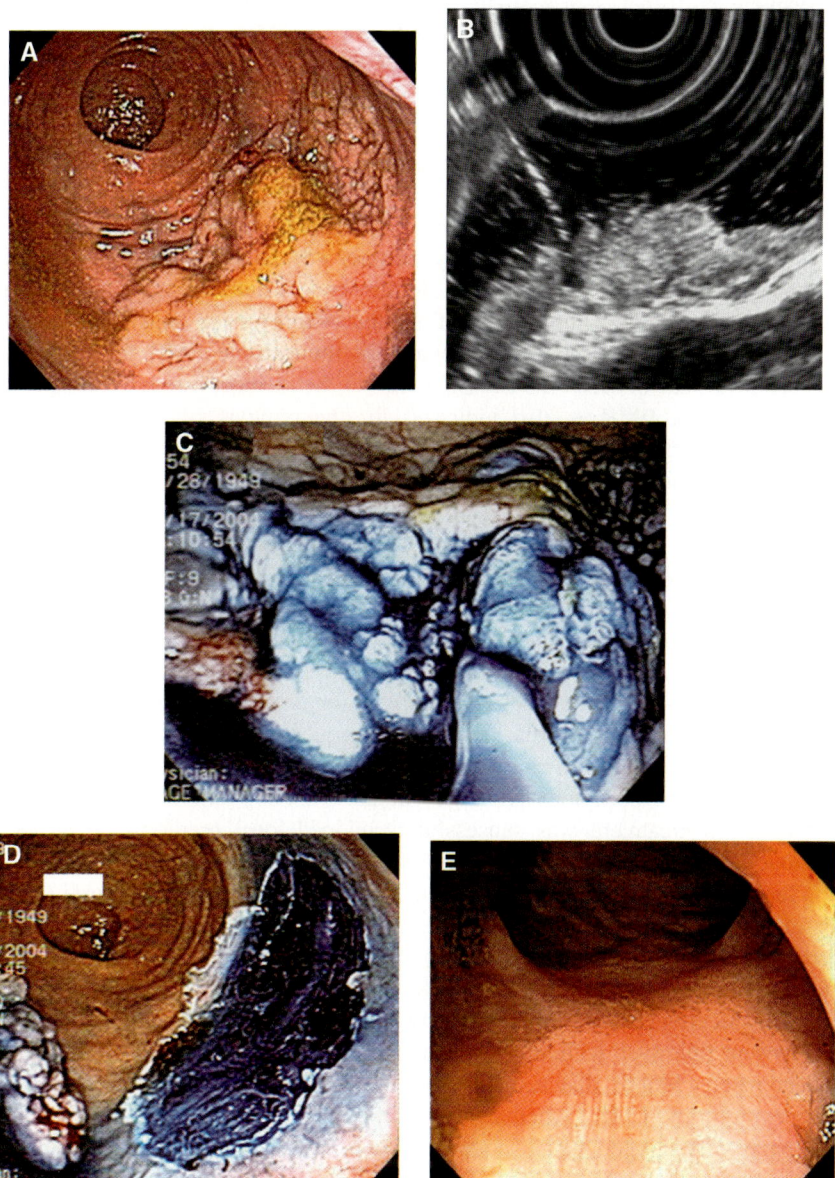

Fig. 5. (*A*) Endoscopic image of a 6 cm villous adenoma with dysplasia located 1 cm from the dentate line. (*B*) Endosonographic view demonstrating the lesion to be confined to the muscularis mucosa. (*C*) Chromoendoscopy with Indigo carmine (0.5%). (*D*) Endoscopic appearance of the mucosectomy site. The blue color of the exposed submucosal tissue is obtained by adding indigo carmine to the solution used to performed submucosal injection. This coloring of the submucosa aids in the assessment of depth during and after resection. (*E*) Appearance of the resection site follow-up endoscopic examination performed 3 months after endoscopic mucosal resection.

invasive even if their size is small compared with IIa and IIb lesions. Opinions differ with regard to the size limit of a lesion for EMR. A representative case of rectal EMR is shown in Fig. 5.

Indications for endoscopic mucosal resection

EMR is indicated in I, IIa, and lateral spreading tumors measuring 3 cm or less and in type IIb tumors (mostly minute, <5 mm). In addition, EMR is indicated for type IIc + IIa and IIa + IIc tumors <10 mm because larger lesions are associated with a high rate of submucosal invasion and lymph node involvement (Table 1) [108]. The outcomes for curative EMR for colorectal cancer with submucosal invasion remain to be demonstrated by long-term follow-up data. EMR is also indicated for the removal of carpet-type adenomatous colonic polyps, which, despite their large size, have a low risk for cancer or invasion [108].

Long-term outcome

Kudo [109] reported his experience of 674 cases of early colorectal cancer on colonoscopy. EMR was performed in 633 cases, and surgery was performed exclusively in 44 patients due to massive submucosal invasion. In the EMR group, 10 patients underwent surgery subsequently because of submucosal invasion; residual tumor tissue in the surgical resection specimens was noted in 20%, and lymph node metastasis was noted in 30%. None of the patients in whom EMR treatment was successful developed local or distant recurrence, although the follow-up period was not specified.

Tanaka et al [110] reported their experience in 81 patients with large carpet lesions (mean diameter 31 mm) who were treated with EMR. En bloc resection was performed in 50%. Minimal submucosal invasion (depth <400 mm) was found in seven patients (8.6%), and surgery was required in three of the seven. Locally recurrent lesions were detected in 6 of the 78 patients (7.7%) who underwent follow-up without additional surgical treatment. All recurrences were adenomatous lesions that accompanied the primary lesions and were treated successfully by EMR. After a mean follow-up of 5 years, none of these 78 patients developed lymph node or distant metastasis or died as a result of the tumor [110].

Duodenum

There are a limited number of studies evaluating the role of EMR for the treatment of duodenal lesions. In a recently published study, 27 patients with duodenal lesions were treated with EMR [111]. The final histologic diagnoses were adenoma in 19 patients, HGD in four patients, benign lesions in two patients, and carcinoid tumor in two patients. Complete resection was achieved in all patients.

Benign and malignant tumors of the papilla of Vater represent a growing indication for duodenal EMR [112]. The indications for endoscopic snare papillectomy of papillary adenomas as suggested by Binmoeller et al [113] are as follows: size <4 cm, no evidence for malignancy based on endoscopic appearance (regular margin, no ulceration, soft consistency), benign histologic findings (minimum of six forceps biopsies), and absence of intraductal involvement as demonstrated by ERCP. These criteria are seen as flexible; for example, tumors larger than 4 cm have been completely resected in a piecemeal fashion during sequential procedures. Malignant transformation is frequently focal, and up to 50% of villous adenomas arising at the papilla contain foci of adenocarcinoma at the time of diagnosis, making impossible to be certain that a lesion is benign by examination of standard forceps biopsy specimens alone [114]. Thus, tumor extension is a much more important criterion than the histologic diagnosis in assessing the feasibility of endoscopic resection. Endoscopic snare papillectomy remains contraindicated when the tumor extends into the biliary or pancreatic duct, which can be evaluated by performing EUS [115,116] or by the use of intraductal ultrasonography [117,118].

Long-term success rates ranging from 70% to 80% have been reported [113,119,120]. In the multicenter study by Catalano et al [120] of 103 patients, which represents the largest experience published to date, smaller lesion size (3.0 cm), older age (>54 years), adjunctive use of thermal ablation, and sporadic adenomas were significantly associated with successful therapeutic results. When a papillary lesion has been resected endoscopically, surveillance duodenoscopy is mandatory because recurrent disease occurs in up to one fourth of the cases [113], although most recurrences have been treated successfully by using endoscopic methods.

Submucosal tumors

EMR has been reported for the diagnosis and treatment of submucosal tumors (SMTs) [121–123]. In this context, Waxman et al [123] described their experience with the use of HFUPS to accurately delineate the depth of penetration of SMTs before endoscopic resection. HFUPS were also used to assess the completeness of tumor detachment from the muscularis propria after submucosal saline injection before resection. Based on this information, EMR was successfully performed in 26 of the 28 (93%) patients with SMTs evaluated without complications. Median tumor diameter was 9 mm (range 3–20 mm). More provocative and innovative techniques to remove larger stromal tumors originating also from the muscularis propria have been described but remain anecdotal [124,125].

Summary

Endoscopic mucosal resection is an exciting new technique that provides heightened levels of diagnostic accuracy and minimally invasive therapy for the management of early cancers of the GI tract. An increasing body of literature suggests that EMR provides comparable outcomes to surgery for selected indications. Current challenges limiting the proliferation of this technique in the United States include lack of training and technique standardization, lack of training in recognition of superficial GI neoplasms and indications for EMR, lack familiarity with principles of GI oncology, and lack of sufficient reimbursement for the procedure. Nevertheless, EMR is here to stay. Significant research efforts in developing uniform techniques and the development of new accessories are ongoing [126–128]. Although current techniques may seem to be rudimentary, they represent the first step into the evolving field of intraluminal endoscopic surgery.

References

[1] Tada M, Murata M, Tamekoto T. The development of "strip-off" biopsy. Gastroenterol Endosc 1984;26:833–9.

[2] Fujii T, Rembacken BJ, Dixon MF, et al. Flat adenomas in the United Kingdom: are treatable cancers being missed? Endoscopy 1998;30:437–43.

[3] Kobayashi K, Sivak Jr MV. Flat adenoma: are western colonoscopists careful enough? Endoscopy 1998;30:487–9.

[4] Shim CS. Staining in gastrointestinal endoscopy: clinical applications and limitations. Endoscopy 1999;31:487–96.

[5] Kiesslich R, Jung M, DiSario JA, et al. Perspectives of chromo and magnifying endoscopy: how, how much, when, and whom should we stain? J Clin Gastroenterol 2004;38:7–13.

[6] Japanese Gastric Cancer Association. Japanese classification of gastric carcinoma: 2nd English edition. Gastric Cancer 1998;1:10–24.

[7] Endo M, Kawano T. Detection and classification of early squamous cell esophageal cancer. Dis Esophagus 1997;10:155–8.

[8] Kudo S, Kashida H, Nakajima T, et al. Endoscopic diagnosis and treatment of early colorectal cancer. World J Surg 1997;21:694–701.

[9] Ell C, May A, Gossner L, Pech O, et al. Endoscopic mucosal resection of early cancer and high-grade dysplasia in Barrett's esophagus. Gastroenterology 2000;118:670–7.

[10] Okabayashi T, Gotoda T, Kondo H, et al. Early carcinoma of the gastric cardia in Japan: is it different from that in the West? Cancer 2000;89:2555–9.

[11] Participants in the Paris Workshop. The Paris endoscopic classification of superficial neoplastic lesions: esophagus, stomach, and colon: November 30 to December 1, 2002. Gastrointest Endosc 2003;58(Suppl):S3–43.

[12] Dawsey SM, Fleischer DE, Wang GQ, et al. Mucosal iodine staining improves endoscopic visualization of squamous dysplasia and squamous cell carcinoma of the esophagus in Linxian, China. Cancer 1998;83:220–31.

[13] Hurlstone DP, Cross SS, Slater R, et al. Detecting diminutive colorectal lesions at colonoscopy: a randomised controlled trial of pan-colonic versus targeted chromoscopy. Gut 2004; 53:376–80.

[14] Canto MI. Methylene blue chromoendoscopy for Barrett's esophagus: coming soon to your GI unit? Gastrointest Endosc 2001;54:403–9.

[15] Lambert R, Rey JF, Sankaranarayanan R. Magnification and chromoscopy with the acetic acid test. Endoscopy 2003;35:437–45.

[16] Hurlstone DP, Cross SS, Brown S, et al. A prospective evaluation of high-magnification chromoscopic colonoscopy in predicting completeness of EMR. Gastrointest Endosc 2004; 59:642–50.

[17] Hurlstone DP, Cross SS, Drew K, et al. An evaluation of colorectal endoscopic mucosal resection using high-magnification chromoscopic colonoscopy: a prospective study of 1000 colonoscopies. Endoscopy 2004;36:491–8.

[18] Dacosta RS, Wilson BC, Marcon NE. New optical technologies for earlier endoscopic diagnosis of premalignant gastrointestinal lesions. J Gastroenterol Hepatol 2002;17(Suppl): S85–104.

[19] Lambert R. Diagnosis of esophagogastric tumors. Endoscopy 2004;36:110–9.

[20] Saitoh Y, Obara T, Einami K, et al. Efficacy of high-frequency ultrasound probes for the preoperative staging of invasion depth in flat and depressed colorectal tumors. Gastrointest Endosc 1996;44:34–9.

[21] Murata Y, Suzuki S, Ohta M, et al. Small ultrasonic probes for determination of the depth of superficial esophageal cancer. Gastrointest Endosc 1996;44:23–8.

[22] Akahoshi K, Chijiiwa Y, Hamada S, et al. Endoscopic ultrasonography: a promising method for assessing the prospects of endoscopic mucosal resection in early gastric cancer. Endoscopy 1997;29:614–9.

[23] Akahoshi K, Chijiwa Y, Hamada S, et al. Pretreatment staging of endoscopically early gastric cancer with a 15 MHz ultrasound catheter probe. Gastrointest Endosc 1998;48:470–6.

[24] Murata Y, Suzuki S, Mitsunaga A, et al. Endoscopic ultrasonography in diagnosis and mucosal resection for early esophageal cancer. Endoscopy 1998;30(Suppl 1):A44–6.

[25] Kida M, Tanabe S, Watanabe M, et al. Staging of gastric cancer with endoscopic ultrasonography and endoscopic mucosal resection. Endoscopy 1998;30(Suppl 1):A64–8.

[26] Yanai H, Matsumoto Y, Harada T, et al. Endoscopic ultrasonography and endoscopy for staging depth of invasion in early gastric cancer: a pilot study. Gastrointest Endosc 1997;46:212–6.

[27] Rembacken BJ, Gotoda T, Fujii T, et al. Endoscopic mucosal resection. Endoscopy 2001;33: 709–18.

[28] Soetikno RM, Gotoda T, Nakanishi Y, et al. Endoscopic mucosal resection. Gastrointest Endosc 2003;57:567–79.

[29] Kato H, Haga S, Endo S, et al. Lifting of lesions during endoscopic mucosal resection (EMR) of early colorectal cancer: implications for the assessment of resectability. Endoscopy 2001; 33:568–73.

[30] Ishiguro A, Uno Y, Ishiguro Y, et al. Correlation of lifting versus non-lifting and microscopic depth of invasion in early colorectal cancer. Gastrointest Endosc 1999;50:329–33.

[31] Uno Y, Munakata A. The non-lifting sign of invasive colon cancer. Gastrointest Endosc 1994;40:485–9.

[32] Tada M. Endoscopic mucosal resection of the stomach: initial description. Gastrointest Endosc Clin N Am 2001;11:499–510.

[33] Lightdale CJ, Larghi A, Rotterdam H, et al. Endoscopic ultrasonography (EUS) and endoscopic mucosal resection (EMR) for staging and treatment of high-grade dysplasia (HGD) and early adenocarcinoma (EAC) in Barrett's esophagus (BE) [abstract]. Gastrointest Endosc 2004;59:AB90.

[34] Shirai M, Nakamura T, Matsuura A, et al. Safer colonoscopic polypectomy with local submucosal injection of hypertonic saline-epinephrine solution. Am J Gastroenterol 1994; 89:334–8.

[35] Yamamoto H, Kawata H, Sunada K, et al. Success rate of curative endoscopic mucosal resection with circumferential mucosal incision assisted by submucosal injection of sodium hyaluronate. Gastrointest Endosc 2002;56:507–12.

[36] Fujishiro M, Yahagi N, Kashimura K, et al. Comparison of various submucosal injection solutions for maintaining mucosal elevation during endoscopic mucosal resection. Endoscopy 2004;36:579–83.

[37] Fujishiro M, Yahagi N, Kashimura K, et al. Different mixtures of sodium hyaluronate and their ability to create submucosal fluid cushions for endoscopic mucosal resection. Endoscopy 2004;36:584–9.

[38] Kanamori T, Itoh M, Yokoyama Y, et al. Injection-incision-assisted snare resection of large sessile colorectal polyps. Gastrointest Endosc 1996;43:189–95.

[39] Tada M, Murakami A, Karita M, et al. Endoscopic resection of early gastric cancer. Endoscopy 1993;25:445–50.

[40] Torii A, Sakai M, Kajiyama T, et al. Endoscopic aspiration mucosectomy as curative endoscopic surgery: analysis of 24 cases of early gastric cancer. Gastrointest Endosc 1995; 42:475–9.

[41] Inoue H, Takeshita K, Hori H, et al. Endoscopic mucosal resection with a capfitted panendoscope for esophagus, stomach, and colon mucosal lesions. Gastrointest Endosc 1993;39: 58–62.

[42] Inoue H, Endo M. Endoscopic esophageal mucosal resection using a transparent tube. Surg Endosc 1990;4:198–201.

[43] Makuuchi H. Esophageal endoscopic mucosal resection (EEMR) tube. Surg Laparosc Endosc 1996;6:160–1.

[44] Makuuchi H. Endoscopic mucosal resection for mucosal cancer in the esophagus. Gastrointest Endosc Clin N Am 2001;11:445–58.

[45] Fleischer DE, Wang GQ, Dawsey S, et al. Tissue band ligation followed by snare resection (band and snare): a new technique for tissue acquisition in the esophagus. Gastrointest Endosc 1996;44:68–72.

[46] Suzuki Y, Hiraishi H, Kanke K, et al. Treatment of gastric tumors by endoscopic mucosal resection with a ligating device. Gastrointest Endosc 1999;49:192–9.

[47] Suzuki H. Endoscopic mucosal resection using ligating device for early gastric cancer. Gastrointest Endosc Clin N Am 2001;11:511–8.

[48] Soehendra N, Binmoeller KF, Bohnacker S, et al. Endoscopic snare mucosectomy in the esophagus without any additional equipment: a simple technique for resection of flat early cancer. Endoscopy 1997;29:380–3.

[49] Inoue H. Endoscopic mucosal resection for the entire gastrointestinal mucosal lesions. Gastrointest Endosc Clin N Am 2001;11:459–78.

[50] Suzuki Y, Hiraishi H, Kanke K, et al. Treatment of gastric tumors by endoscopic mucosal resection with a ligating device. Gastrointest Endosc 1999;49:192–9.

[51] Gotoda T, Kondo H, Ono H, et al. A new endoscopic mucosal resection procedure using an insulation-tipped electrosurgical knife for rectal flat lesions: report of two cases. Gastrointest Endosc 1999;50:560–3.

[52] Miyamoto S, Muto M, Hamamoto Y, et al. A new technique for endoscopic mucosal resection with an insulated-tip electrosurgical knife improves the completeness of resection of intramucosal gastric neoplasms. Gastrointest Endosc 2002;55:576–81.

[53] Kodama M, Kakegawa T. Treatment of superficial cancer of the esophagus: a summary of responses to a questionnaire on superficial cancer of the esophagus in Japan. Surgery 1998; 123:432–9.

[54] Binmoeller KF, Bohnacker S, Seifert H, et al. Endoscopic snare excision of "giant" colorectal polyps. Gastrointest Endosc 1996;43:183–8.

[55] Raju GS, Gajula L. Endoclips for GI endoscopy. Gastrointest Endosc 2004;59:267–79.

[56] Binmoeller KF, Thonke F, Soehendra N. Endoscopic hemoclip treatment for gastrointestinal bleeding. Endoscopy 1993;25:167–70.

[57] Parra-Blanco A, Kaminaga N, Kojima T, et al. Hemoclipping for postpolypectomy and postbiopsy colonic bleeding. Gastrointest Endosc 2000;51:37–41.

[58] Shioji K, Suzuki Y, Kobayashi M, et al. Prophylactic clip application does not decrease delayed bleeding after colonoscopic polypectomy. Gastrointest Endosc 2003;57:691–4.

[59] Inoue H. Endoscopic mucosal resection for esophageal and gastric mucosal cancers. Can J Gastroenterol 1998;12:355–9.

[60] Izumi Y, Inoue H, Kawano T, et al. Endosonography during endoscopic mucosal resection to enhance its safety: a new technique. Surg Endosc 1999;13:358–60.

[61] Binmoeller KF, Grimm H, Soehendra N. Endoscopic closure of a perforation using metallic clips after snare excision of a gastric leiomyoma. Gastrointest Endosc 1993;39:172–4.

[62] Yoshikane H, Hidano H, Sakakibara A, et al. Endoscopic repair by clipping of iatrogenic colonic perforation. Gastrointest Endosc 1997;46:464–6.

[63] Kim HS, Lee DK, Jeong YS, et al. Successful endoscopic management of a perforated gastric dysplastic lesion after endoscopic mucosal resection. Gastrointest Endosc 2000;51:613–5.

[64] Conio M, Sorbi D, Batts KP, et al. Endoscopic circumferential esophageal mucosectomy in a porcine model: an assessment of technical feasibility, safety, and outcome. Endoscopy 2001;33:791–4.

[65] Katada C, Muto M, Manabe T, et al. Esophageal stenosis after endoscopic mucosal resection of superficial esophageal lesions. Gastrointest Endosc 2003;57:165–9.

[66] Raju GS, Waxman I. High-frequency US probe sonography-assisted endoscopic mucosal resection. Gastrointest Endosc 2000;52(Suppl):S39–49.

[67] Seewald S, Groth S, Brand B, et al. Circumferential EMR-Future endoscopic management of HGIN and IMC in Barrett's esophagus? Preliminary results of an ongoing study [abstract]. Gastrointest Endosc 2004;59:AB101.

[68] Yoshida M, Hanashi T, Momma K, et al. Endoscopic mucosal resection for radical treatment of esophageal cancer. Gan To Kagaku Ryoho 1995;22:847–54.

[69] Makuuchi H, Machimura T, Mizutani K, et al. Controversy in the treatment of superficial esophageal carcinoma–indications and problems of the procedures. Nippon Geka Gakkai Zasshi 1992;93:1059–62.

[70] Watanabe H, Komokai S, Ajioka Y, et al. Histopathology of m3 and sm1 invasive squamous cell carcinoma of the esophagus with special reference to endoscopic resection. Stomach Intest 1998;33:1001–9.

[71] Clark G, Peters J, Ireland A, et al. Nodal metastasis and sites of recurrence after en bloc esophagectomy for adenocarcinoma. Ann Thorac Surg 1994;58:646–53.

[72] Rice TW, Zuccaro Jr G, Adelstein DJ, et al. Esophageal carcinoma: depth of tumor invasion is predictive of regional lymph node status. Ann Thorac Surg 1998;65:787–92.

[73] Nigro JJ, Hagen JA, DeMeester TR, et al. Prevalence and location of nodal metastases in distal esophageal adenocarcinoma confined to the wall: implications for therapy. J Thorac Cardiovasc Surg 1999;117:16–23.

[74] Stein HJ, Feith M, Mueller J, et al. Limited resection for early adenocarcinoma in Barrett's esophagus. Ann Surg 2000;232:733–42.

[75] Lambert R. Endoscopic treatment of esophagogastric tumors. Endoscopy 1998;30:80–93.

[76] May A, Gossner L, Pech O, et al. Intraepithelial high-grade neoplasia and early adenocarcinoma in short-segment Barrett's esophagus (SSBE): curative treatment using local endoscopic treatment techniques. Endoscopy 2002;34:604–10.

[77] May A, Gossner L, Pech O, et al. Local endoscopic therapy for intraepithelial high-grade neoplasia and early adenocarcinoma in Barrett's oesophagus: acute-phase and intermediate results of a new treatment approach. Eur J Gastroenterol Hepatol 2002;14:1085–91.

[78] Seewald S, Akaraviputh T, Seitz U, et al. Circumferential EMR and complete removal of Barrett's epithelium: a new approach to management of Barrett's esophagus containing high-grade intraepithelial neoplasia and intramucosal carcinoma. Gastrointest Endosc 2003;57: 854–9.

[79] Giovannini M, Bories E, Pesenti C, et al. Circumferential endoscopic mucosal resection in Barrett's esophagus with high-grade intraepithelial neoplasia or mucosal cancer: preliminary results in 21 patients. Endoscopy 2004;36:782–7.

[80] Shimizu Y, Tsukagoshi H, Fujita M, et al. Long-term outcome after endoscopic mucosal resection in patients with esophageal squamous cell carcinoma invading the muscularis mucosae or deeper. Gastrointest Endosc 2002;56:387–90.

[81] Nijhawan PK, Wang KK. Endoscopic mucosal resection for lesions with endoscopic features

suggestive of malignancy and high-grade dysplasia within Barrett's esophagus. Gastrointest Endosc 2000;52:328–32.

[82] Waxman I, Saitoh Y. Clinical outcome of endoscopic mucosal resection for superficial GI lesions and the role of high-frequency US probe sonography in an American population. Gastroenterol Endosc 2000;52:322–7.

[83] Buttar NS, Wang KK, Lutzke LS, et al. Combined endoscopic mucosal resection and photodynamic therapy for esophageal neoplasia within Barrett's esophagus. Gastrointest Endosc 2001;54:682–8.

[84] Pacifico RJ, Wang KK, Wongkeesong L, et al. Combined endoscopic mucosal resection and photodynamic therapy versus esophagectomy for management of early adenocarcinoma in Barrett's esophagus. Clin Gastroenterol Hepatol 2003;1:252–7.

[85] Pech O, May A, Gossner L, et al. Long-term results of local endoscopic therapy for intra-epithelial high-grade neoplasia and early adenocarcinoma in Barrett's esophagus [abstract]. Gastrointest Endosc 2003;57:110.

[86] Sano T, Kobori O, Muto T. Lymph node metastasis from early gastric cancer: endoscopic resection of tumour. Br J Surg 1992;79:241–4.

[87] Yamao T, Shirao K, Ono H, et al. Risk factors for lymph node metastasis from intramucosal gastric carcinoma. Cancer 1996;77:602–6.

[88] Okamura T, Tsujitani S, Korenaga D, et al. Lymphadenectomy for cure in patients with early gastric cancer and lymph node metastasis. Am J Surg 1988;155:476–80.

[89] Noguchi Y, Imada T, Matsumoto A, et al. Radical surgery for gastric cancer: a review of the Japanese experience. Cancer 1989;64:2053–62.

[90] Takekoshi T. General view of gastric cancer with depth invasion into muscle layer (m cancer) from a survey of reports of the Japanese Research Society for Gastric Cancer. J Gastroenterol Mass Survey 1994;32:94–132.

[91] Ishigami S, Hokita S, Natsugoe S, et al. Carcinomatous infiltration into the submucosa as a predictor of lymph node involvement in early gastric cancer. World J Surg 1998;22:1056–9.

[92] Kurihara N, Kubota T, Otani Y, et al. Lymph node metastasis of early gastric cancer with submucosal invasion. Br J Sur 1998;85:835–9.

[93] Yasuda K, Shiraishi N, Suematsu T, et al. Rate of detection of lymph node metastasis is correlated with the depth of submucosal invasion in early stage gastric carcinoma. Cancer 1999;85:2119–23.

[94] Makuuchi H, Kise Y, Shimada H, et al. Endoscopic mucosal resection for early gastric cancer. Semin Surg Oncol 1999;17:108–16.

[95] Noda M, Kodama T, Atsumi M, et al. Possibilities and limitations of endoscopic resection for early gastric cancer. Endoscopy 1997;29:361–5.

[96] Amano Y, Ishihara S, Amano K, et al. An assessment of local curability of endoscopic surgery in early gastric cancer without satisfaction of current therapeutic indications. Endoscopy 1998;30:548–52.

[97] Inoue H, Tani M, Nagai K, et al. Treatment of esophageal and gastric tumors. Endoscopy 1999;31:47–55.

[98] Gotoda T, Yanagisawa A, Sasako M, et al. Incidence of lymph node metastasis from early gastric cancer: estimation with a large number of cases at two large centers. Gastric Cancer 2000;3:219–25.

[99] Kojima T, Parra-Blanco A, Takahashi H, et al. Outcome of endoscopic mucosal resection for early gastric cancer: review of the Japanese literature. Gastrointest Endosc 1998;48:550–4.

[100] Ono H, Kondo H, Gotoda T, et al. Endoscopic mucosal resection for treatment of early gastric cancer. Gut 2001;48:225–9.

[101] Kudo S. Endoscopic mucosal resection of flat and depressed types of early colorectal cancer. Endoscopy 1993;25:455–61.

[102] Haggitt RC, Glotzbach RE, Soffer EE, et al. Prognostic factors in colorectal carcinomas arising in adenomas: implications for lesions removed by endoscopic polypectomy. Gastroenterology 1985;89:328–36.

[103] Waye JD, Haggitt RC. Controversies, dilemmas, and dialogues: when is colonoscopic resection of an adenomatous polyp containing a "malignancy" sufficient? Am J Gastroenterol 1990;85:1564–8.

[104] Kodaira S, Yao T, Nakamura K. The incidence of lymph node metastasis of submucosal colorectal carcinomas in each submucosal invasion depth degree: results from a questionnaire survey (in Japanese with English abstract). Stomach Intest 1994;29:1137–42.

[105] Yokoyama J, Ajioka Y, Watanabe H, et al. lymph node metastasis and micrometastasis of submucosal invasive colorectal carcinoma: an indicator of the curative potential of endoscopic treatment. Acta Med Biol 2002;50:1–8.

[106] Aoki R, Tanaka S, Haruma K, et al. MUC-1 expression as a predictor of the curative endoscopic treatment of submucosally invasive colorectal carcinoma. Dis Colon Rectum 1998;41: 1262–72.

[107] Kudo S, Tamegai Y, Yamano H, et al. Endoscopic mucosal resection of the colon: the Japanese technique. Gastrointest Endosc Clin N Am 2001;11:519–35.

[108] Kudo S, Kashida H, Tamura T, et al. Colonoscopic diagnosis and management of nonpolypoid early colorectal cancer. World J Surg 2000;24:1081–90.

[109] Kudo S. Endoscopic mucosal resection of flat and depressed types of early colorectal cancer. Endoscopy 1993;25:455–61.

[110] Tanaka S, Haruma K, Oka S, et al. Clinicopathologic features and endoscopic treatment of superficially spreading colorectal neoplasms larger than 20 mm. Gastrointest Endosc 2001; 54:62–6.

[111] Ahmad NA, Kochman ML, Long WB, et al. Efficacy, safety, and clinical outcomes of endoscopic mucosal resection: a study of 101 cases. Gastrointest Endosc 2002;55:390–6.

[112] Kim MH, Lee SK, Seo DW, et al. Tumors of the major duodenal papilla. Gastrointest Endosc 2001;54:609–20.

[113] Binmoeller KF, Boaventura S, Ramsperger K, et al. Endoscopic snare excision of benign adenomas of the papilla of Vater. Gastrointest Endosc 1993;39:127–31.

[114] Sakorafas GH, Friess H, Dervenis CG. Villous tumors of the duodenum: biologic characters and clinical implications. Scand J Gastroenterol 2000;35:337–44.

[115] Tio TL, Mulder CJ, Eggink WF. Endosonography in staging early carcinoma of the ampulla of Vater. Gastroenterology 1992;102:1392–5.

[116] Walsh RM, Connelly M, Baker M. Imaging for the diagnosis and staging of periampullary carcinomas. Surg Endosc 2003;17:1514–20.

[117] Itoh A, Goto H, Naitoh Y, et al. Intraductal ultrasonography in diagnosing tumor extension of cancer of the papilla of Vater. Gastrointest Endosc 1997;45:251–60.

[118] Menzel J, Hoepffner N, Sulkowski U, et al. Polypoid tumors of the major duodenal papilla: preoperative staging with intraductal US, EUS, and CT: a prospective, histopathologically controlled study. Gastrointest Endosc 1999;49:349–57.

[119] Norton ID, Gostout CJ, Baron TH, et al. Safety and outcome of endoscopic snare excision of the major duodenal papilla. Gastrointest Endosc 2002;56:239–43.

[120] Catalano MF, Linder JD, Chak A, et al. Endoscopic management of adenoma of the major duodenal papilla. Gastrointest Endosc 2004;59:225–32.

[121] Kawamoto K, Yamada Y, Furukawa N, et al. Endoscopic submucosal tumorectomy for gastrointestinal submucosal tumors restricted to the submucosa: a new form of endoscopic minimal surgery. Gastrointest Endosc 1997;46:311–7.

[122] Kojima T, Takahashi H, Parra-Blanco A, et al. Diagnosis of submucosal tumor of the upper GI tract by endoscopic resection. Gastrointest Endosc 1999;50:516–22.

[123] Waxman I, Saitoh Y, Raju GS, et al. High-frequency probe EUS-assisted endoscopic mucosal resection: a therapeutic strategy for submucosal tumors of the GI tract. Gastrointest Endosc 2002;55:44–9.

[124] Kim TI, Park YS, Choi EH, et al. Endoscopic resection of a large leiomyoma of the esophagus. Gastrointest Endosc 2004;59:129–33.

[125] Park YS, Park SW, Kim TI, et al. Endoscopic enucleation of upper-GI submucosal tumors by using an insulated-tip electrosurgical knife. Gastrointest Endosc 2004;59:409–15.

[126] Dye C, Blanchard P, Waxman I. Fluidjet technology-assisted endoscopic mucosal resection (FJT-EMR): preliminary results of a novel technology [abstract]. Gastrointest Endosc 2002; 55:AB96.

[127] Dye C, Kinney T, Chi K, et al. Holmium Laser Assisted Mucosectomy (HLAM) [abstract]. Gastrointest Endosc 2004;59:AB90.

[128] Rajan E, Gostout CJ, Feitoza AB, et al. Widespread EMR: a new technique for removal of large areas of mucosa. Gastrointest Endosc 2004;60:623–7.

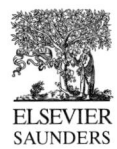

ELSEVIER
SAUNDERS

Gastrointest Endoscopy Clin N Am
15 (2005) 455–466

GASTROINTESTINAL
ENDOSCOPY CLINICS
OF NORTH AMERICA

Endoscopic Approach to Gastrointestinal Stromal Tumors

Nicholas Nickl, MD

Department of Medicine, University of Kentucky Medical Center, 800 Rose Street, Room MN 649, Lexington, KY 40536, USA

The scenario is unfortunately all too common. Evaluating a patient for dyspepsia, the endoscopist is surprised to discover a submucosal mass in the stomach. It is obviously unrelated to the patient's complaint and probably benign—but then again, maybe not. The ensuing encounter with the patient ends unsatisfactorily amid confusion and alarm: Is it causing my symptoms? Is it cancer? Why don't you just take it out? Unrevealing CT scans and ambiguous surveillance endoscopies fuel rising frustration for patient and physician. When the curtain finally rings down on this drama—if it ever does–the plot is often left unresolved. Fortunately, a revision of this sad script is at hand because several recent developments have added considerably to our understanding of submucosal masses and the stromal cell tumors often lurking within them.

Evaluation of submucosal tumors

Background

Mesenchymal tumors of the gastrointestinal (GI) tract arise from the embryologic mesoderm and as such usually occupy a position within the wall of the GI tract. They often protrude into the lumen of the hollow viscus, where they can be seen on endoscopic or radiographic studies. Such an appearance is referred to as a "submucosal tumor," which is a somewhat confusing term because not all such lesions arise within the submucosal layer. A large variety of lesions originating in several locations can present such an appearance, some of which are

E-mail address: nickl@pop.uky.edu

doi:10.1016/j.giec.2005.04.001
giendo.theclinics.com

Table 1
Classification of submucosal tumors of the GI tract

	Non neoplasms	Neoplasms
Extramural position	Cyst of adjacent organ (pancreas, liver) Organomegaly	Primary or metastatic neoplasm of adjacent organ including lymph nodes
Intramural position	Intramural cyst varices Pancreatic rest	GI stromal tumor Lipoma Granular cell tumor Glomus tumor Metastatic malignancy

listed in Table 1. Whenever a submucosal tumor is encountered, the alert endo-scopist bears in mind all the possibilities.

Prior studies of submucosal tumors (SMTs) have suggested that as many as half are extramural structures. These include normal organs such as the liver, spleen, gallbladder, and kidney; enlargement of these adjacent organs (organo-megaly); abnormal structures such as aneurysms, cysts, and pseudocysts; and neoplasms of adjacent organs [1–3]. Among the intramural non-neoplastic le-sions, varices are likely the most common but are easily recognized by endo-scopic appearance and clinical circumstances. A few other non-neoplastic masses, such as pancreatic rests and duplication cysts, may occasionally be seen.

What are left, after these have all been excluded, are the mesenchymal neoplasms. This group comprises a confusing array of obscure and infrequent tumors, many of which are listed in Table 2. GI stromal tumors (GISTs) are the most frequently encountered tumors on this list [4], and all GISTs contain potential for malignant behavior. For this reason, a discussion of SMTs almost always evolves promptly into a discussion of GIST.

Of lumps and bumps: initial characterization

When a submucosal tumor is encountered on visual endoscopy, the first step is to characterize it with respect to several parameters. The important considerations include location, size, shape, number, color, overlying mucosa, and compression characteristics. Other specific features, such a pedunculation, may occasionally be relevant. Table 3 lists the parameters that may characterize each of these features.

Table 2
Mesenchymal tumors of the GI tract

Tumor type	Examples
Stromal tumor	GI stromal tumor, smooth muscle tumor (true leiomyoma or leiomyosarcoma), glomus tumor
Lipocytic tumor	Lipoma, liposarcoma
Vascular tumor	Hemangioma, hemangiosarcoma, Kaposi's sarcoma
Neural tumor	Neuroma/neurofibroma
Miscellaneous tumors	Granular cell tumor, inflammatory fibroid polyp, fibrovascular polyp

Table 3
Features of submucosal tumors and examples

Feature	Characterizations	Examples
Location	Organ, site	Granular cell tumors are typically esophageal.
Size	In two dimensions	Certain lesions, such as granular cell tumors, rarely exceed 1–2 cm.
Shape/contour	Smooth, lumpy, oval, irregular	GISTs are typically oval and smooth. Primary malignancies and metastases may be lumpy.
Color	Yellow, blue, pale, pink	Lipomas and granular cell tumors are often yellow. Vascular lesions are often blue.
Number	Single, multiple	Granular cell tumors are sometimes multiple.
Overlying mucosa	Ulcerated, dimpled, normal, erythematous	GISTs typically have normal mucosa but may be dimpled or ulcerated. Pancreatic rests are typically dimpled. Malignancies are often dimpled or ulcerated.
Compression characteristics	Firm, soft	Lipomas and vascular lesions are easily compressible. GISTs and pseudocysts are usually firm.
Miscellaneous	Sessile/pedunculated Bleeding Motion	Lipomas and varices are sometimes pedunculated. Extramural structures often move relative to the mucosa with respiration or pulse.

Abbreviation: GIST, gastrointestinal stromal tumor.

It is difficult to overstate the importance of this type of basic endoscopic characterization. Because mucosal pinch biopsies rarely yield diagnostic material, the endoscopic appearance and clinical circumstances usually determine which such lesions deserve further evaluation. It may be necessary to use special techniques: Compression with a biopsy forceps is often helpful even when no biopsies are intended, and side-viewing endoscopy using a duodenoscope is regularly needed to fully characterize duodenal SMTs. A few extra minutes of study while peristalsis changes the perspective can be invaluable.

Endoscopic ultrasound (EUS) is usually the next diagnostic step. Although not every lump and bump deserves such examination, several features can be suggested to identify those that need further testing, including size >1 cm, dimpled or ulcerated surface, lumpy or irregular shape, multiple lesions, a hard or firm texture, and a personal history of malignancy. Lesions that are obviously lipomas (small, soft, yellow, smooth) or granular cell tumors (small, esophageal, yellow, round) usually do not need further diagnostic testing. Lesions with obvious mucosal involvement, as may be indicated by an adenomatous surface, are not truly submucosal tumors; these are typically best managed by aggressive efforts to obtain diagnostic tissue by conventional biopsy before EUS.

The role of endoscopic ultrasound

Having determined that a given SMT deserves further attention, what should be done? New CT imaging methods are able to identify lesions as small as 1 cm, but further useful characterization has not been described [5]. Nevertheless, CT is

Table 4
Endoscopic ultrasound characterization of intramural tumors

Characteristic	Descriptors
Size	Cross-sectional diameters
Shape	Round, oval, triangular, irregular
Margin definition	Well defined (distinct), poorly defined (indistinct)
Margin contour	Smooth, irregular
Wall layer	relative to five-layer wall structure
Background echogenicity	Anechoic, hypoechoic, hyperechoic
Focal echogenicity	Hypoechoic foci, anechoic foci, hyperechoic foci

a reasonable next step for large lesions (2–3 cm or bigger) not least because, if nothing abnormal is seen, extrinsic compression by extraluminal organs becomes a strong consideration.

EUS has become the most important next step in evaluating submucosal tumors. Normal and abnormal extramural structures and organs are readily identified as the cause of extrinsic compression into the GI lumen [6]. More importantly, EUS can characterize intramural lesions with respect to a number of features helpful in suggesting pathologic diagnoses (Table 4). In addition, for tumors that are invasive, the degree of invasion (tumor T stage) can be described.

The accuracy of such characterizations and their relationship to various pathologic types has been examined. Rosch et al [4], in a study that included 102 intramural lesions, described the appearance of stromal tumors, lipomas, varices, and other entities. Yasuda [7] also described such findings in 210 submucosal tumors. Rosch [4] reported diagnostic accuracy figures ranging from 80% to 90% for various types of lesions.

Fig. 1 shows the typical appearance of an esophageal granular cell tumor. These benign lesions are usually found in the distal esophagus and are characteristically under 2 cm in size. Most are asymptomatic, although dysphagia may occasionally be present. Multiple lesions are not uncommon. They may be of Schwann cell origin, although the pathogenesis is uncertain. The endoscopic

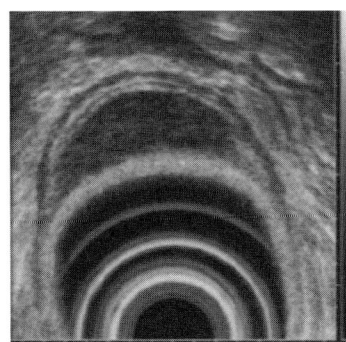

Fig. 1. EUS appearance of a granular cell tumor. The tumor is located within the submucosa, and the muscularis propria layer is intact.

appearance is of a flattish pale yellow oval submucosal lesion without overlying mucosal abnormality. Endosonographically, they appear as hypoechoic round or oval masses arising within the submucosal layer. The ground glass echostructure usually does not contain internal features. Because they do not seem to have a malignant form, they may be safely left in situ unless they are symptomatic.

Fig. 2 shows the typical EUS appearance of a submucosal lipoma. In this case, the neoplasm is pedunculated. Lipomas consist of clustered adiposites and seem to arise from the submucosa. They are most common in the stomach, duodenum, and colon but can be found anywhere in the GI tract. Although they are usually asymptomatic, they may cause obstruction if located at a narrow area, especially if they are large. Ulceration with chronic GI blood loss is occasionally seen. Endoscopically, lipomas are soft yellowish masses that deform easily on palpation with an instrument. They are typically round or oval and have normal overlying mucosa. On EUS examination, lipomas are brightly echogenic structures arising from the third echo layer (the submucosa). They have well-defined and smooth margins and have an oval shape. Almost all are benign. A malignant form (the liposarcoma) has been described, but the EUS appearance of such a lesion has not been reported. Unless the lesion is large, symptomatic, or shows unusual alarming features, it may be safely left in situ.

Fig. 3 shows the EUS appearance of a GIST. Endoscopically, stromal tumors appear as rounded firm smooth masses. The overlying mucosa is usually normal, although dimpling or even frank ulceration is common. GISTs are most common in the stomach but have been described throughout the GI tract. On EUS evaluation, these lesions usually seem to arise from the fourth echo layer (the muscularis propria) and to be contiguous with it. They may appear within the second echo layer. Regardless of the origin layer, the surrounding layers are usually well preserved (unless the tumor is malignant) and can be demonstrated by careful imaging. The parenchyma of GISTs are hypoechoic but not anechoic,

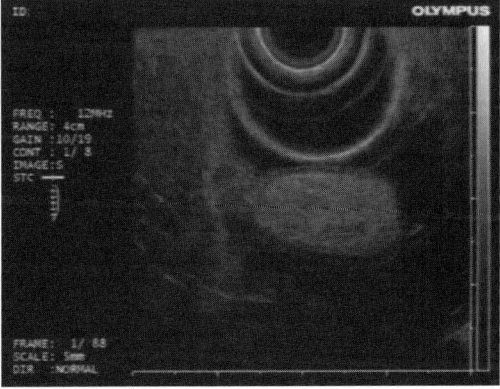

Fig. 2. EUS appearance of a pedunculated duodenal lipoma. The tumor is brightly echogenic due to the fat content, but the first two echo layers are preserved.

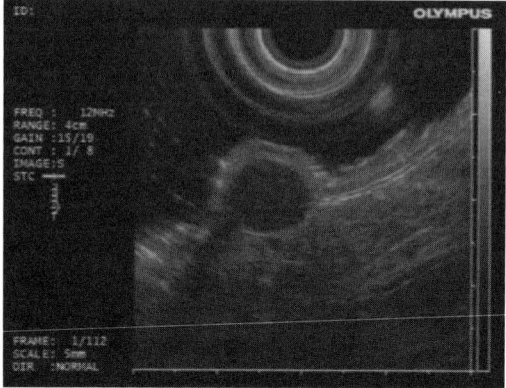

Fig. 3. A benign GIST of the stomach. Note the small size, round shape, and well-defined and smooth margins. This lesion contains no internal hyperechoic or hypoechoic foci.

appearing as a "ground glass" echodensity. Foci within this background are often seen and may be hypoechoic, anechoic, or hyperechoic (Fig. 4).

Although GISTs are the largest category of lesions demonstrating this appearance, several other entities can do so. Granular cell tumors are oval hypoechoic masses; so are carcinoids, lymphomas, pancreatic rests, and metastatic malignancies. Clinical setting and endoscopic appearance usually allow these to be distinguished.

Several features have been examined that may provide clues about benign versus malignant pathology when GISTs are seen. Large size and irregular or knobby margins are alarm signs (Fig. 5), and these are relatively objective fea-

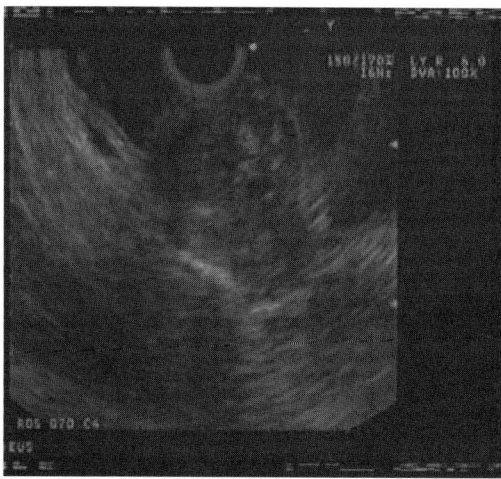

Fig. 4. A hypoechoic intramural tumor showing hypoechoic and hyperechoic internal foci. This lesion proved to be a carcinoid tumor on resection.

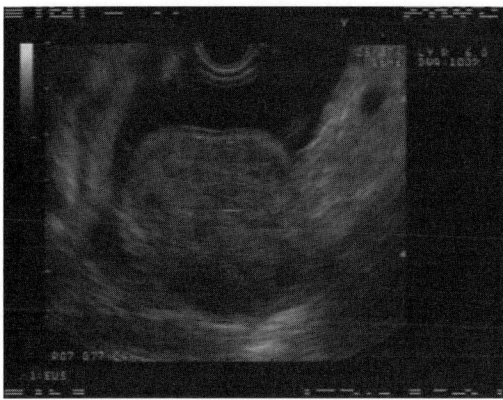

Fig. 5. A GIST showing signs for possible malignancy. Note the large size, irregular shape, and lumpy (although well-defined) margins.

tures [8]. Internal hyperechoic, hypoechoic, and anechoic ("cystic") foci have been proposed as features of malignant risk, but validation of these features has been much more difficult. Although Tsai et al [9] demonstrated that such features were statistically associated with malignancy, the diagnostic accuracy was suboptimal. Chak et al [10], in a retrospective videotape study, found good association of these features with malignancy. However, a recent large, multicenter, prospective study of 198 tumors could validate only the association of size >3 cm, surface ulceration, non-oval shape, and irregular or indistinct margins with malignancy. Hypoechoic and hyperechoic internal foci were unassociated with pathology [11]. In this same study, one or more of the associated features was present in all lesions that were malignant or had significant malignant potential; however, the specificity was relatively low. Surface ulceration and EUS characterization of size, shape, and margin features should be considered valid indicators of malignant risk, whereas internal hyperechoic or hypoechoic foci should not, by themselves, prompt resection.

Gastrointestinal stromal tumors: new insights

Several developments during the last decade have provided significant insights which improve our understanding of GISTs.

The pathology problem: new diagnostic criteria

A major stumbling block regarding GISTs has been the problem of characterizing benign and malignant tumors. In most other neoplasms, benign is benign, malignant is malignant, and that's that: Benign adenomatous colon polyps, once removed, are no longer a problem, whereas colon cancer, untreated, will promptly kill you. It has long been known, however, that for GISTs the histology only imperfectly predicts clinical behavior: Tumors with frightening histology do not always locally invade or metastasize, whereas histologically "benign" tumors are occasionally described as showing these malignant behaviors. Under such circumstances, the meanings of the terms "benign" and "malignant" are vague.

One reflection of this problem was the difficulty in identifying and validating the specific pathologic and histologic parameters useful in characterizing benign and malignant GIST. One of the heretofore most widely used systems relied on size plus six other histologic features as risk factors; those lacking all the features were benign, those with two or more were malignant, and those with one were of "indeterminate" malignant risk [12]. Many resected tumors fell into the vague "indeterminate" category; moreover, many of the features, such as epithelioid pattern or pleomorphism, were fairly subjective, limiting the usefulness of this system.

A recent NIH consensus conference has developed new guidelines for GIST histologic classification (Table 5) [13,14]. The guidelines incorporate two innovations. First, only two criteria are used: size and mitotic index, the latter defined as the number of mitotic figures seen in 50 high-power fields. These criteria are objective and are reasonably well validated with respect to malignant behavior compared with the other histologic features previously used. The second innovation is that tumors are no longer classified as "benign" or "malignant" but rather according to four levels of risk for malignant behavior, ranging from "very low risk" to "high risk." This system emphasizes that, for even the most innocent GIST, the malignant risk is low but not zero, whereas even the ugliest histology is not a guarantee of malignant behavior. The consensus group agreed that smaller size thresholds are probably justified for lesions arising in locations other than the stomach but did not specify such sizes. These criteria do not apply to GISTs, which are already locally invasive or metastatic; these are definitely malignant. The system does retain the troublesome "intermediate" category, but further improvement in GIST pathologic characterization will likely require the emergence of new knowledge about the tumor, probably requiring biochemical markers.

Table 5
NIH criteria for malignant risk in gastrointestinal stromal tumors

Risk level	Size (cm)	Mitoses/50 HPF
Very low risk	<2	<5
Low risk	2–5	<5
Intermediate risk	<5	6–10
	5–10	<5
High risk	>5	>5
	>10	Any rate
	Any size	>10

Abbreviation: HPF, high-power field.

Proto-oncogenes in the genesis of gastrointestinal stromal tumors

Other recent work has shed light on the pathogenesis of GISTs. Originally, the tumors were thought to be of smooth muscle origin, in part because they arise predominantly from the muscle layers of the GI tract wall and in part because, microscopically, the sheets of uniform eosinophilic spindle cells resemble muscle tissue. For this reason, the terms "GIST" and "leiomyoma" were sometimes used interchangeably. In 1998, Sarlomo-Rikala et al [15] reported that the majority of GISTs express a specific tyrosine kinase receptor (KIT). This receptor, originally also called CD117, mediates several cellular growth functions. In the GI tract, it is normally expressed by the interstitial cells of Cajal (ICC), giving rise to the current prevailing theory that GISTs arise from or are related to ICC. When stimulated by stem cell factor, KIT stimulates a variety of cellular proliferative mechanisms, including antiapoptotic pathways, transcription proteins, and other cascades. The result is cellular proliferation, inhibition of apoptosis, and other growth functions [16]. The interesting feature of KIT expression in GISTs is that the receptor has a gain-of-function abnormality resulting from a mutation in the corresponding gene [17]. The abnormal KIT expressed in GISTs allows initiation of the cell proliferative pathways without stimulation by stem cell factor, resulting in unregulated growth—an obvious step in the development of a neoplastic tumor. Several gene mutations, usually acquired, have been identified in GISTs, and all seem to be capable of initiating the cell-proliferative cascades, although to different degrees. More recent research has identified a second tyrosine kinase receptor mutation present in many malignant GISTs that are KIT negative. The abnormal platelet-derived growth factor alpha (PDGF-α) receptor present in these tumors also contains a gain-of-function mutation and is capable of initiating many of the same cell proliferation pathways as KIT [18].

The current theory of the pathogenesis of GISTs is that a mutation (acquired as a result of unidentified factors) to ICC or ICC progenitor cells results in expression of gain-of-function tyrosine kinase receptors associated with cell proliferation. A variety of mutations in genes for at least two such receptors, KIT and PDGF-α, are known. The abnormal receptor promotes unregulated cell proliferation resulting in tumor formation. Additional unknown factors concurrently or subsequently promote frank malignant behavior in at least some such tumors.

Imatinib: hope for the hopeless

The incidence of frankly malignant GISTs is fortunately low because, although the tumor is slow growing, it is relentlessly progressive and has been resistant to all conventional treatment regimens. Progress in this area has been made during the last decade, and effective treatment for even this hopeless cancer is now emerging. The pathophysiology centering on disordered tyrosine kinase receptor function has led to the development of an agent that specifically inhibits this activity. Imatinib (Gleevec; Novartis, Basel, Switzerland) is a selective competitive inhibitor of the KIT receptor and downregulates the abnormal cell pro-liferative activity caused by the oncogene expression. Two clinical studies have shown impressive results. In a European study of 36 subjects, 32 halted tumor progression while on the drug, and 25 showed tumor regression. Similar find-ings were seen in an American study of 147 patients. Over half of patients showed tumor regression (more than 50% reduction in tumor bulk), and in most of the remainder of patients no further progression occurred on therapy. Although no complete regression (ie, cure) was seen, these results are never-theless highly meaningful.

Additional work has shown correlation between imatinib response and the specific mutations involved. The most common mutation in the c-KIT oncogene was also the phenotype that responded best to imatinib, and other c-KIT muta-tions responded less well. Tumors associated with mutations in PDGF-α receptor also responded less well, although the response was suggested to vary depend-ing on the specific mutation. Tumors that had mutations of neither c-KIT nor PDGF-α receptor responded poorly to imatinib.

The management of hypoechoic intramural tumors

The question usually confronting the endoscopist and patient with a hypo-echoic intramural tumor not obviously malignant is less "Where did it come from?" and more "What to do about it?" The choices are two: ignore it, or resect it. A third choice—watch it (by surveillance examinations)—ultimately results in one of the two primary choices. How to go about deciding?

Specific EUS criteria (size, shape, ulceration, and margins), although in-completely validated, seem to be capable of identifying lesions suspicious for malignancy or malignant risk. Although the sensitivity of these criteria is probably high, the specificity may be low. The prospective study of 198 tumors suggested that well over half of hypoechoic intramural tumors will meet at least one of these criteria and merit resection [11]. Part of the problem is that the exact risk of malignant behavior in "indeterminate risk" GISTs is unknown, and there is not even a consensus about whether all such lesions deserve resection. If one assumes that the prudent physician (and patient) would want such a tumor out, then a specificity figure of around 50% might be ascribed to the EUS criteria. This figure, combined with sensitivity exceeding 90% is, if not optimal, at least not unreasonable. Mollifying the distaste of resection with such an indifferent degree of discrimination is the emergence of laparoscopic approaches that have been shown to be technically successful and safe in several case series [19,20].

For lesions that do not clearly require resection, surveillance examination (by, presumably, EUS) seems attractive. However, the evidence suggests that this middle-ground management strategy is almost certainly unsatisfactory. In the Hypoechoic Intramural Tumor Study, approximately half of enrolled subjects were assigned to annual surveillance EUS spanning a 3-year period. At follow-

up, fewer than one third could be persuaded to return for even a single surveillance examination [11]. Moreover, the surveillance examinations that were
performed yielded not a single additional malignant-risk lesion in the series. The
disappointing surveillance rate is commensurate with other recent data indicating
poor compliance with surveillance endoscopy. In a study of patients with
Barrett's esophagus, only 42% were compliant with a surveillance program [21],
and in a study of colorectal cancer screening, similarly low compliance rates were
documented [22]. Although surveillance may be appropriate in highly selected
circumstances, these findings suggest that, on an intention-to-treat basis, the
sensitivity of surveillance as a management strategy is unlikely to be satisfactory
when cancer is on the line.

The decision to dismiss a submucosal tumor without resection or further
follow-up takes courage. Yet, it is neither wise clinical practice nor prudent
stewardship of medical resources to refer every bump for EUS, and little is to be
gained by further examination of those meeting clinical and endoscopic criteria
for benign appearance. When EUS is performed, trust should be invested in the
findings, and the clinician should rest secure that the criteria as we understand
them seem to be sufficiently conservative that little dangerous pathology will
slip through the net.

The last decade has seen remarkable progress in nearly all areas related to
SMTs and GISTs: new diagnostic modalities, new pathophysiologic understanding, and new treatments. Much work remains, and the script contains several
unfinished scenes. Nevertheless, we have reason to hope that the unfortunate
theater we witnessed at the opening of this article will, with the new plot outline
now available, eventually vanish from the medical stage.

References

[1] Motoo Y, Okai T, Ohta H, et al. Endoscopic ultrasonography in the diagnosis of extraluminal
compressions mimicking gastric submucosal tumors. Endoscopy 1994;26:239–42.

[2] Nickl N, Bhutani M, Catalano M, et al. Clinical implications of endoscopic ultrasound: the
American Endosonography Club study. Gastrointest Endosc 1996;44:371–7.

[3] Allgayer H. Cost-effectiveness of endoscopic ultrasonography in submucosal tumors. Gastrointest Endosc Clin N Am 1995;5:625–9.

[4] Rosch T, Kapfer B, Will U, et al. Accuracy of endoscopic ultrasonography in upper gastrointestinal submucosal lesions: a prospective multicenter study. Scand J Gastroenterol 2002;37:
856–62.

[5] Nishida T, Kumano S, Sugiura T, et al. Multidetector CT of high risk patients with occult
gastrointestinal stromal tumors. AJR Am J Roentgenol 2003;180:185–9.

[6] Allgayer H. Cost effectiveness of endoscopic ultrasonography in submucosal tumors. Gastrointest Endosc Clin N Am 1995;5:625–9.

[7] Yasuda K, Cho E, Nakamima M, et al. Diagnosis of submucosal lesions of the upper
gastrointestinal tract by endoscopic ultrasonography. Gastrointest Endosc 1990;36:S17–20.

[8] Rosch T, Lorenz R, Dancygier H, et al. Endosonographic diagnosis of submucosal upper
gastrointestinal tract tumors. Scand J Gastroenterol 1992;27:1–8.

[9] Tsai TL, Changchien CS, Hu TH, et al. Differentiation of benign and malignant gastric stromal
tumors using endoscopic ultrasonography. Chang Gung Med J 2001;24:167–73.

[10] Chak A, Canto MI, Rosch T, et al. Endosonographic differentiation of benign and malignant stromal tumors. Gastrointest Endosc 1997;45:468–73.
[11] Nickl N, Gress F, McClave S, et al. Hypoechoic intramural tumor study: final report. Gastrointest Endosc 2002;55:AB98.
[12] Lewin K, Riddel RH, Weinstein WM. Mesenchymal tumors. In: Gastrointestinal pathology and its clinical implications. New York: Igaku-Shoin; 1992. p. 284–341.
[13] Berman JJ, O'Leary TJ. Gastrointestinal stromal tumor workshop. Hum Pathol 2001;32:578–82.
[14] Fletcher CD, Berman JJ, Corless C, et al. Diagnosis of gastrointestinal stromal tumors: a consensus approach. Hum Pathol 2002;33:459–65.
[15] Sarlomo-Rikala M, Kovatich AJ, Barusevicius A, et al. CD117: a sensitive marker for gastrointestinal stromal tumors that is more specific than CD34. Mod Pathol 1998;11:728–34.
[16] Duffaud F, Blay JY. Gastrointestinal stromal tumors: biology and treatment. Oncology 2003; 65:187–97.
[17] Hirohita S, Osizaki K, Moriyama Y. Gain of function mutations of c-kit in human gastrointestinal stromal tumors. Science 1998;279:577–80.
[18] Heinrich MD, Corless CL, Duensing A, et al. PDGFRA activating mutations in gastrointestinal stromal tumors. Science 2003;299:708–10.
[19] Pross M, Wolff S, Schubert D, et al. Combined minimal-invasive procedures for resection of benign gastric wall tumors. Zentralbl Chir 2003;128:191–4.
[20] Walsh RM, Ponsky J, Brody F, et al. Combined endoscopic/laparoscopic intragastric resection of gastric stromal tumors. J Gastrointest Surg 2003;7:386–92.
[21] Eckardt VF, Kanzler G, Bernhard G. Life expectancy and cancer risk in patients with Barrett's esophagus: a prospective controlled investigation. Am J Med 2001;111:33–7.
[22] Schoen RE, Weisswfeld JL, Trauth JM, et al. A population-based, community estimate of total colon examination: the impact on compliance with screening for colorectal cancer. Am J Gastroenterol 2002;97:446–51.

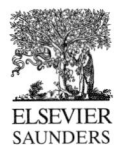
ELSEVIER
SAUNDERS

Gastrointest Endoscopy Clin N Am
15 (2005) 467–484

GASTROINTESTINAL
ENDOSCOPY CLINICS
OF NORTH AMERICA

Endoluminal Palliation

Dia T. Simmons, MD, Todd H. Baron, MD, FACP*

Division of Gastroenterology and Hepatology, Mayo Clinic College of Medicine,
Rochester, MN 55905, USA

An estimated 14,520 new cases of esophageal cancer are expected in the United States in 2005. The number of expected deaths from this disease exceeds 13,500 [1]. In the United States, the incidence of adenocarcinoma of the esophagus has been increasing, with a dwindling incidence of squamous cell carcinoma. Other regions, such as Asia, Northern Africa, and Iran, have comparatively higher incidences of squamous cell cancer of the esophagus.

Esophageal cancer is associated with significant mortality, with an estimated 5-year relative survival of 14.9%. With distant spread, this survival decreases to 2.7% [2]. Although surgery can be used in a curative approach to early-stage cancers, locally advanced and metastatic esophageal cancer is unresectable.

With advanced disease, the focus of care shifts to preserving and improving quality of life. Obstruction of the esophageal lumen by tumor leads to substantial dysphagia and poor nutritional status. Such patients are also at risk for aspiration pneumonia.

Endoscopic methods for palliation of malignant dysphagia are aimed at debulking or displacing obstructing tumors to improve swallowing and decrease the risk of aspiration (Box 1). Thermal and nonthermal endoscopic ablative therapies may be applied to tumors within the esophageal lumen but have no role in the palliation of dysphagia from extrinsic causes [3,4]. Endoscopically placed stents apply internal radial forces to the esophagus, mechanically widening the esophageal lumen. Stents are useful for palliating malignant dysphagia resulting from tumors within the esophagus and from malignant processes that cause external compression of the esophagus, such as extra-esophageal cancers and lymphadenopathy.

* Corresponding author. 200 1st Street SW, Charlton 8, Rochester, MN 55905.
E-mail address: baron.todd@mayo.edu (T.H. Baron).

1052-5157/05/$ – see front matter © 2005 Elsevier Inc. All rights reserved.
doi:10.1016/j.giec.2005.03.005   *giendo.theclinics.com*

Box 1. Methods of endoluminal palliation of esophageal cancer

Ablative

• Laser
• Argon beam plasma coagulation
• Photodynamic therapy
• Brachytherapy catheter placement
• Alcohol injection
• Chemotherapy injection

Stents

• Rigid plastic (traditional non-expanding)
• Self-expandable metal
• Self-expandable plastic

Endoscopically placed stents provide an alternative to surgery for the palliation of inoperable cancers involving the esophagus or gastric cardia. Unlike feeding tubes, the use of stents can result in palliation of dysphagia, allowing peroral nutrition. Covered metal stents are considered to be the nonsurgical treatment of choice in the management of tracheoesophageal fistulas [5].

Self-expandable metal stents (SEMS) have largely replaced conventional plastic stents. The fixed diameters of rigid plastic stents limit their usefulness in treating significant esophageal strictures, and the placement of rigid plastic stents in the esophagus is associated with considerable discomfort and the need for aggressive dilation. This may necessitate general anesthesia for placement and increases the risk of perforation. SEMS have the advantage of a thin wall and collapsed design that allows expansion to a larger, suitable diameter after deployment. The lower cost of plastic stents allows them to be used in regions where resources are limited or where esophageal malignancy is encountered infrequently. One institution reported that deployment of SEMS was six times as costly as deployment of plastic stents [6].

De Palma et al [7] published a randomized controlled trial of plastic versus gelatin-covered SEMS for palliation of esophageal cancer in 39 patients. Patients with esophagorespiratory fistulas were excluded. Both stents were placed using fluoroscopic guidance. Plastic stents were placed after Savary dilation. Both devices were similar in technical success (>90%), and both stents resulted in immediate significant improvement in dysphagia. General anesthesia was required for plastic stent placement in 60% of patients. Twenty-two percent of patients who received a plastic stent suffered early severe complications, including perforation, bleeding, and death. No early complications developed in the metal stent group. Four instances of late stent obstruction were seen in each group. Tumor ingrowth was observed in two patients with SEMS. This study helped demonstrate the superiority of SEMS over plastic stents regarding insertion complications. Despite this, the late complications of SEMS may offset their early benefits as compared with plastic stent [8].

Efficacy of self-expandable metal stents for malignant dysphagia

Dysphagia has been shown to be effectively and reliably relieved after insertion of SEMS. In a review of 121 patients who received covered and uncovered SEMS for malignant esophageal obstruction dysphagia, scores improved in 95% [9]. Six patients required two stents to fully cover the tumor. Overall complications occurred in 20% of patients. Stent collapse, food impaction, and bleeding occurred in 2.5% of patients; stent migration occurred in six patients (5%); tumor overgrowth occurred in six patients; and tumor ingrowth occurred in seven patients, all of whom had received uncovered stents. Overall tumor ingrowth and overgrowth occurred in 11% of subjects. There were no procedure-related deaths.

The incidence of esophageal malignancies involving the gastric cardia or the distal esophagus is increasing. Although dysphagia from these inoperable cancers can be effectively managed with SEMS that traverse the gastroesophageal junction, their placement results in free reflux of stomach contents into the esophagus. These patients are at high risk for reflux esophagitis and aspiration. Although proton pump inhibitors (PPIs) raise gastric pH, they do not provide a barrier to reflux or regurgitation of gastric contents. Adaptations to standard SEMS have been proposed to address stent-related reflux. Dua et al [10] published a pilot study of polyurethane-coated SEMS (Z-stents) equipped with an anti-reflux valve in 11 patients. The valve attached at the distal end of the stent was functional for the prevention of reflux at normal intragastric pressure. At elevated intragastric pressures over 48 cm H_2O, such as that associated with vomiting, the valve inverted into the stent, allowing expulsion of gastric contents. Patients could evert the valve back into the stomach by drinking a small amount of water. They found no significant difference in quality of life score. Dysphagia scores improved significantly, and heartburn was effectively prevented. One randomized trial of traditional open stents versus anti-reflux stents across the gastroesophageal junction has been published. Twenty-four of 25 patients (96%) with standard open stents had symptoms of esophageal reflux; 19 (76%) of 25 patients required treatment. Three of 25 patients (12%) with antireflux stents (Dua; Wilson-Cook Medical, Winston-Salem, North Carolina) reported esophageal reflux; 1 of 25 patients (4%) required treatment ($P < 0.001$). There was no significant difference in survival, complications, or reintervention rate among the groups [11].

Early complications after esophageal stent placement include perforation, aspiration, chest pain, and malpositioning of the stent (Box 2). Perforations, especially in the mid- and upper esophagus, are usually related to the use of excessive force in dilation or guidewire trauma. Treatment measures include na-

---

Box 2. Complications of expandable metal esophageal stents

Early

- Perforation
- Chest pain
- Bleeding (almost always mild)
- Airway obstruction
- Aspiration

Late

- Perforation
- Tracheoesophageal fistula
- Obstruction due to tumor ingrowth
- Obstruction due to tumor overgrowth
- Obstruction due to tissue hyperplasia
- Food impaction
- Reflux with aspiration, esophagitis
- Bleeding (often massive)
- Migration

---

sogastric tube suction, antibiotics, and surgery. Whenever possible, surgery is avoided in this palliative patient group. Transient (up to 1 week) chest pain is expected and is best treated with narcotic analgesics. More prolonged or severe, intractable chest pain may occur after uncomplicated stent placement, but an evaluation to exclude a procedural-related complication should be instituted. Partial stent malpositioning during initial placement can be managed by stent repositioning if possible or by the placement of a second, overlapping stent. Airway obstruction can occur in the presence of a large mediastinal mass that impinges upon an area at or near the trachea or tracheal bifurcation. It can be managed with emergent stent removal or with mechanical intubation and subsequent airway stent placement [12].

Late esophageal stent complications may occur as a result of SEMS placement (see Box 2) [13]. These may include gastroesophageal reflux and aspiration if the stent traverses the gastroesophageal junction. Such patients should be placed on high-dose PPI therapy indefinitely. Additional precautions should be taken, such as elevating the head of the bed and avoiding recumbency within 3 hours of a meal. Patients should be counseled regarding nutrition and choosing food of appropriate consistency to avoid food impaction. Chest pain may result from gastroesophageal reflux. Stent occlusion may result from an impacted food bolus, which can be dislodged endoscopically. Tissue-related stent occlusion may be due to tumor ingrowth, tumor overgrowth, or tissue hyperplasia. Treatment

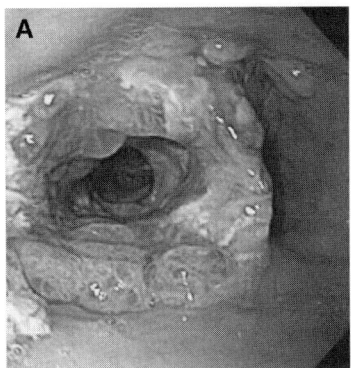
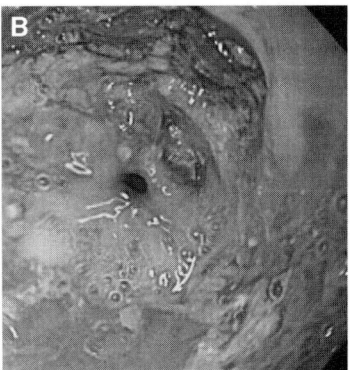
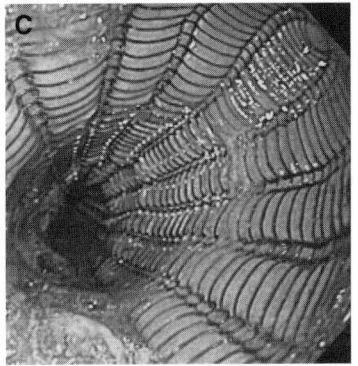

Fig. 1. Endoscopic photos taken 6 weeks after initial placement of expandable metal stent in the mid-esophagus. The patient returned due to recurrent dysphagia. (*A*) View of the proximal end of the stent demonstrates significant tumor ingrowth. (*B*) View of the distal esophagus reveals tumor overgrowth and stricture. (*C*) Successful deployment of additional expandable metal stent through the previous stent.

options to restore luminal patency include placing a new stent through the previous stent (Fig. 1), ablative techniques such as argon beam plasma co-agulation, and mechanical debridement. Covered metal stents are associated with less tumor ingrowth than uncovered stents but are more prone to migration [14]. Major bleeding can result from erosion of the stent through the esophagus and into a major vessel such as the aorta. Tracheoesophageal fistula can result from stent erosion into the respiratory tree.

When selecting a method of endoscopic palliation, it is important to consider the patient's life expectancy. If a patient is not expected to live more than 6 months, then SEMS may be more appropriate than chemo or radiation therapy.

Types of stents

There are a variety of FDA-approved stents available for palliation of malignant dysphagia (Fig. 2) [15]. These devices differ by the type of alloy,

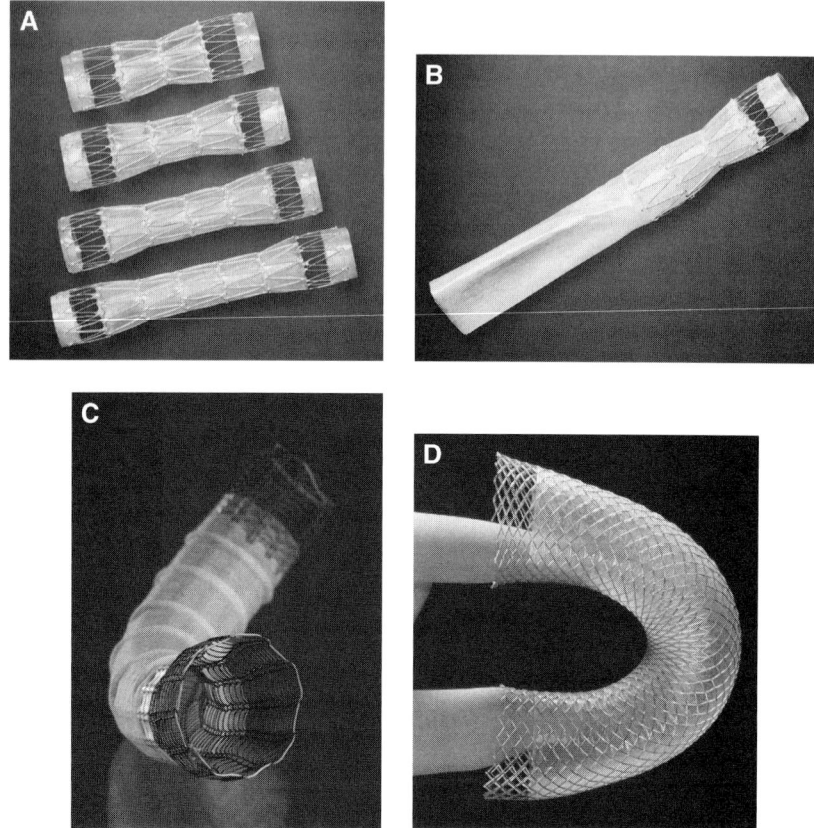

Fig. 2. Commercially available esophageal SEMS. (*A*) Z stent (Wilson-Cook, Winston-Salem, North Carolina). (*B*) Dua Anti-reflux (Wilson-Cook). (*C*) Ultraflex II (Boston Scientific, Natick, Massachusetts). (*D*) Wallstent II (Boston Scientific).

delivery system, type and extent of covering, luminal diameter, degree of shortening after deployment, and presence or absence of an antireflux valve. The few published comparative studies suggest there is little difference in clinical outcomes [16–18].

Ablative therapy

Thermal and nonthermal ablative therapies are available as independent or as adjunctive modalities to stent placement for palliation of malignant dysphagia. Several studies have addressed the use of laser therapy, brachytherapy, and photodynamic therapy for obstructive esophageal malignancies.

Self-expandable metal stents versus laser ablative therapy for malignant dysphagia

Dallal et al [19] randomized 65 patients with malignant esophagogastric strictures who had similar pretreatment dysphagia scores to SEMS ($n = 31$) versus thermal tumor ablation ($n = 34$) with laser photoablation (Nd:YAG or argon diode laser) and in a few cases argon beam plasma coagulation. Uncovered stents were used except in suspected esophageal perforation or suspected tracheo-esophageal fistula, where covered metal stents were used. Dysphagia scores and health-related quality of life were measured. Recurrent dysphagia in both groups was treated with crossover. Thirteen serious complications or recurrent/persistent dysphagia requiring additional therapy occurred in the thermal tumor ablation group. Twelve serious complications or dysphagia requiring additional treatment occurred in the stent group. There were no differences in dysphagia scores between the two groups at 1 month. A longer median survival was seen in the thermal tumor ablation group (125 days) compared with the stent group (68 days), which may be due to a tumor debulking effect of ablation therapy. This study suggests that these therapies are complementary and that the treatment approach individualized, although the SEMS therapy may have been more effective had covered SEMS been used.

Brachytherapy

Brachytherapy is performed by passing radiation catheters under endoscopic and fluoroscopic guidance into the esophageal lumen to deliver high doses of radiation [20]. One study of 232 patients with advanced squamous cell esophageal cancer followed to death randomized patients to different dosing strategies [21]. One group received two fractions of therapy over 3 days, and the other group received three fractions over 5 days. Overall survival was 7.9 months, with a dysphagia-free survival of 7.1 months. No deaths were attributable to the intervention. Median survival for all patients was 237 days. Strictures developed in 25 patients (11.3%) and required dilation, whereas 28 patients (12.6%) did not experience an improvement in dysphagia and subsequently underwent external beam radiation therapy; fistula formation occurred in 23 patients. Although brachytherapy seems to be effective with long-lasting palliation, multiple sessions are required, and strictures or fistulae occur in a modest number of patients.

Brachytherapy versus self-expandable metal stents

In a randomized controlled trial of palliation of inoperable esophageal cancer, 209 patients were randomized. SEMS were placed in 108 patients, and single-dose brachytherapy was used in 101 patients [22]. Postprocedure follow-up data were collected at 2 weeks, 1 month, and monthly for the first year and then every 3 months. Major complications occurred significantly more often in the SEMS group (25%); complications included bleeding, perforation, fistula, and severe pain compared with the brachytherapy group (13%, $P = 0.02$). Approximately 40% of patients in both treatment groups required retreatment for tumor recurrence, stent migration, and food bolus obstruction in the SEMS group and for tumor recurrence or persistent dysphagia in the brachytherapy group. There was no difference in median survival between the two arms (155 days brachytherapy; 145 days stents). Although there was more immediate improvement in dysphagia in the SEMS group, by 1 month the dysphagia scores were similar in the SEMS and brachytherapy groups. By 150 days, dysphagia scores were better in the brachytherapy group. Therefore, SEMS provide superior immediate relief of dysphagia compared with brachytherapy, but this superiority diminishes over time.

Photodynamic therapy

Photodynamic therapy (PDT) is a nonthermal ablative process used to treat luminal malignancies because of its tumor-debulking properties and its ability to treat bleeding. It can be used to treat tumor overgrowth or ingrowth complicated SEMS placement. PDT can be applied under conscious sedation. An intravenous photosensitizer is administered approximately 48 hours before the endoscopic application of an activating light source (laser light) at the site of tumor. Disadvantages of PDT are that the symptomatic improvement is not immediate, several sessions may be required, it is not useful for relieving dysphagia due to extrinsic compression, it is expensive, and strict precautions are needed to avoid sunlight or significant sunburn. Luketich et al [23] reported a single center's experience of 77 patients treated with photodynamic therapy for palliation of obstruction or bleeding from inoperable esophageal cancer. Patients with bronchoscopic evidence of tracheo/bronchial esophageal fistulae were excluded. Thirty-two patients received photodynamic therapy for the management of tumor ingrowth or overgrowth from stent. Thirty-three (43%) had received prior chemotherapy or radiation. Intravenous Photofrin, a porfimer sodium photosensitizer, was administered (1.5–2.0 mg/kg), followed by endoscopic light application using a 630 nm red dye laser. Additional treatment included endoscopic mechanical debridement and balloon dilation. A 90% efficacy was seen at 4 weeks as defined by significant improvement in dysphagia scores and control of all bleeding. Twenty-nine patients (38%) required retreatment. Mean dysphagia-free interval was 80.3 ± 58.2 days. Median survival was 5.9 months after initial PDT. Complications included sunburn (mostly first degree) in 10%, esophageal stricture requiring balloon dilation in 4.8%, candida esophagitis in 3.2%, symptomatic pleural effusion in 3.2%, and aspiration pneumonia in 1.6%. Perforation, attributed to balloon dilation, occurred in 2.4%. The 30-day mortality rate was 3.9%. Another published review from the same institution included 215 patients treated with PDT for palliation of esophageal cancer [24]. Palliation of dysphagia was achieved in 85%. The mean dysphagia-free interval was 66 days. Complications included stricture in 2%, perforation in 1.6% (possibly associated with balloon dilation), sunburn in 6%, and pleural effusion in 3.5%. The median survival from the initial PDT was 4.8 months. Thirty-day procedure mortality was 1.8% (4/215). Thus, palliation is achievable in these patients using PDT, although the data suggest that it is superior to other therapies, with the exception perhaps of the ability to palliate bleeding.

Photodynamic therapy versus Nd:YAG laser

Lightdale et al [25] reported the results of a large, multicenter, randomized trial of PDT with porfimer sodium versus Nd:YAG laser for palliation of esophageal cancer. Two hundred twenty-six patients were randomized. Efficacy was similar for PDT and laser, but there were more minor and major complications as a result of laser therapy. Fewer esophageal perforations occurred with PDT (1%) compared with laser (7%). These data formed the basis of the FDA approval for PDT for the palliation of malignant dysphagia of esophageal cancer.

Brachytherapy combined with laser therapy versus laser therapy alone

In a randomized study from the United Kingdom, the outcome of brachytherapy combined with Nd:YAG laser was compared with laser therapy alone for palliation of dysphagia due to adenocarcinoma of the esophagus and cardia [26]. Only patients with exophytic tumors who had not received prior radiation, chemotherapy, surgery, or stents were included. Patients with fistulas were excluded. Laser treatment generally required two or three sessions performed several days apart. Only the 20 patients who had reasonable swallowing after laser therapy and who were tolerating a soft diet were randomized to a single dose of brachytherapy or no brachytherapy. Similar median survival was seen in both groups—20 weeks for laser alone and 26 weeks for laser plus brachytherapy. There was a significant difference in median time to recurrence of dysphagia; 5 weeks for those treated with laser therapy alone versus 19 weeks for those receiving brachytherapy and laser treatment. Thirty-day mortality from time of first treatment was 0%. No complications developed from laser therapy alone. Three patients developed odynophagia after brachytherapy, which resolved with antacids. This study confirms the short-term nature of treatment response seen with laser therapy, which can be significantly lengthened by the addition of single-dose brachytherapy.

Chemotherapeutic agent injection to the esophagus

A variety of caustic agents, including ethanol, have been injected into esophageal tumors to induce necrosis, causing a debulking effect. A few studies have been published on the intramural injection of combination cisplatin/epinephrine injectable gel. The gel formulation allows delivery of high-concentration chemotherapy directly to the tumor, with the goal of debulking. Harbord et al [27] published a multicenter (Europe and the United States), open-label study of the efficacy of cisplatin/epinephrine injectable gel for advanced malignant dysphagia. The study included only patients with endoscopically accessible exophytic tumors and excluded patients with fistulae or externally compressing lesions. Chemotherapeutic gel was injected (0.5–1.0 µL) and was repeated weekly. Patients received up to six injections in 8 weeks. The efficacy was low: Although eight patients reported improved quality of swallowing (ie, lack of pain), only four of 18 patients had improvement of dysphagia lasting between 30 and 45 days. Eleven patients had no change in dysphagia, and three patients experienced worsening dysphagia. Eight of 18 patients had measurable decrease in the size of the exophytic tumor. Lumen patency improved in six patients and stabilized in 10 patients.

In summary, the appropriate choice of endoscopic therapy for palliation is patient dependent, and the life expectancy of the patient influences the treatment choice. The precise location of tumors also influences the treatment approach. For example, patients with lesions in the most proximal cervical esophagus do not usually tolerate stent placement. Extrinsic lesions cannot be managed by ablative techniques. Consideration must be given to the potential need for repeated therapies and the necessity for general anesthesia. The availability of palliative endoscopic modalities varies by medical center and local expertise.

Self-expandable plastic stents

Recently, a self-expandable plastic stent has been developed for relief of malignant dysphagia. The potential advantages of the stent over SEMS are its removability, avoidance of erosive complications (fistula), and decrease in tissue hyperplasia. Two single-arm studies from outside the United States suggest that this stent is useful for palliation of malignant dysphagia [28,29], but comparative studies with SEMS are needed.

Enteral self-expandable metal stents

Gastroduodenal and colonic SEMS are referred to as enteral stents. Commercially available enteral SEMS are depicted in Fig. 3.

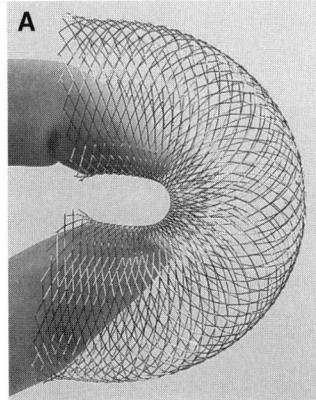

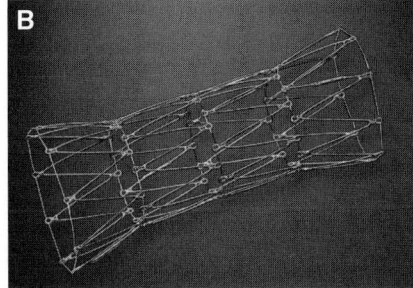

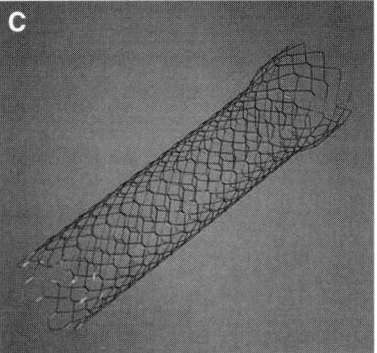

Fig. 3. Commercially available enteral SEMS. (*A*). Enteral Wallstent (Boston Scientific, Natick, Massachusetts). (*B*) Colonic Z stent (Wilson-Cook, Winston-Salem, North Carolina). (*C*) Precision Colonic (Boston Scientific).

Malignant gastric outlet obstruction

Gastric outlet obstruction (GOO) may result from malignancies of the antrum, duodenum, pancreas, or bile ducts or may result from metastasis from distant organs. Common presenting symptoms of malignant GOO include postprandial abdominal pain, early satiety, vomiting, and intolerability of oral intake. Truong [30] first reported the use of SEMS for malignant GOO in 1992. Since that time, there have been numerous publications describing the efficacy of SEMS for palliating GOO. The types of stents and technique for placement have been described elsewhere [31]. Dorman et al [32] recently published a systematic review of 32 case series, including 10 prospective series, of the efficacy of SEMS for gastroduodenal malignancies. The majority of malignancies included were gastric and pancreatic in origin. In all, 606 patients underwent attempted stent placement. Technical success, defined as successful stent placement and deployment, was achieved in 589 patients (97%). Technical failure was attributed to severe obstruction, difficult anatomy, malpositioning, and one failed delivery. Clinical success, defined as relief of symptoms and improved oral intake, occurred in 89% of the technical successes. Clinical failures were due to early stent migration (20%), disease progression (61%), and procedural complications (15%), such as a malpositioned stent or a partially expanded stent. Severe complications included bleeding (1%). There were no procedural-related deaths. Nonsevere complications occurred in 27% of attempted stent placements. The most commonly reported nonsevere complication was stent obstruction (17%) primarily caused by tumor growth or obstruction away from the stent. Migration occurred in 5% of subjects, which was generally managed with additional stent placement. Pain was reported in 2% of subjects. Evidence of biliary obstruction after stent placement was noted in 1% of subjects. The mean survival was 12.1 weeks. In summary, severe complications occurred in 1.2%, and nonsevere complications occurred in 27%. The majority of nonsevere complications were related to stent obstruction.

Adler and Baron [33] reviewed the experience in 36 patients who received stents for palliation of malignant GOO at a single center. Symptoms were assessed with a gastric outlet obstruction scoring system (GOOSS) regarding diet tolerability. In most cases, enteral Wallstents were used. Technical success was achieved in 100%. Eight patients (25%) required reintervention for recurrent obstruction-related symptoms. There was a statistically significant improvement in GOOSS scores after stent placement. No perforations or clinically significant bleeding occurred. Two stents failed to deploy but were subsequently successfully placed. Fifty-eight percent of patients resumed oral intake within 24 hours of stent placement. Improvement in dietary performance was noted in 86% of patients. Forty-one percent developed biliary obstruction. This study emphasizes the need to consider a prophylactic biliary stent before gastroduodenal stent if there is concern for future biliary obstruction because the papilla becomes inaccessible once the gastroduodenal stent has been placed (Fig. 4).

Surgical gastroenterostomy (bypass) is an alternative for palliation of malignant GOO, but this approach may not be suitable for patients with a limited life expectancy. Surgically placed feeding tubes are an option but do not allow peroral nutrition. Fiori et al [34] recently published results of a small, randomized, prospective trial of 18 patients comparing the efficacy of open gastroenterostomy versus endoscopic SEMS for palliation of unresectable malignant antro-pyloric stenosis. Stent placement was successful in 100%. Mean time to oral intake was 6.3 days for surgical patients and 2.1 days for patients treated with a stent ($P<0.0001$). Median length of hospital stay was 10 days in the surgical group, compared with 3.1 days in the stent group. Mean procedure time was twice as long compared with the endoscopy group. Stent dislocation occurred in the stent group, and postoperative hemorrhage occurred in the surgery group. No differences in morbidity and mortality were reported.

Mittal et al [35] reported outcomes of open gastrojejunostomy, laparoscopic gastrojejunostomy, and endoscopically placed SEMS for palliation of malignant GOO. This review included 181 patients treated between 1989 and 2002. Adenocarcinoma of the stomach and pancreas were the most common causes

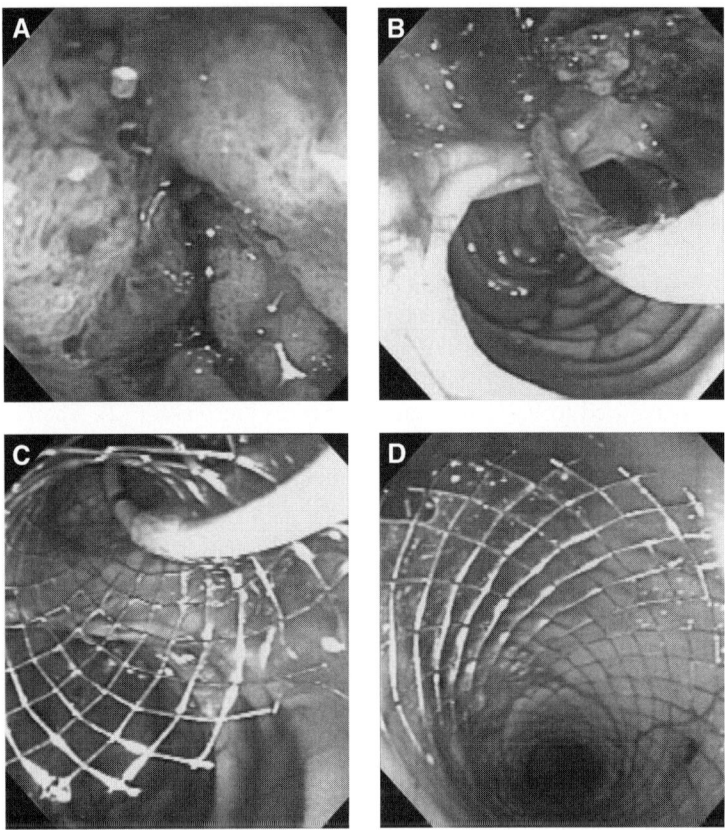

Fig. 4. Double stenting of ampullary tumor with duodenal bulb stricture. (*A*) Endoscopic view of a tumor obstructing the duodenum. (*B*) After dilating the duodenal stricture. The ampullary mass is seen with a pre-deployed biliary Wallstent. (*C*) Immediately after deployment of biliary Wallstent. (*D*) Immediately after deployment of enteral Wallstent in the duodenum.

of GOO in this review. Patients who underwent endoscopic or laparoscopic palliation were matched with those who underwent open gastrojejunostomy for age, presenting symptoms, location of obstruction, and American Society of Anesthesiologists classification. Time to ingestion of liquids and light-consistency diet and postprocedure length of hospital stay were significantly shorter in the endoscopic stent group compared with both surgical groups. Mean survival was longer in the surgically palliated group (199 days), compared with the endoscopically palliated group (59 days, $P = 0.031$). Postprocedural and procedural costs were 1.9 times higher in the laparoscopic gastrojejunostomy group and 2.3 times higher in the open gastrojejunostomy group as compared with the endoscopic group. The complication rate was 0% in the endoscopic group, 37.5% in the open gastrojejunostomy group, and 42.9% in the laparoscopic group. The most frequent complication was pneumonia. There was no significant difference in the need for biliary intervention among the groups.

These findings suggest that endoscopic placement of expandable metal stents provides at least equal palliation of symptoms at a lower cost, less morbidity and mortality, earlier per oral intake, and shorter hospital stay compared with open or laparoscopic gastrojejunostomy for palliation of malignant GOO.

Self-expandable metal stents for palliation of colonic and rectal tumors

In the United States, approximately 104,950 colon cancer cases and 40,340 new rectal cancer cases are estimated for 2005 [1]. In the same year, combined deaths due to colon and rectal cancer are expected to reach 56,290. The overall 5-year relative survival for colon and rectal cancer is 64.1% [2]. Five-year survival is reduced to 9.7% if distant metastases are present [2]. The mortality associated with acute colonic obstruction is high, and colonic obstruction due to malignancy is the number one cause of emergency large bowel surgery [36].

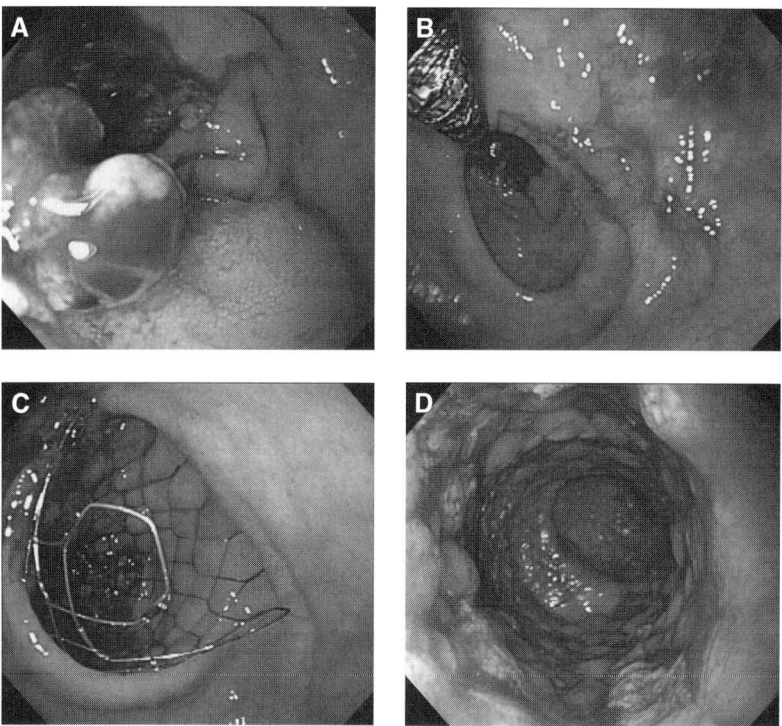

Fig. 5. Stenting of tumor at the recto-sigmoid junction. (*A*) Endoscopic view of partially obstructing tumor at the recto-sigmoid junction. (*B*) View of pre-deployed Ultraflex precision colonic stent advanced proximal to the stricture. (*C*) View of distal end of deployed expandable metal stent immediately after successful deployment. (*D*) Immediately after successful deployment of expandable metal stent through the obstruction.

Endoscopically placed stents are placed for several indications in patients with obstructive colorectal malignancies [37]. The methods of colorectal stent placement have been described in detail elsewhere [37]. Stents can be used for temporary decompression before resection of operable colonic tumors. This decompression may permit a one-stage bowel resection operation, versus a two-stage operation for an unprepared colon. The two-stage operation includes resection of involved bowel and the creation of a colostomy, followed by colostomy takedown and reanastomosis of the colon, which is necessary if the colon has not been cleansed. Second, stents can be used for palliation of inoperable obstructive colorectal malignancies (Fig. 5). Extrinsic compression from pelvic malignancies and lymphadenopathy may also be palliated with stents. Finally, covered stents can be placed in the rectum to seal fistulas to the vagina and bladder [38].

Colorectal palliation

Sebastian et al [39] recently published a comprehensive report on the efficacy and safety of SEMS for malignant colorectal obstruction based on studies published from 1990 and 2003. No randomized trials were identified. Fifty-four case series comprising 1198 patients were included in this pooled analysis; 791 of the patients had undergone stent placement for palliation. In the remaining patients, stenting was performed as a bridge to surgery. Of the patients treated palliatively, technical success in stent placement was achieved in 93%, and clinical success was achieved in 91% (cumulative rates). Perforations, predominantly in the rectosigmoid region, occurred in 3.8% of patients. Of those, 64% required emergency surgery. In 17.7% of perforations, predilation was thought to be a causative factor. The use of laser therapy in the pre-stent setting was thought to contribute to perforation in a few cases. Perforations were attributed to balloon dilation, stent wires, and guide wires. Migration in technically successful stent placements occurred in 11.8% of cases, two thirds of which occurred within the first week. Most migration was distal (94.7%). Fifteen percent of the palliative stents migrated, compared with 3.9% of the stents used as bridge to surgery. The cumulative procedure-related mortality rate for all stent placements was 0.58%. The majority of these deaths were patients receiving palliative therapy. Re-obstruction was noted in 7.3% of patients at a median time of 24 weeks. Re-obstruction was due to tumor ingrowth in most cases. Other causes of obstruction, such as fecal impaction, mucosal prolapse, tumor overgrowth, and peritoneal seeding, occurred less frequently. Laser, argon plasma coagulation, stent replacement, and surgery were among the modalities used to treat re-obstruction. These studies demonstrate that SEMS are safe and effective in the palliation of malignant colorectal obstruction to avoid an ostomy and are useful in the majority of cases in avoiding the need for a temporary colostomy by allowing resection and re-anastomosis at an initial operation.

Box 3. Complications of expandable metal gastroduodenal stents and colonic stents

- Perforation: immediate/delayed
- Obstruction due to tumor ingrowth
- Obstruction due to tumor overgrowth
- Obstruction due to tissue hyperplasia
- Bleeding
- Migration
- Tenesmus, incontinence, and pain (distal rectal placement)

Placement of gastroduodenal and colonic (enteral) SEMS is not without risk. Complications after placement of these devices are listed in Box 3.

Summary

Endoluminal palliation of the esophagus can be achieved in several ways, including SEMS placement, laser ablation, photodynamic therapy, and injection therapy. There are few comparative studies to guide optimal palliative therapy for malignant dysphagia, although stents are effective and widely available. SEMS placement is the only endoscopic management option that restores luminal continuity in patients with malignant gastroduodenal and colonic obstruction.

References

[1] Jemal A, Murray T, Ward E, et al. Cancer statistics, 2005. CA Cancer J Clin 2005;55:10–30.
[2] Reis LAG, Eisner MP, Kosary CL, et al. SEER Cancer Statistics Review, 1975–2002. Bethesda: National Cancer Institute. Available at: www.seer.cancer.gov/csr/1975_2002/. Accessed April 25, 2005.
[3] Luketich JD, Meehan M, Nguyen NT, et al. Minimally invasive surgical staging for esophageal cancer. Surg Endosc 2000;14:700–2.
[4] Adler DG, Baron TH. Endoscopic palliation of malignant dysphagia. Mayo Clin Proc 2001;76: 731–8.
[5] Baron TH. Expandable metal stents for the treatment of cancerous obstruction of the gastrointestinal tract. N Engl J Med 2001;344:1681–7.
[6] Szentpali K, Palotas A, Lazar G, et al. Endoscopic intubation with conventional plastic stents: a safe and cost-effective palliation for inoperable esophageal cancer. Dysphagia 2004;19:22–7.
[7] De Palma GD, Di Matteo E, Romano G, et al. Plastic prosthesis versus expandable metal stents for palliation of inoperable esophageal thoracic carcinoma: a controlled prospective study. Gastrointest Endosc 1996;43:478–82.
[8] Kozarek RA, Ball TJ, Brandabur JJ, et al. Expandable versus conventional esophageal prostheses: easier insertion may not preclude subsequent stent-related problems. Gastrointest Endosc 1996;43:204–8.

[9] O'Sullivan GJ, Grundy A. Palliation of malignant dysphagia with expanding metallic stents. J Vasc Interv Radiol 1999;10:346–51.

[10] Dua KS, Kozarek R, Kim J, et al. Self-expanding metal esophageal stent with anti-reflux mechanism. Gastrointest Endosc 2001;53:603–13.

[11] Laasch HU, Marriott A, Wilbraham L, et al. Effectiveness of open versus antireflux stents for palliation of distal esophageal carcinoma and prevention of symptomatic gastroesophageal reflux. Radiology 2002;225:359–65.

[12] Sihoe AD, Wan IY, Yim AP. Airway stenting for unresectable esophageal cancer. Surg Oncol 2004;13:17–25.

[13] Wang MQ, Sze DY, Wang ZP, et al. Delayed complications after esophageal stent placement for treatment of malignant esophageal obstructions and esophagorespiratory fistulas. J Vasc Interv Radiol 2001;12:465–74.

[14] Vakil N, Morris AI, Marcon N, et al. A prospective, randomized, controlled trial of covered expandable metal stents in the palliation of malignant esophageal obstruction at the gastro-esophageal junction. Am J Gastroenterol 2001;96:1791–6.

[15] Baron TH. A practical guide for choosing an expandable metal stent for GI malignancies: is a stent by any other name still a stent? Gastrointest Endosc 2001;54:269–72.

[16] Sabharwal T, Hamady MS, Chui S, et al. A randomised prospective comparison of the Flamingo Wallstent and Ultraflex stent for palliation of dysphagia associated with lower third oesophageal carcinoma. Gut 2003;52:922–6.

[17] Siersema PD, Hop WC, van Blankenstein M, et al. A comparison of 3 types of covered metal stents for the palliation of patients with dysphagia caused by esophagogastric carcinoma: a prospective, randomized study. Gastrointest Endosc 2001;54:145–53.

[18] Riccioni ME, Shah SK, Tringali A, et al. Endoscopic palliation of unresectable malignant oesophageal strictures with self-expanding metal stents: comparing Ultraflex and Esophacoil stents. Dig Liver Dis 2002;34:356–63.

[19] Dallal HJ, Smith GD, Grieve DC, et al. A randomized trial of thermal ablative therapy versus expandable metal stents in the palliative treatment of patients with esophageal carcinoma. Gastrointest Endsoc 2001;54:549–57.

[20] Sur RK, Donde B, Levin VC, et al. Fractionated high dose rate intraluminal brachytherapy in palliation of advanced esophageal cancer. Int J Radiat Oncol Biol Phys 1998,40.447–53.

[21] Sur RK, Levin CV, Donde B, et al. Prospective randomized trial of HDR brachytherapy as a sole modality in palliation of advanced esophageal carcinoma: an International Atomic Energy Agency study. Int J Radiat Oncol Biol Phys 2002;53:127–33.

[22] Homs MY, Essink-Bot ML, Borsboom GJ, et al. Quality of life after palliative treatment for oesophageal carcinoma: a prospective comparison between stent placement and single dose brachytherapy. Dutch SIREC Study Group. Eur J Cancer 2004;40:1862–71.

[23] Luketich JD, Christie NA, Buenaventura PO, et al. Endoscopic photodynamic therapy for obstructing esophageal cancer: 77 cases over a 2-year period. Surg Endosc 2000;14:653–7.

[24] Litle VR, Luketich JD, Christie NA, et al. Photodynamic therapy as palliation for esophageal cancer: experience in 215 patients. Ann Thorac Surg 2003;76:1687–92.

[25] Lightdale CJ, Heier SK, Marcon NE, et al. Photodynamic therapy with porfimer sodium versus thermal ablation therapy with Nd:YAG laser for palliation of esophageal cancer: a multicenter randomized trial. Gastrointest Endsoc 1995;42:507–12.

[26] Spencer GM, Thorpe SM, Blackman GM, et al. Laser augmented by brachytherapy versus laser alone in the palliation of adenocarcinoma of the oesophagus and cardia: a randomised study. Gut 2002;50:224–7.

[27] Harbord M, Dawes RF, Barr H, et al. Palliation of patients with dysphagia due to advanced esophageal cancer by endoscopic injection of cisplatin/epinephrine injectable gel. Gastrointest Endsc 2002;56:644–51.

[28] Dormann AJ, Eisendrath P, Wigginghaus B, et al. Palliation of esophageal carcinoma with a new self-expanding plastic stent. Endoscopy 2003;35:207–11.

[29] Costamagna G, Shah SK, Tringali A, et al. Prospective evaluation of a new self-expanding plastic stent for inoperable esophageal strictures. Surg Endosc 2003;17:891–5.

[30] Truong S, Bohndorf V, Geller H, et al. Self-expanding metal stents for palliation of malignant gastric outlet obstruction. Endoscopy 1992;24:433–5.

[31] Baron TH, Schofl R, Puespoek A, et al. Expandable metal stent placement for gastric outlet obstruction. Endoscopy 2001;33:623–8.

[32] Dormann A, Meisner S, Verin N, et al. Self-expanding metal stents for gastroduodenal malignancies: systematic review of their clinical effectiveness. Endoscopy 2004;36:543–50.

[33] Adler DG, Baron TH. Endoscopic palliation of malignant gastric outlet obstruction using self-expanding metal stents: experience in 36 patients. Am J Gastroenterol 2002;97:72–8.

[34] Fiori E, Lamazza A, Volpino P, et al. Palliative management of malignant antro-pyloric strictures: gastroenterostomy vs. endoscopic stenting. A randomized prospective trial. Anticancer Res 2004;24:269–71.

[35] Mittal A, Windsor J, Woodfield J, et al. Matched study of three methods for palliation of malignant pyloroduodenal obstruction. Br J Surg 2004;91:205–9.

[36] Baron TH. Benign and malignant colorectal strictures. In: Waye JD, Rex DK, Williams CB, editors. Colonoscopy: principles and practice. 1st edition. Boston: Blackwell Publishing; 2003. p. 611–23.

[37] Baron TH, Rey JF, Spinelli P. Expandable metal stent placement for malignant colorectal obstruction. Endoscopy 2002;34:823–30.

[38] Repici A, Reggio D, Saracco G, et al. Self-expanding covered esophageal Ultraflex stent for palliation of malignant colorectal anastomotic obstruction complicated by multiple fistulas. Gastrointest Endosc 2000;51:346–8.

[39] Sebastian S, Johnston S, Geoghegan T, et al. Pooled analysis of the efficacy and safety of self-expanding metal stenting in malignant colorectal obstruction. Am J Gastroenterol 2004; 99:2051–7.

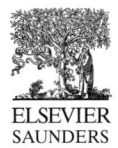

ELSEVIER
SAUNDERS

Gastrointest Endoscopy Clin N Am
15 (2005) 485–496

GASTROINTESTINAL
ENDOSCOPY CLINICS
OF NORTH AMERICA

Approach to Cystic Pancreatic Lesions

William R. Brugge, MD

*Massachusetts General Hospital, Gastrointestinal Unit, Blake 4, 55 Fruit Street,
Boston, MA 02114, USA*

Cystic neoplasms of the pancreas represent the best example of a malignant precursor in the pancreas. There are many parallels between pancreatic cystic neoplasms and the colon polyp-cancer sequence. In the past, cystic neoplasms of the pancreas were thought to be relatively rare, composing less than 10% of cancers of the pancreas. With the greater use of cross-sectional imaging, an increasing number of these neoplasms are being seen.

The malignancies represented by cystic neoplasms of the pancreas range from benign lesions to premalignant and malignant cystic lesions. In general, from a clinical and operational perspective, it is useful to divide cystic neoplasms into nonmucinous (nonmalignant) and mucinous (premalignant and malignant) [1]. Nonmucinous cystic lesions are represented by serous cystadenomas. There are two types of mucinous lesions: the mucinous cystic neoplasm (MCN) and the closely related lesion, the intraductal papillary mucinous tumor (IPMT). Both types of lesions may be benign, contain a focus of malignancy, or be frankly malignant. Incidentally noted early pancreatic cancers in autopsy studies are frequently mucinous cystic neoplasms [2].

Epidemiology

The prevalence of pancreatic cysts has been examined with cross-sectional imaging studies in the United States and autopsy studies in Japan, with similar results. In clinical studies of CT and MR imaging, the prevalence of cystic lesions has been estimated to be between 1% to 2% [3]. Small cystic lesions in 1374 autopsied pancreata from elderly patients were analyzed histologically [4]. The cysts were located throughout the pancreatic parenchyma and were not

E-mail address: wbrugge@partners.org

related to the presence of chronic pancreatitis. The epithelium of the cysts displayed a range of early malignancy, including atypia (2.4%) and carcinoma in situ (0.6%). The malignant epithelium was more commonly found in small cystic lesions rather than large lesions. These lesions most likely represent early forms of IPMTs.

Clinical epidemiology

MCNs account for approximately 2% to 5% of all exocrine pancreatic tumors and are the more common type of cystic lesion. Women are affected far more commonly than men (9:1 ratio), with a mean age at diagnosis in the fifth decade.

IPMTs share many of the features of MCNs. Their true incidence is uncertain, but estimates range from 1% to 8% of all pancreatic tumors. IPMTs affect men and women equally or men predominantly, depending on the reported series, and they tend to occur in an older age group than MCNs.

Serous cystadenomas have been estimated to account for about 25% of all cystic neoplasms of the pancreas [5]. Serous cystadenomas were not established as an independent clinical or pathologic entity until 1978 when the unique bland, cuboidal, periodic acid Schiff-positive epithelial features that distinguish them from mucinous cystic tumors were accepted. Estimates of the incidence and prevalence vary. Using surgical pathology studies, it has been estimated that serous cystadenomas account for about 1% to 2% of all exocrine pancreatic neoplasms.

Serous cystadenomas occur in adults with a median age in the sixth or seventh decade. The vast majority of patients with serous cystadenomas are female [6]. About half of these tumors are discovered as incidental findings during abdominal imaging, surgery, or at autopsy.

Pathology

Detailed histologic studies of cystic lesions of the pancreas can accurately predict the biologic behavior of the tumor and are predictive of patient survival. In general, small, superficial malignancies are rarely associated with metastases or poor prognosis [7]. Invasive malignancies confer a poor prognosis similar to the prognosis seen with solid tumors of the pancreas.

Serous cystadenomas (Fig. 1) are benign, solitary, cystic tumors that arise from centro-acinar cells with an even distribution through the gland [8]. Although the majority of serous cystadenomas have microcystic morphology, there are two other variants based on growth pattern: (1) macrocystic and (2) solid. Microcystic serous cystadenomas are composed of a well-defined lesion with a honeycomb-like appearance on cross-section. Microcystic serous cystadenomas may grow to a large diameter over the long term, and the large lesions often have a complex fibrotic or calcified center. The parenchyma of the lesions is vascular with multiple, small, vessels coursing through the lesion. Macrocystic serous

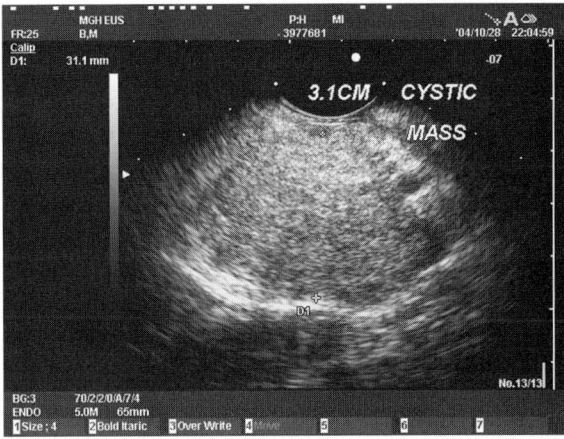

Fig. 1. Linear EUS image of serous cystadenoma. Note the microcystic morphology.

cystadenomas are composed of far fewer cyst cavities, and the diameter of each cavity varies from a few millimeters to large cavities [9]. The presence of discrete, large cystic cavities mimics the appearance of mucinous lesions. The cyst fluid from serous cystadenomas is nonviscous and clear, and contains no mucin.

The epithelial cells of all types of serous cystadenomas are similar. The cells are small and cuboidal and contain glycogen-rich, clear-cytoplasm, and small centrally located nuclei [10]. Small surface microvilli are apparent on electron microscopy. The appearance of the surrounding stroma is variable and ranges from highly vascular to fibrotic.

MCNs (Fig. 2) are composed of discrete individual locules that vary in diameter. MCNs are lined by mucin-producing cells arising from a columnar epithelium. The World Health Organization classification catalogs MCNs into

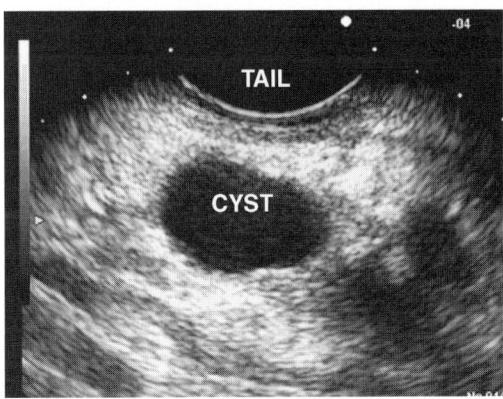

Fig. 2. Linear EUS image of a mucinous cystic neoplasm. Note the macrocystic morphology. The FNA demonstrated atypical cells and the cyst fluid CEA was > 1000 ng/mL.

three types, based on the degree of epithelial dysplasia: benign, borderline, and malignant. The degree of atypia of the tumor is classified according to the most advanced degree of dysplasia/carcinoma present.

MCNs of the pancreas are often surrounded by a unique, highly cellular (so-called "ovarian") stroma. It occurs almost exclusively in female patients, although rare cases of MCNs with ovarian stroma in male patients have been encountered. Many classifications have restricted the definition of MCNs to include only MCNs that contain ovarian stroma. The cyst fluid from MCNs is often viscous and translucent.

IPMTs are similar to MCNs in that they are cystic tumors that secrete mucin (Fig. 3). However, IPMTs are characterized by a unique papillary epithelium and arise from ductal epithelium. The presence of a papillary neoplasm produces dilatation of the ducts as a result of tumor growth. In many centers, this lesion is the most commonly resected cystic lesion of the pancreas [11]. The degree of ductal ectasia produced varies with degree of mucin production, but duct dilatation great enough to be seen on imaging studies or gross pathologic examination is a sine qua non of the diagnosis. Mucin production may be so exuberant that extrusion from the papilla of Vater is seen. The degree of dysplasia exhibited by the epithelium may range from mild to moderate to severe (carcinoma in situ), and the entire tumor is classified according to the greatest degree of dysplasia present [12].

Cystic neoplasms that are composed of neuroendocrine elements are rare and comprise 0.5% to 4% of all primary pancreatic neoplasms. The classic cystic neuroendocrine tumor is a solitary lesion lined with small, granular cells that are stainable for immunoreactive hormones, chromogranin, and synaptophysin [13]. It is rare for the cystic endocrine tumors to produce sufficient hormones to be clinically active. These lesions do not have a true epithelium; the neuroendocrine cells are present on the basis of a solid mass, and central necrosis is the

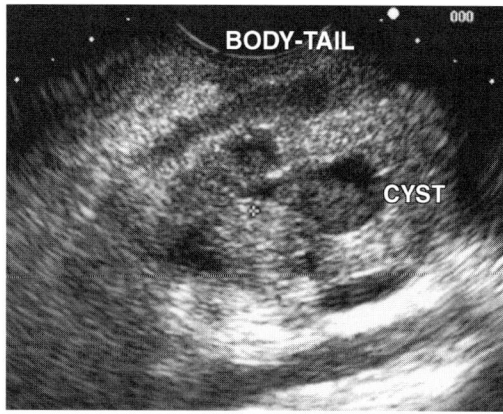

Fig. 3. Linear EUS image of an intraductal papillary mucinous tumor. Note the complex cystic and mass-like morphology. FNA demonstrated benign epithelial cells and a CEA >2500 ng/mL.

origin of the cystic space. Cystic endocrine tumors are seen in association with Von Hippel-Lindau (VHL) syndrome [14]. A related cystic lesion, the solid pseudopapillary tumor is most commonly found in young women [15]. The lesion is composed of neuroendocrine-like cells with a low malignant potential. The tumor often contains areas of hemorrhage and necrosis, a unique feature of this tumor. The cytologic findings of pseudopapillary tumors are highly characteristic, and a diagnosis can often be rendered on the basis of the aspiration cytology [16].

Pathogenesis

The pathogenesis of cystic neoplasms of the pancreas does not seem to be dietary or environmental (Fig. 4). The genetic pathways leading to malignancy have been examined in serous and mucinous lesions [17]. Serous cystadenomas are strongly associated with mutations of the VHL gene, located on chromosome 3p25 [18]. The VHL gene is likely to play an important role in the pathogenesis of sporadic serous cystadenomas. In one study, 70% of the sporadic serous cystadenomas studied demonstrated loss of heterozygosity (LOH) at 3p25 with a VHL gene mutation in the remaining allele [19]. The mutations in the VHL gene probably affect most commonly the centro-acinar cell and result in hamartomatous proliferation of these small cuboidal cells. K-ras mutations are rarely seen in serous cystadenomas [17]. There are fewer than 10 case reports in the literature of serous cystadenomas with malignant features [17,20].

The pathogenesis of mucinous cystic and IPMTs is most likely different compared with serous cystadenomas. K-ras mutation is the most common mutation found in MCNs. Using microarray analysis, a large number of genes associated with MCNs have been reported [21]. A single pattern of K-ras oncogene mutation and mutations of the p53 tumor suppressor gene increases with increasing degrees of dysplasia in the neoplasm [22]. DpC4 is highly associated with invasive malignancy [23]. The frequency of K-ras mutation in mucinous cystic neoplasms is linearly related to the grades of atypia [24]. The degree of atypia in IPMT does not seem to correlate with the presence of k-ras mutations. LOH of the p16 gene was observed with increasing degrees of histologic atypia in IPMT, whereas LOH of the p53 gene was seen only in invasive carcinomas. The distribution of LOH in 9p21(p16) and 17p13(p53) of IPMT lesions is mostly clonal, without the presence of the genetic alterations. The identical genetic statuses in the precursor lesions are consistent with the presence of clonal progression during the development of this tumor [25].

Diagnostic tests

MCNs are commonly diagnosed with CT and MR scanning based on the imaging characteristics of the cyst [26]. CT is a popular diagnostic test for cys-

Progression model for pancreatic cancer

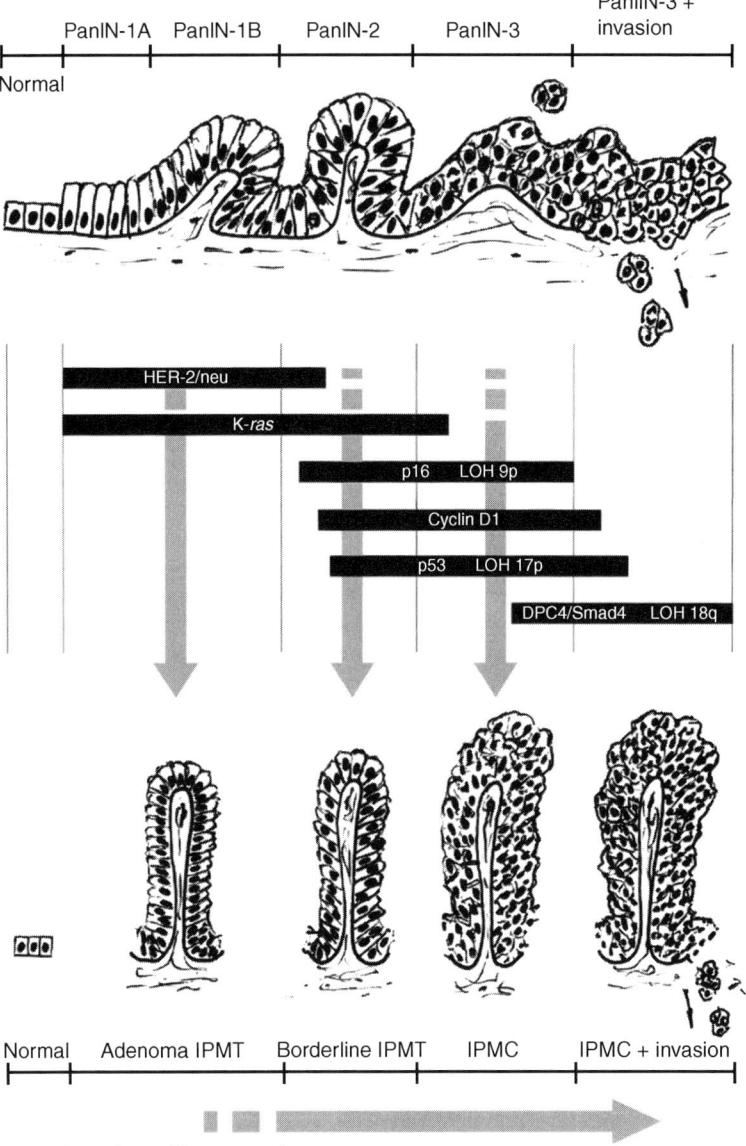

Fig. 4. Progression model for IPMT. The progression from histologically normal epithelium to invasive carcinoma (*left to right*) is associated with the accumulation of specific genetic alterations. (*From* Biankin AV, Biankin SA, Kench JG, et al. Aberrant p16INK4A and *DPC4*/Smad4 expression in intraductal papillary mucinous tumours of the pancreas is adenocarcinoma. Gut 2002;50:861–8; with permission.)

tic lesions of the pancreas because of its widespread availability and ability to detect cysts [27]. MRI is used increasingly because of the lack of radiation exposure and the ability to image the pancreatic duct with MR cholangiopancreatography (MRCP) [28]. Transabdominal ultrasonography may aid in differentiating between solid and cystic lesions, but complete evaluation of the pancreas is often difficult due to overlying bowel gas [29].

Although it is seen in less than 20% of lesions, demonstration of a central area of fibrosis by CT or MRI is a highly diagnostic feature of a serous cystadenoma [30]. The honeycombed or microcystic appearance of the lesion is commonly used to provide an imaging diagnosis. However, macrocystic serous cystadenomas are difficult to diagnose with cross-sectional imaging because of the morphologic similarities with mucinous lesions [31]. The lack of wall enhancement and a lobular contour are features seen in serous cystadenomas [32]. Mucinous cystic neoplasms, in contrast, are commonly diagnosed with CT based on the unilocular or macrocystic morphologic characteristics [33]. Although not frequently seen, the finding of peripheral egg shell calcification by CT is highly specific for a mucinous cystic neoplasm [34]. IPMTs may involve the main pancreatic duct exclusively, a side-branch duct, or both ductal systems. MRCP can demonstrate the diagnostic findings of pancreatic duct dilation, mural nodules, and cyst-ductal connection better than endoscopic retrograde cholangiopancreatography (ERCP) [28]. Mural nodules, a sign of intraductal malignancy, can be demonstrated on MRCP and CT scanning as small, round isodense foci [35]. For CT and MRCP monitoring of patients with IPMT, a change in the diameter of the main duct or a peripheral cystic lesion is used to predict the development of malignancy [30].

Despite these imaging features, the ability to accurately diagnose a specific cystic lesion and to determine whether malignancy is present by CT and MRI remains uncertain [36]. Furthermore, pseudocysts may present with many of the same imaging features of MCNs and IPMTs. Pancreatic pseudocysts appear as unilocular fluid-filled cavities associated with parenchymal changes such as calcifications and atrophy. The diagnosis of a pancreatic pseudocyst is more dependent upon the clinical history and the associated findings of chronic pancreatitis.

Endoscopic retrograde cholangiopancreatography

Retrograde injection into the pancreatic duct provides detailed imaging of the pancreatic ductal system and involvement by IPMT [37]. The presence of intraductal filling defects and cystic lesions filling on retrograde injection are highly suggestive of IPMT [38]. Although ERCP is highly sensitive for the presence of intraductal papillary mucinous neoplasia of the main pancreatic duct, it is difficult to obtain diagnostic tissue from ductal brushing or aspirations [39]. Ductal communication by a serous cystadenoma or a MCN is rare and raises the possibility of malignancy. ERCP-directed pancreatoscopy can demonstrate the papillary features of IPMT but is not used routinely.

Endoscopic ultrasound

The high-frequency imaging by endoscopic ultrasound (EUS) provides detailed information regarding the morphology of cystic lesions. In the first study of EUS of pancreatic cystic lesions, Koito [40] performed retrospective correlations between pathologic and radial EUS findings from 52 patients with solitary pancreatic cystic tumors. Six major morphologic features were identified for the cystic lesions: thick walls, tumor protrusion, thick septations, microcystic, thin septations, and simple unilocularity. All neoplastic cysts demonstrated a number of these features, including a thick wall, protruding tumor, thick septations, and microcystic morphology. All non-neoplastic cysts exhibited morphologic findings of thin septations and simple unilocular compartments. The accuracy of EUS for differentiating benign and malignant tumors was estimated at 96% and 92%, respectively, by two observers.

Gress [41] has further characterized the EUS appearances of cystic neoplasms by examining a number of EUS findings in a variety of cystic lesions. Thirty-five consecutive cases of cystic tumors of the pancreas with an established pathologic diagnosis were analyzed for characteristic radial EUS features. Mucinous cystadenocarcinomas were more likely to be characterized by an associated mass or complex cyst and caused associated pancreatic duct obstruction. The EUS appearance of benign mucinous duct ectasia (IPMT) included a diffusely dilated main pancreatic duct with thickened walls. Malignancy arising from intraductal papillary carcinoma was seen as a complex mass with a thickened wall, septations, or intra-ductal nodules. These findings suggested that EUS might be used to differentiate between solid and cystic malignancies of the pancreas.

One of the major issues of EUS is whether this imaging modality alone is capable of differentiating between benign and malignant cystic lesions. Ahmad [42] evaluated 48 patients with a cystic lesion, basing the diagnosis on the results of surgical pathology of resected lesions. The original endosonographic images were reviewed by two endosonographers who were blinded to each other's interpretation and to the surgical and pathologic interpretation. Several key components of the EUS findings were examined to see if they could differentiate benign and malignant lesions: (1) wall thickness, (2) the presence of a solid component, (3) the presence of septations, (4) the presence of lymphadenopathy, and (5) number of cysts (Fig. 5). No EUS finding was found to be predictive of a malignancy.

EUS-guided fine needle aspiration (EUS-FNA) of a cystic lesion may improve the accuracy of EUS through the use of cyst fluid analysis and cytology. In the study by Frossard [43], 67 patients with pancreatic cystic lesions were prospectively studied for cytologic and histologic analysis and for biochemical and tumor markers analysis. The quality of FNA was sufficient to provide a diagnosis in 98 cases (77%). When the results of EUS and EUS-FNA were compared with the final diagnosis (67 cases), EUS correctly identified 49 cases (73%), whereas FNA correctly identified 65 cases (97%). This study demon-

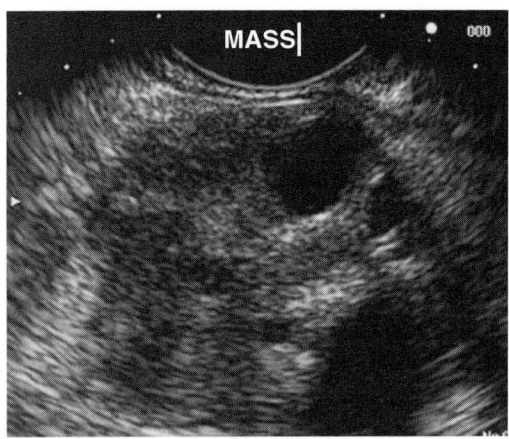

Fig. 5. Linear EUS image of a malignant mucinous cystic tumor. Note the presence of an irregular, hypoechoic mass surrounding the cystic lesion. The FNA demonstrated malignant epithelial cells.

strates the ability of a careful cytologic analysis to provide a definitive diagnosis, using a dedicated cytologist.

In the Cooperative Pancreatic Cyst study, 341 patients underwent EUS and FNA of a pancreatic cystic lesion; 112 of these patients underwent surgical resection, providing a histologic diagnosis of the cystic lesion (68 mucinous, 7 serous, 27 inflammatory, 5 endocrine, and 5 other) [44]. Receiver-operator curve analysis of the tumor markers demonstrated that cyst fluid carcinoembryonic antigen (CEA) (optimal cutoff of 192 ng/mL) demonstrated the greatest area under the curve (0.79) for differentiating mucinous versus nonmucinous cystic lesions. The accuracy of CEA (88 of 111, 79%) was significantly greater than the accuracy of EUS morphology (57 of 112, 51%) or cytology (64 of 109, 59%). There was no combination of tests that provided greater accuracy than cyst fluid CEA alone. Based on these findings, cyst fluid CEA seems to be the best test available for differentiating between mucinous and nonmucinous lesions (Table 1).

Table 1
Key factors of the most common cystic lesions of the pancreas

	Morphology	Location	Cytology	CEA
Serous	Microcystic	Evenly distributed	Bland PAS+	<0.5
Mucinous	Macrocystic	Tail	Mucinous	>200
IPMT	Mixed	Head	Mucinous	>200
Pseudocyst	Unilocular	Evenly distributed	Pigmented histiocytes	<200

Abbreviations: CEA, carcinoembryonic antigen; IPMT, intraductal papillary mucinous tumor; PAS, periodic acid Schiff.

Management

Surgical resection is the only treatment available for the management of patients with a cystic neoplasm. The timing and selection of patients has not been well defined except for good surgical candidates who have evidence of an early malignancy. The factors that need to be considered in the management of cystic tumors of the pancreas include age and surgical risk of the patient and location and size of the lesion. The results of CT, EUS, and cyst fluid analysis can be useful to guide management toward observation in lesions with minimal malignant potential or to resection in lesions with substantial risk of cancer.

The recent declines in surgical morbidity and mortality have expanded the role of surgery for the treatment of benign and premalignant cystic lesions. Because most MCNs are located in the tail of the pancreas, a distal pancreatectomy provides a low-risk, curative treatment. IPMTs are more frequently located in the head of the pancreas and therefore require a pancreatoduodenectomy for definitive resection. Because IPMTs tend to grow longitudinally along ducts rather than radially into the parenchyma, it is important that resection margins of IPMTs be examined with frozen section during surgery to confirm clearance of the tumor. A small percentage of patients requires a total pancreatectomy to remove the entire lesion.

With the exception of mucinous cystic tumors with malignant invasion through the cyst wall, the prognosis for resected cystic tumors of the pancreas is excellent (nearly 100%) [45]. Even for IPMTs containing invasive carcinoma, the 5-year survival was 36% in one series [46].

The recommendations for patient management are limited by the inability to reliably distinguish benign from potentially malignant mucinous lesions and by the poor understanding of the natural history of these tumors. It is likely that patients with a mucinous lesion that have a low likelihood of malignant change can be managed with monitoring. In contrast, young patients with a MCN or IPMT should be managed with resection because of the long-term risk of the development of malignancy.

Summary

Pancreatic cystic tumors represent the best-described precursor to pancreatic cancer. The lesions can be readily identified by cross-sectional imaging, and EUS-FNA can provide cytologic and biochemical evidence of premalignant and malignant lesions.

References

[1] Brugge WR, Lauwers GY, Sahani D, et al. Cystic neoplasms of the pancreas. N Engl J Med 2004;351:1218–26.

[2] Kimura W, Morikane K, Esaki Y, et al. Histologic and biologic patterns of microscopic pancreatic ductal adenocarcinomas detected incidentally at autopsy. Cancer 1998;82:1839–49.

[3] Spinelli KS, Fromwiller TE, Daniel RA, et al. Cystic pancreatic neoplasms: observe or operate. Ann Surg 2004;239:651–7 [discussion 657–9].

[4] Kimura W. How many millimeters do atypical epithelia of the pancreas spread intraductally before beginning to infiltrate? Hepatogastroenterology 2003;54:2218–24.

[5] Compton CC. Serous cystic tumors of the pancreas. Semin Diagn Pathol 2000;17:43–55.

[6] Bassi C, Salvia R, Molinari E, et al. Management of 100 consecutive cases of pancreatic serous cystadenoma: wait for symptoms and see at imaging or vice versa? World J Surg 2003; 27:319–23.

[7] Wilentz RE, Albores-Saavedra J, Zahurak M, et al. Pathologic examination accurately predicts prognosis in mucinous cystic neoplasms of the pancreas. Am J Surg Pathol 1999;23:1320–7.

[8] Kosmahl M, Wagner J, Peters K, et al. Serous cystic neoplasms of the pancreas: an immuno-histochemical analysis revealing alpha-inhibin, neuron-specific enolase, and MUC6 as new markers. Am J Surg Pathol 2004;28:339–46.

[9] Khurana B, Mortele KJ, Glickman J, et al. Macrocystic serous adenoma of the pancreas: radiologic-pathologic correlation. AJR Am J Roentgenol 2003;181:119–23.

[10] Santos LD, Chow C, Henderson CJ, et al. Serous oligocystic adenoma of the pancreas: a clini-copathological and immunohistochemical study of three cases with ultrastructural findings. Pathology 2002;34:148–56.

[11] Kosmahl M, Pauser U, Peters K, et al. Cystic neoplasms of the pancreas and tumor-like lesions with cystic features: a review of 418 cases and a classification proposal. Virchows Arch 2004; 445:168–78.

[12] Hruban RH, Takaori K, Klimstra DS, et al. An illustrated consensus on the classification of pancreatic intraepithelial neoplasia and intraductal papillary mucinous neoplasms. Am J Surg Pathol 2004;28:977–87.

[13] Kann P, Bittinger F, Engelbach M, et al. Endosonography of insulin-secreting and clinically non-functioning neuroendocrine tumors of the pancreas: criteria for benignancy and malignancy. Eur J Med Res 2001;6:385–90.

[14] Marcos HB, Libutti SK, Alexander HR, et al. Neuroendocrine tumors of the pancreas in von Hippel-Lindau disease: spectrum of appearances at CT and MR imaging with histopathologic comparison. Radiology 2002;225:751–8.

[15] Ferlan-Marolt V, Pleskovic L, Pegan V. Solid papillary-cystic tumor of the pancreas. Hepato-gastroenterology 1999;46:2978–82.

[16] Pettinato G, Di Vizio D, Manivel JC, et al. Solid-pseudopapillary tumor of the pancreas: a neoplasm with distinct and highly characteristic cytological features. Diagn Cytopathol 2002; 27:325–34.

[17] Kim SG, Wu TT, Lee JH, et al. Comparison of epigenetic and genetic alterations in mucinous cystic neoplasm and serous microcystic adenoma of pancreas. Mod Pathol 2003;16:1086–94.

[18] Moore PS, Zamboni G, Brighenti A, et al. Molecular characterization of pancreatic serous microcystic adenomas: evidence for a tumor suppressor gene on chromosome 10q. Am J Pathol 2001;158:317–21.

[19] Hammel PR, Vilgrain V, Terris B, et al. Pancreatic involvement in von Hippel-Lindau disease. The Groupe Francophone d'Etude de la Maladie de von Hippel-Lindau. Gastroenterology 2000; 119:1087–95.

[20] Abe H, Kubota K, Mori M, et al. Serous cystadenoma of the pancreas with invasive growth: benign or malignant? Am J Gastroenterol 1998;93:1963–6.

[21] Fukushima N, Sato N, Prasad N, et al. Characterization of gene expression in mucinous cystic neoplasms of the pancreas using oligonucleotide microarrays. Oncogene 2004;23:9042–51.

[22] Uemura K, Hiyama E, Murakami Y, et al. Comparative analysis of K-ras point mutation, telomerase activity, and p53 overexpression in pancreatic tumours. Oncol Rep 2003;10:277–83.

[23] Iacobuzio-Donahue CA, Wilentz RE, Argani P, et al. Dpc4 protein in mucinous cystic neoplasms of the pancreas: frequent loss of expression in invasive carcinomas suggests a role in genetic progression. Am J Surg Pathol 2000;24:1544–8.

[24] Yoshizawa K, Nagai H, Sakurai S, et al. Clonality and K-ras mutation analyses of epithelia in intraductal papillary mucinous tumor and mucinous cystic tumor of the pancreas. Virchows Arch 2002;441:437–43.

[25] Wada K, Takada T, Yasuda H, et al. Does "clonal progression" relate to the development of intraductal papillary mucinous tumors of the pancreas? J Gastrointest Surg 2004;8:289–96.

[26] Gritzmann N, Macheiner P, Hollerweger A, et al. CT in the differentiation of pancreatic neoplasms: progress report. Dig Dis 2004;22:6–17.

[27] Fernandez-del Castillo C, Targarona J, Thayer SP, et al. Incidental pancreatic cysts: clinico-pathologic characteristics and comparison with symptomatic patients. Arch Surg 2003;138: 427–33 [discussion 433-4].

[28] Sahani D, Prasad S, Saini S, et al. Cystic pancreatic neoplasms evaluation by CT and magnetic resonance cholangiopancreatography. Gastrointest Endosc Clin N Am 2002;12:657–72.

[29] Rickes S, Wermke W. Differentiation of cystic pancreatic neoplasms and pseudocysts by conventional and echo-enhanced ultrasound. J Gastroenterol Hepatol 2004;19:761–6.

[30] Irie H, Yoshimitsu K, Aibe H, et al. Natural history of pancreatic intraductal papillary mucinous tumor of branch duct type: follow-up study by magnetic resonance cholangiopancreatography. J Comput Assist Tomogr 2004;28:117–22.

[31] Torresan F, Casadei R, Solmi L, et al. The role of ultrasound in the differential diagnosis of serous and mucinous cystic tumours of the pancreas. Eur J Gastroenterol Hepatol 1997;9:169–72.

[32] Cohen-Scali F, Vilgrain V, Brancatelli G, et al. Discrimination of unilocular macrocystic serous cystadenoma from pancreatic pseudocyst and mucinous cystadenoma with CT: initial observations. Radiology 2003;228:727–33.

[33] Chatelain D, Hammel P, O'Toole D, et al. Macrocystic form of serous pancreatic cystadenoma. Am J Gastroenterol 2002;97:2566–71.

[34] Scott J, Martin I, Redhead D, et al. Mucinous cystic neoplasms of the pancreas: imaging features and diagnostic difficulties. Clin Radiol 2000;55:187–92.

[35] Fukukura Y, Fujiyoshi F, Hamada H, et al. Intraductal papillary mucinous tumors of the pancreas: comparison of helical CT and MR imaging. Acta Radiol 2003;44:464–71.

[36] Visser BC, Muthusamay VR, Mulvihill SJ, et al. Diagnostic imaging of cystic pancreatic neoplasms. Surg Oncol 2004;13:27–39.

[37] Telford JJ, Carr-Locke DL. The role of ERCP and pancreatoscopy in cystic and intraductal tumors. Gastrointest Endosc Clin N Am 2002;12:747–57.

[38] Yamao K, Nakamura T, Suzuki T, et al. Endoscopic diagnosis and staging of mucinous cystic neoplasms and intraductal papillary-mucinous tumors. J Hepatobiliary Pancreat Surg 2003;10: 142–6.

[39] Madura JA, Wiebke EA, Howard TJ, et al. Mucin-hypersecreting intraductal neoplasms of the pancreas: a precursor to cystic pancreatic malignancies. Surgery 1997;122:786–92 [discussion 792–3].

[40] Koito K, Namieno T, Nagakawa T, et al. Solitary cystic tumor of the pancreas: EUS-pathologic correlation. Gastrointest Endosc 1997;45:268–76.

[41] Gress F, Gottlieb K, Cummings O, et al. Endoscopic ultrasound characteristics of mucinous cystic neoplasms of the pancreas. Am J Gastroenterol 2000;95:961–5.

[42] Ahmad NA, Kochman ML, Lewis JD, et al. Can EUS alone differentiate between malignant and benign cystic lesions of the pancreas? Am J Gastroenterol 2001;96:3295–300.

[43] Frossard JL, Amouyal P, Amouyal G, et al. Performance of endosonography-guided fine needle aspiration and biopsy in the diagnosis of pancreatic cystic lesions. Am J Gastroenterol 2003;98: 1516–24.

[44] Brugge WR, Lewandrowski K, Lee-Lewandrowski E, et al. Diagnosis of pancreatic cystic neoplasms: a report of the cooperative pancreatic cyst study. Gastroenterology 2004;126:1330–6.

[45] Suzuki Y, Atomi Y, Sugiyama M, et al. Cystic neoplasm of the pancreas: a Japanese multi-institutional study of intraductal papillary mucinous tumor and mucinous cystic tumor. Pancreas 2004;28:241–6.

[46] Chari ST, Yadav D, Smyrk TC, et al. Study of recurrence after surgical resection of intraductal papillary mucinous neoplasm of the pancreas. Gastroenterology 2002;123:1500–7.

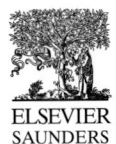

ELSEVIER
SAUNDERS

Gastrointest Endoscopy Clin N Am
15 (2005) 497–511

GASTROINTESTINAL
ENDOSCOPY CLINICS
OF NORTH AMERICA

The Role of Endoscopic Ultrasonography in the Evaluation of Pancreatico-Biliary Cancer

Shyam Varadarajulu, MD,
Mohamad A. Eloubeidi, MD, MHS*

Department of Gastroenterology and Hepatology and the Pancreatico-biliary Center, the University of Alabama at Birmingham, 1530 3rd Ave. S. - ZRB 636, Birmingham, AL 35294-0007, USA

Pancreatic cancer is the fourth leading cause of cancer-related deaths in the United States and develops in approximately 30,000 people annually. The disease is associated with a high mortality rate and a median survival of approximately 4 months in untreated patients. Data from the National Cancer Database show the 5-year survival rate after surgery to be 3% [1]. If surgery achieves clear margins and negative lymph nodes, the 5-year survival rate approaches 25%. Most patients diagnosed with pancreatic cancer present at an advanced stage of the disease when surgical cure is no longer possible. When the cancer is unresectable, chemotherapy, radiation therapy, or a combination of the two may improve overall survival and quality of life.

The regional anatomy of the pancreas is complex, making procurement of cytologic samples difficult without exploratory laparotomy. Traditionally, CT-guided fine-needle aspiration (FNA) has been used for biopsy of the pancreas. This technique is associated with a risk of peritoneal dissemination of cancer cells and has a false-negative rate of up to 20% [2,3]. Endoscopic retrograde cholangiopancreatography (ERCP) brush cytology has a false-negative rate of nearly 30% [4].

With endoscopic ultrasonography (EUS), it is possible to position the transducer in direct proximity to the pancreas by means of the stomach and duodenum. The high-frequency transducer enables production of detailed high-resolution images of the pancreas that far surpass those of CT or MRI. The high

---

* Corresponding author.
E-mail address: meloubeidi@uabmc.edu (M.A. Eloubeidi).

1052-5157/05/$ – see front matter © 2005 Elsevier Inc. All rights reserved.
doi:10.1016/j.giec.2005.03.002

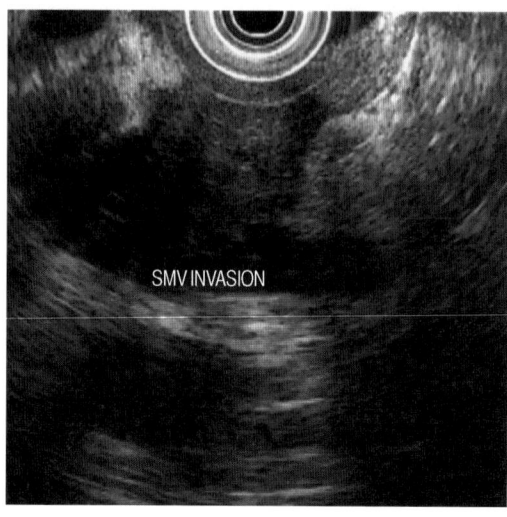

Fig. 1. Radial EUS image (Olympus GF-UM 130; range 6 cm, frequency 7.5 Mhz) of a patient
with pancreatic head mass invading the superior mesenteric vein (SMV).

resolution of these images allows identification of lesions as small as 2 to 3 mm
and their relationship to adjacent blood vessels, such as the portal vein and
mesenteric vasculature (Fig. 1). An added advantage of EUS is the ability to
perform FNA. Compared with other imaging modalities, the results of EUS-FNA
of pancreatic masses are excellent, with a sensitivity of 85% to 90% and a
specificity of virtually 100% [5–7]. The procedure is safe, with reported complication rates being <1% [8]. EUS-guided therapies, such as celiac plexus
neurolysis for pain control and direct injection of cytotoxins into malignant
lesions, are becoming important adjuncts in the management of patients with
surgically unresectable disease. This article focuses on the role of EUS in the
diagnosis and staging of malignant pancreatic lesions.

Pancreatic adenocarcinoma

Accuracy of staging by endoscopic ultrasonography

EUS staging of pancreatic and other tumors follows the (T)umor, (N)ode
(M)etastasis system of the American Joint Committee on Cancer (AJCC). In
2002, the AJCC modified the T staging system for pancreatic cancer to classify
tumors invading the portal venous (superior mesenteric vein or portal vein)
(see Fig. 1) system as T3 (these were previously staged as T4) and tumors
invading the celiac or superior mesenteric artery as T4 (Fig. 2). Although this
change is likely to result in decreased reported accuracy for EUS, it remains
unclear if surgical therapy is beneficial compared with radiochemotherapy for

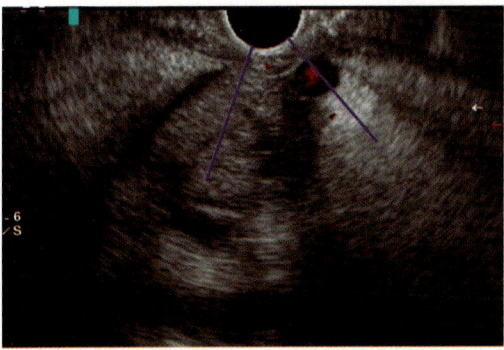

Fig. 2. Curvilinear echoendoscope image (Olympus UC-30 P, scanning at 5 Mhz) with Doppler reveals mass in pancreatic body with splenic artery invasion.

tumors invading the portal venous system. Most literature is based on the previous AJCC staging system, in which all mesenteric vascular invasion (venous or arterial) were staged T4.

Many large series have found T-stage accuracy to range from approximately 78% to 94% and nodal (N)-stage accuracy to range from 64% to 82% [9–12]. Lower accuracy has also been described. In a study of 89 patients in whom EUS was compared with surgical and histopathologic TNM staging [13], the overall accuracy of EUS for T and N staging was 69% and 54%, respectively. Only 46% of tumors believed to be resectable by EUS were found to be resectable during laparotomy. Staging accuracy of EUS can be influenced by several factors, including the experience level of the endosonographer, imaging artifacts, and the endosonographer's knowledge of the results of previous imaging tests. In general, T-stage accuracy for EUS is highest in patients with smaller tumors, whereas helical CT is more accurate in staging larger tumors [14–16]. The accuracy of EUS for detecting invasion into the superior mesenteric artery and vein is lower than that for detecting portal or splenic vein invasion [17,18].

A recent review [19] that pooled data from four studies comparing the accuracy of EUS with helical CT in the evaluation of pancreatic cancer found that EUS detected more tumors (97% versus 73%), was more accurate for determining tumor resectability (91% versus 83%), and was more sensitive for detecting vascular invasion (91% versus 64%). When the data were interpreted individually, two of the reports concluded that CT and EUS were approximately equivalent in detecting the primary tumors [14,20], whereas the other two found EUS to be superior [21,22]. Several features of the individual reports may account for these variable conclusions, including differences in the gold standards, variations in the specific techniques used for helical CT, and the proportion of patients with advanced disease in each study. A reasonable conclusion from these data and from clinical experience is that EUS and helical CT are complementary for staging pancreatic cancer. EUS is a more accurate modality for local T staging and for predicting vascular invasion, especially in tumors

<3 cm, whereas helical CT is better for the evaluation of distant metastasis and for staging larger tumors. Similar to CT, studies comparing MRI with EUS suggest that EUS may be more sensitive for detecting small tumors while providing complementary information regarding resectability [23].

Recent advances in CT technology, including the development of spiral scanners and more recently multidetector CT (MDCT) scanners, and the development of three-dimensional (3D) imaging software have improved the ability of CT to image the pancreas and to evaluate a wide range of pancreatic pathology. In most of the published series, older dynamic scanners or single-row spiral scanners were used, and 3D imaging was not included. With the narrow collimation and faster scanning possibilities with new MDCT scanners, it is likely that the CT accuracy for detecting pancreatic tumor will improve. In a recently published study by McNulty et al [24] using MDCT, 27 of 28 pancreatic cancers were detected. This progress will continue as manufacturers introduce the next generation of scanners, which can acquire up to 32 slices per second with faster scan times. The impact of these new scanners on diagnostic accuracy will need to be carefully evaluated.

Several studies have compared the accuracy of angiography and EUS for determining vascular invasion [17,18,25]. Although the results varied, a general conclusion is that EUS is as accurate or more accurate for determining vascular invasion, with the exception of some tumors that invade the superior mesenteric artery. In a study of 21 patients with pancreatic cancer who underwent EUS and angiography before an attempt at curative resection, EUS was more sensitive than angiography for detecting vascular invasion (86% versus 21%). The specificity and accuracy of EUS were 71% and 81%, respectively, compared with 71% and 38% for angiography [23].

Role of endoscopic ultrasonography-guided fine-needle aspiration in pancreatic cancer

EUS has an important role in guiding a biopsy needle into lesions that are too small to be identified by CT or MRI or too well encased by surrounding vascular structures to safely allow percutaneous biopsy (Figs. 3 and 4) [26]. The impact of EUS-FNA was studied by Chang et al [27] in a series of 44 patients. EUS-FNA had an accuracy rate of 95% for pancreatic lesions and 88% for lymph nodes. Three patients had enlarged celiac nodes on EUS that showed malignancy on FNA. FNA precluded surgery in 41% of the patients, avoided the need for further diagnostic tests in 57%, and influenced clinical decisions in 68% of the patients, thus providing substantial cost savings. Gress et al [26] examined the role of EUS-FNA in patients with suspected pancreatic cancer after a negative CT-guided FNA or ERCP brush cytology. Of 102 patients, 57 had positive cytology on EUS-FNA, and 37 had negative cytology. The examination was inconclusive in eight patients. After a median follow-up of 24 months, all 57 patients with positive cytology on EUS-FNA had verification of the diagnosis of pancreatic cancer. Of the 45 patients with negative or inconclusive cytology on

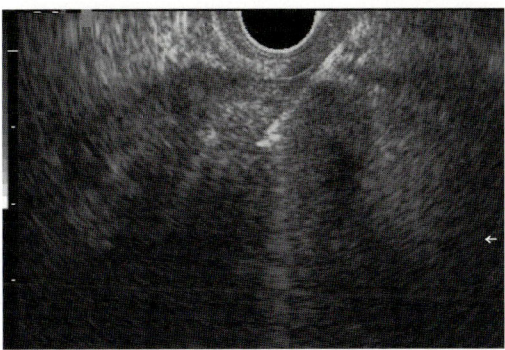

Fig. 3. Linear EUS image (Olympus UC-30 P, scanning at 5 Mhz) of a patient with pancreatic head mass undergoing EUS-FNA.

EUS-FNA, 41 had no evidence of pancreatic malignancy at follow-up. One important application of EUS-FNA is the detection of malignant lymph nodes. FNA has been demonstrated to increase the accuracy of lymph node staging and thereby reduce the number of unnecessary surgical explorations by identifying patients with surgically incurable disease [27].

Lesions located in the uncinate process of the pancreas are the most difficult to puncture. To access a mass in the uncinate process, the echoendoscope must

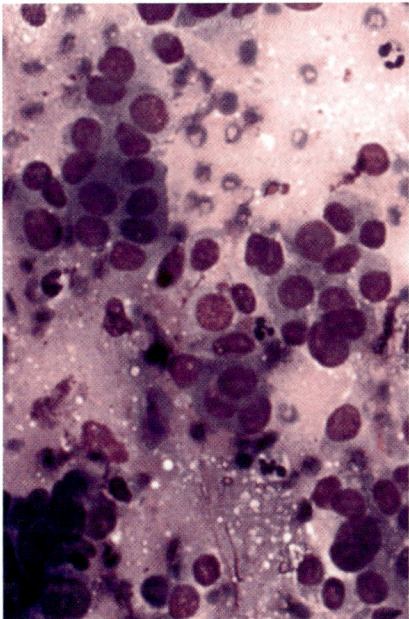

Fig. 4. Cytologic features consistent with malignancy (Papanicoulou stain 40×).

be advanced into the duodenal C-loop in the "long" position. This exerts substantial angulation and torque on the FNA needle. The needle is more difficult to advance, and the procedure causes a "bowed shape" in the needle. This altered shape can result in mistargeting. Lesions in the pancreatic isthmus pose a similar challenge in that the echoendoscope is usually in the "long" scope position with the tip in the gastric antrum.

A transgastric approach can be more difficult than the transduodenal approach due to the laxity and redundancy of the gastric wall and the capaciousness of the stomach. Lacking anchorage, the echoendoscope tends to displace during advancement of the FNA needle.

A controversial issue is identifying who should undergo EUS-FNA (Box 1). There is general consensus that it is reasonable to obtain a tissue diagnosis in patients suspected of having pancreatic cancer who are poor surgical candidates. Histologic confirmation in such patients can be helpful in deciding on chemotherapy or radiotherapy. More controversial is the role of EUS-FNA in patients suspected of having pancreatic cancer who seem to be resectable on other imaging studies. One view is that a tissue diagnosis does not alter management and is therefore unnecessary. This argument is supported by the recognition that the sensitivity of EUS-FNA is in the range of 85% to 90%, thereby potentially leading to false-negative results in up to 15% of patients. An argument can be made for EUS-FNA in such patients when the establishment of a histologic diagnosis before surgery may alter management because other types of malignancy involving the pancreas can mimic adenocarcinoma (eg, lymphoma). Therapy for these tumors may not include surgery. Some patients and physicians want to know definitively whether cancer is present before undergoing a surgical resection. When the FNA is negative, some patients may be willing to accept the 15% chance of missing a diagnosis of cancer rather than undergoing surgery. This is especially true when there is concurrent acute or chronic pancreatitis that may mimic a focal pancreatic cancer.

Box 1. Indications for the use of EUS-FNA

- To document a diagnosis of malignancy in a patient with an unresectable mass as a prerequisite for adjuvant chemotherapy or radiation therapy
- To exclude other tumor types, such as lymphoma, small-cell metastasis, or neuroendocrine cancer, that may require a different management strategy
- To determine a diagnosis in patients who are reluctant to undergo major surgery without a definitive diagnosis
- To document the absence of malignancy when the pretest probability of malignancy is low

Role of endoscopic ultrasonography in metastatic pancreatic cancer

An emerging role for EUS is the detection of small, occult liver metastases in patients with pancreatic tumors. Although EUS is best suited for loco-regional staging, its high resolution and proximity to the left lobe and inferior right lobe of the liver has led to detection of small liver metastases [28,29]. The ability to perform immediate EUS-FNA allows accurate distinction of benign from malignant lesions. A recent study reported the results of EUS-FNA of liver lesions in 167 patients (including 62 with pancreatic cancer), all of whom had negative or equivocal CT or ultrasound (US) of the liver. EUS-FNA was highly accurate, with a complication rate of 4%. One death occurred when EUS-FNA of a liver lesion was performed in the setting of an obstructed biliary stent, leading to cholangitis. Antibiotic prophylaxis and biliary drainage should be used in conjunction with EUS-FNA of liver lesions in the setting of obstructing pancreatic tumors [29].

Another emerging role of EUS is the identification of small, occult pancreatic tumors in the patients with liver metastases of "unknown" primary. In the report by ten-Berge et al [29], EUS identified a pancreatic tumor in 17 of 33 patients whose CT showed only metastatic tumor of unknown primary. The identification of a pancreas primary allowed pancreas-specific chemotherapy to be administered in each of these cases.

Safety and complications of endoscopic ultrasonography-guided fine-needle aspiration

The safety of EUS-FNA for evaluating pancreatic lesions is well established [30,31]. Rare complications include pancreatitis, infection, and bleeding. In a multicenter study evaluating the safety of EUS-FNA of solid pancreatic masses, 14 of 4958 patients developed pancreatitis [30]. In another study involving EUS-FNA of pancreatic cystic lesions, 1 of 81 patients developed an infected cystadenoma after EUS-FNA [31]. This patient did not receive prophylactic antibiotics before the procedure. The current standard of care includes routine administration of antibiotics for patients undergoing FNA of pancreatic cystic lesions.

Management of pancreatic focal solid masses

Accurate staging of patients with pancreatic cancer is critical to avoid the expense, morbidity, and mortality related to unnecessary surgery. Although several tests are available for assessing such patients, consensus has not been achieved on the optimal approach. Thus, the role of EUS and EUS-FNA varies among treatment centers. EUS has a more prominent role at our institution (Fig. 5). We recommend that helical CT be performed initially to evaluate for the presence of a pancreatic mass. EUS is most clearly indicated when no clear tumor or only equivocal changes are seen on CT. If metastatic disease is evident,

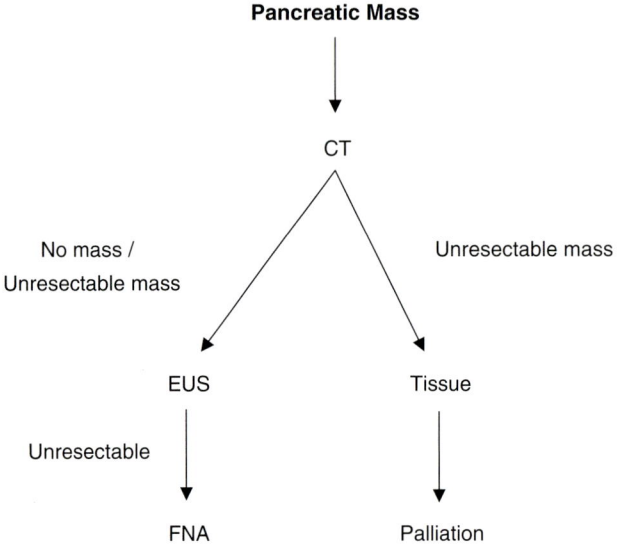

Fig. 5. Algorithm for management of pancreatic cancer.

EUS or CT-guided biopsy can establish the diagnosis. If the helical CT is negative for metastatic disease or an obvious mass, EUS should be performed to further evaluate the pancreas (if the clinical suspicion is high for pancreatic cancer) followed by EUS-FNA of any apparent mass noted.

Neuroendocrine tumors

Pancreatic endocrine tumors are often small and hard to detect by radiologic techniques. Since the original description of gastrinomas in 1955 by Zollinger and Ellison [32], multiple imaging modalities have been evaluated to localize pancreatic neuroendocrine lesions for surgical resection. Studies have shown that CT, MRI, and conventional US detect tumors in less than 50% of patients [33]. Somatostatin receptor scintigraphy (SRS) is reported to have the highest sensitivity for gastrinomas but is less accurate for detecting insulinomas [34]. The optimal algorithm for staging pancreatic neuroendocrine tumors is unknown. Issues important for clinical management include (1) Is the tumor localized to the region of the pancreas (including gastrinoma triangle) or metastatic? (2) Is the tumor unifocal or multifocal within the pancreas? and (3) Is it functional or nonfunctional, benign or malignant?

To determine whether a tumor is localized or metastatic, cross-sectional imaging and SRS are likely more accurate than EUS due to their ability to image broad areas [35]. For imaging within the pancreas, EUS provides superior resolution and accuracy compared with CT scan. In a study of 82 patients, Anderson et al [35] identified 100 tumors in 54 patients, emphasizing the frequency of multifocal tumors. EUS accurately localized the tumor in 93% of patients and had a specificity of 95%, which was higher than CT or transabdominal US. EUS was not reliable for detection of extra-pancreatic tumors. Zimmer et al [36] compared EUS with CT, SRS, US, and MRI in 40 patients with neuroendocrine tumors. EUS had the highest overall accuracy for gastrinomas and insulinomas but missed 50% of extra pancreatic tumors. In a report of patients who had negative ultrasonography and CT scans, EUS detected endocrine tumors in the pancreas with high sensitivity (82%) and specificity (95%) [37].

In patients with nonfunctioning neuroendocrine tumors where the risk of surgery is high, it is useful to distinguish benign from malignant neuroendocrine tumors. In two studies, EUS was able to accurately distinguish malignant lesions based on the presence of an irregular inhomogeneous hypoechoic mass or on invasion and obstruction of the pancreatic duct [38,39]. Tumors without these features were almost always benign.

Intraductal ultrasonography and neuroendocrine tumors

Intraductal endoscopic ultrasonography (IDUS) involves the insertion of an ultra-thin (2 mm) US probe directly into the pancreatic duct during ERCP. Preliminary experience suggests that it may be more accurate than standard EUS for the detection of neuroendocrine tumors. Although experience with IDUS is limited, initial data suggest that IDUS may improve the evaluation of these patients and lead to the identification of tumors arising within the pancreas that have gone unrecognized by other techniques [40,41]. In one study, IDUS was able to identify the presence of an islet cell tumor in seven of seven patients [41]. In one of these patients who had multifocal disease, IDUS accurately determined the number of tumors, whereas EUS failed to detect all lesions. The distance from the tumors to the main pancreatic duct was accurately determined, thus aiding preoperative planning of wedge resection, which was possible in two patients.

EUS can be useful for preoperative localization of pancreatic endocrine tumors by its ability to tattoo lesions by fine-needle injection using India ink [42]. This may shorten operative time because it obviates the need to localize the tumor by palpation and intraoperative US. This technique may have the potential to facilitate tumor resection by less invasive methods, such as laparoscopic enucleation.

These data suggest that EUS serves an important role in localizing tumors within the pancreas, detecting multifocal tumors, and distinguishing benign from malignant tumors. In addition, EUS should be used with cross-sectional imaging and SRS to identify extra-pancreatic tumors or metastases.

Cholangiocarcinoma

Cholangiocarcinoma is a difficult neoplasm to diagnose non-operatively. Although ERCP remains the modality of choice for characterizing common bile duct strictures, a definitive histologic diagnosis of a neoplastic stricture is not made in many patients despite aggressive endoscopic techniques, including the combination of brushings, biopsy, and FNA [43–46]. Without a histologic or cytologic diagnosis of cancer, potentially beneficial therapy may be inappropriately withheld. Left untreated, more than 95% of afflicted patients die within 1 to 2 years. To achieve the best survival rates, complete radical tumor resections, including major partial hepatectomies, are usually required. These procedures remain challenging, with a mortality rate of 8% to 10% and a complication rate of 37% to 64% [47–49]. Because of the therapeutic dilemma and technical challenges of radical surgery, patients need to be chosen carefully because only 20% to 49% fulfill the criteria for resectability to undergo radical surgery and because about 20% may have diagnoses other than cholangiocarcinoma, and surgery might not be the first choice for therapy in these patients [50,51]. Therefore, it seems preferable to have a histologic diagnosis available before attempting curative surgical resection so that individualized treatment can be provided.

Accuracy of endoscopic ultrasonography-guided fine-needle aspiration in cholangiocarcinoma

Although EUS can identify biliary strictures, tissue diagnosis is crucial for differentiation of malignant versus benign lesions. Two prospective studies have evaluated the role of EUS-FNA in biliary strictures (Fig. 6). In the first study, 44 patients with strictures at the liver hilum underwent EUS-FNA. The accuracy, sensitivity, and specificity for diagnosis of cholangiocarcinoma were 91%, 89%, and 100%, respectively. EUS and EUS-FNA changed the pre-planned surgical approach in 27 of 44 patients [52]. In the second study, 28 patients with

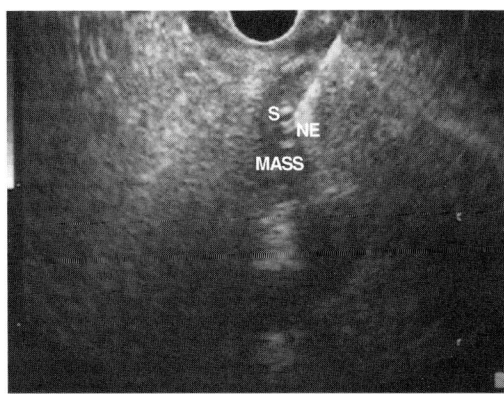

Fig. 6. Linear EUS-image of a patient with cholangiocarcinoma undergoing EUS-FNA (Olympus UC-140T, scanning at 5 Mhz). FNA needle (NE) is advanced into a hypoechoic mass that is associated with the bile duct containing a biliary stent (S).

previously failed tissues diagnosis underwent EUS-FNA of biliary strictures [53]. The sensitivity, specificity, positive predictive value, negative predictive value, and accuracy of EUS-FNA were 86%, 100%, 100%, 57%, and 88%, respectively. EUS-FNA had a positive impact on patient management in 84% of patients: preventing surgery for tissue diagnosis in patients with inoperable disease ($n = 10$), facilitating surgery in patients with unidentifiable cancer by other modalities ($n = 8$), and avoiding surgery in benign disease ($n = 4$). No major complications were reported in either study. Both studies were done at tertiary referral centers by expert endosonographers. It remains to be seen whether these results can be replicated and reproduced in other settings. EUS is most optimal for lesions in the mid- or distal bile duct. Hilar lesions, when not visualized by EUS, can usually be seen using the IDUS probes with the caveat that tissue procurement is not possible.

Technique of endoscopic ultrasonography-guided fine-needle aspiration

The technique of EUS-FNA of biliary lesions is more difficult and slightly different from FNA of pancreatic mass lesions. Evaluation of the bile duct is usually started with the echo endoscope positioned at the papilla. By gradually withdrawing and rotating the instrument cephalad into the duodenal bulb and pylorus region, the common bile duct up to the proximal part can be visualized. A stent, when present, serves as a guide to follow the bile duct. When the tip of the scope is placed and bent posteriorly just beyond the pylorus, the hepatic hilum can be well identified, with the tumor appearing as an echo-poor transductal lesion. This enables assessment of the biliary lesion, its spread in the liver and relation to portal vein and hepatic arteries, and the presence and status of lymph nodes. Color Doppler US is useful to verify the different vessels in or in relation to the liver because the anatomy of the hepatic arteries can vary. While the hilar area is imaged, the echoendoscope often tends to slip back into the stomach and needs frequent repositioning; this is of concern, particularly when performing FNA of hilar lesions. To circumvent the problem, the scope can be brought into a "long position" to allow the wall of the greater curve to provide support for the force exerted when the needle is advanced into the tumor.

Intraductal Ultrasound

The IDUS probe used for local staging of biliary strictures can be inserted into the bile duct at ERCP over a guide wire. Although initial studies suggested a need for biliary sphincterotomy, a new small-diameter IDUS probe has been developed that obviates the need for sphincterotomy [54]. Its small diameter and monorail design allows insertion over a 0.035-inch guidewire and greatly simplifies IDUS. The IDUS image of the normal bile duct wall comprises two or three sonographic layers: An outer hyperechoic layer represents the adipose layer of the subserosa, the serosa, and the interface echo between serosa and surrounding organs. Occasionally a third inner hyperechoic layer is identified and represents an interface echo.

IDUS criteria that suggest malignancy include a hypoechoic mass, especially if it is infiltrating surrounding tissues, heterogeneity of the internal echo pattern, notching or irregularity of the outer border, a papillary surface, and disruption of the normal sonographic structure of the duct [55,56]. In a study by Menzel et al [56] that included 56 consecutive patients with bile duct strictures and obstructive jaundice, IDUS was more accurate than EUS (89% versus 76%, $P < 0.002$) for determining the nature of the bile duct strictures. IDUS was also better for determining the resectability of bile duct tumors (82% versus 76%, $P < 0.0002$) and T stage (78% versus 54%, $P < 0.001$). Although IDUS does not reliably determine the nature of a stricture in all cases, the findings may be useful in directing management. As suggested by Tamada et al [55], when IDUS identifies disruption of the wall layers by a protruding tumor, surgical exploration is indicated, even in the absence of tissue confirmation of malignancy. When IDUS demonstrates a localized tumor or polypoid lesion in the presence of a normal-appearing wall, directed biopsy specimens should be obtained. If a polypoid mass identified by IDUS is >8 mm in diameter, even when the wall layers are preserved, malignancy is likely. When IDUS fails to identify a localized intraductal lesion, even if cholangiography suggests irregularity of the duct, the need for further diagnostic evaluation becomes less certain.

IDUS improves the accuracy of local tumor staging of bile duct carcinomas. One study found that local tumor staging by IDUS was accurate in 77% of patients compared with 54% for staging by EUS [56]. The benefit of IDUS over EUS may be even greater for tumors arising from mid-duct to bifurcation. The limited depth of penetration restricts the value of IDUS for assessing tumor extension outside the hepatoduodenal ligament and precludes assessment of distant metastasis (M-stage). The utility of IDUS for lymph node assessment (N-stage) is uncertain and likely limited by the inability to perform FNA.

Bile duct wall thickening may result from tumor spread or inflammation, and IDUS cannot reliably distinguish both in all instances. This is relevant in patients with prior biliary stents. One study found that the presence of a bile duct stent for at least 14 days correlated with the development of wall thickening, possibly as the result of inflammation [57]. Hence, a better understanding of the factors that influence bile duct wall thickening would be helpful.

Summary

EUS is now established as an accurate method for staging malignancies of the pancreatico-biliary system. The most valuable role of EUS is the ability to identify patients unlikely to be cured from surgical excision due to vascular invasion or regional nodal metastasis. The ability to obtain tissue confirmation plays a critical role in identifying those patients unsuitable for surgical therapy but would benefit from palliation. EUS and EUS-FNA are invaluable additions to our armamentarium for the management of pancreatico-bilary cancers.

References

[1] Stephens J, Kuhn J, O'Brien J, et al. Surgical morbidity, mortality, and long-term survival in patients with peripancreatic cancer following pancreaticoduodenectomy. Am J Surg 1997; 174:600–4.

[2] Murr MM, Sarr MG, Oishi AJ, van Heerden JA. Pancreatic cancer. CA Cancer J Clin 1994;44: 304–18.

[3] Bret PM, Nicolet V, Labadie M. Percutaneous fine-needle aspiration biopsy of the pancreas. Diagn Cytopathol 1986;2:221–7.

[4] Lee JG, Leung J. Tissue sampling at ERCP in suspected pancreatic cancer. Gastrointest Endosc Clin North Am 1998;8:221–35.

[5] Eloubeidi MA, Jhala D, Chhieng DC, et al. Yield of endoscopic ultrasound-guided fine-needle aspiration biopsy in patients with suspected pancreatic carcinoma. Cancer 2003;99:285–92.

[6] Gress F, Gottlieb K, Sherman S, et al. Endoscopic ultrasonography- guided fine-needle aspiration biopsy of suspected pancreatic cancer. Ann Intern Med 2001;134:459–64.

[7] Harewood GC, Wiersema MJ. Endosonography-guided fine needle aspiration biopsy in the evaluation of pancreatic masses. Am J Gastroenterol 2002;97:1386–91.

[8] Wiersema MJ, Vilmann P, Giovannini M, et al. Endosonography guided fine-needle aspiration biopsy: diagnostic accuracy and complication assessment. Gastroenterology 1997;112:1087–95.

[9] Rosch T, Lorenz R, Braig C, et al. Endoscopic ultrasound in pancreatic tumor diagnosis. Gastrointest Endosc 1991;37:347–52.

[10] Palazzo L, Roseau G, Gayet B, et al. Endoscopic ultrasonography in the diagnosis and staging of pancreatic adenocarcinoma: results of a prospective study with comparison to ultrasonography and CT scan. Endoscopy 1993;25:143–50.

[11] Gress FG, Hawes RH, Savides TJ, et al. Role of EUS in the preoperative staging of pancreatic cancer: a large single-center experience. Gastrointest Endosc 1999;50:786–91.

[12] Yasuda K, Mukai H, Nakajima M, et al. Staging of pancreatic carcinoma by endoscopic ultrasonography. Endoscopy 1993;25:151–5.

[13] Ahmad NA, Lewis JD, Ginsberg GG, et al. EUS in preoperative staging of pancreatic cancer. Gastrointest Endosc 2000;52:463–8.

[14] Legmann P, Vignaux O, Dousset B, et al. Pancreatic tumors: comparison of dual phase helical CT and endoscopic sonography. Am J Roentgenol 1998;170:1315–22.

[15] Yasuda K, Mukai H, Fujimoto S, et al. The diagnosis of pancreatic cancer by endoscopic ultrasonography. Gastrointest Endosc 1988;34:1–8.

[16] Nakaizumi A, Uehara H, Iishi H, et al. Endoscopic ultrasonography in diagnosis and staging of pancreatic cancer. Dig Dis Sci 1995;40:696–700.

[17] Rosch T, Dittler HJ, Strobel K, et al. Endoscopic ultrasound criteria for vascular invasion in the staging of cancer of the head of the pancreas: a blind reevaluation of videotapes. Gastrointest Endosc 2000;52:469–77.

[18] Brugge WR, Lee MJ, Kelsey PB, et al. The use of EUS to diagnose malignant portal venous system invasion by pancreatic cancer. Gastrointest Endosc 1996;43:561–7.

[19] Hunt GC, Faigel DO. Assessment of EUS for diagnosing, staging, and determining resectability of pancreatic cancer: a review. Gastrointest Endosc 2002;55:232–7.

[20] Midwinter MJ, Beveridge CJ, Wilsdon JB, et al. Correlation between spiral computed tomography, endoscopic ultrasonography and findings at operation in pancreatic and ampullary tumours. Br J Surg 1999;86:189–93.

[21] Mertz HR, Sechopoulos P, Delbeke D, et al. EUS, PET, and CT scanning for evaluation of pancreatic adenocarcinoma. Gastrointest Endosc 2000;52:367–71.

[22] Harewood GC, Wiersema MJ. Endosonography-guided fine needle aspiration biopsy in the evaluation of pancreatic masses. Am J Gastroenterol 2002;97:1386–91.

[23] Ahmad NA, Lewis JD, Siegelman ES, et al. Role of endoscopic ultrasound and magnetic resonance imaging in the preoperative staging of pancreatic adenocarcinoma. Am J Gastroenterol 2000;95:1926–31.

[24] McNulty NJ, Francis IR, Platt JF, et al. A multi-detector row helical CT of the pancreas: effect of contrast-enhanced multiphasic imaging on enhancement of the pancreas, peri-pancreatic vasculature, and pancreatic adenocarcinoma. Radiology 2001;220:97–102.

[25] Ahmad NA, Kochman ML, Lewis JD, et al. Endosonography is superior to angiography in the preoperative assessment of vascular involvement among patients with pancreatic carcinoma. J Clin Gastroenterol 2001;32:54–8.

[26] Gress F, Gottlieb K, Sherman S, et al. Endoscopic ultrasonography- guided fine-needle aspiration biopsy of suspected pancreatic cancer. Ann Intern Med 2001;134:459–64.

[27] Chang KJ, Nguyen P, Erickson RA, et al. The clinical utility of endoscopic ultrasound-guided fine-needle aspiration in the diagnosis and staging of pancreatic carcinoma. Gastrointest Endosc 1997;45:387–93.

[28] Prasad P, Schmulewitz N, Patel A, et al. Detection of occult liver metastases during EUS for staging of malignancies. Gastrointest Endosc 2004;59:49–53.

[29] tenBerge J, Hoffman BJ, Hawes RH, et al. EUS-guided fine needle aspiration of the liver: indications, yield, and safety based on an international survey of 167 cases. Gastrointest Endosc 2002;55:859–62.

[30] Eloubeidi M, Gress FG, Savides TJ, et al. Acute pancreatitis after EUS-guided FNA of solid pancreatic masses: a pooled analysis from (EUS) centers in the United States. Gastrointest Endosc 2004;60:385–9.

[31] Fickling W, Madani N, Hoffman B, et al. Endoscopic ultrasound fine-needle aspiration of cystic lesions of the pancreas: a safe procedure? [abstract]. Gastrointest Endosc 2002;56:S150.

[32] Zollinger RM, Ellison EH. Primary peptic ulcerations of the jejunum associated with islet cell tumors of the pancreas. Ann Surg 1955;142:709–23.

[33] Prinz RA. Localization of gastrinomas. Int J Pancreatol 1996;19:79–91.

[34] Jensen RT, Gibril F, Termanini B. Definition of the role of somatostatin receptor scintigraphy in gastrointestinal neuroendocrine tumor localization. Yale J Biol Med 1997;70:481–500.

[35] Anderson MA, Carpenter S, Thompson NW, et al. Endoscopic ultrasound is highly accurate and directs management in patients with neuroendocrine tumors of the pancreas. Am J Gastroenterol 2000;95:2271–7.

[36] Zimmer T, Scherubl H, Faiss S, et al. Endoscopic ultrasonography of neuroendocrine tumors. Digestion 2000;62(Suppl 1):45–50.

[37] Rosch T, Lightdale CJ, Botet JF, et al. Localization of pancreatic endocrine tumors by endoscopic ultrasonography. N Engl J Med 1992;326:1721–6.

[38] Sugiyama M, Abe N, Izumisato Y, et al. Differential diagnosis of benign versus malignant nonfunctioning islet cell tumors of the pancreas: the role of EUS and ERCP. Gastrointest Endosc 2002;55:115–9.

[39] Kann P, Bittinger F, Engelbach M, et al. Endosonography of insulin-secreting and clinically non-functioning neuroendocrine tumors of the pancreas: criteria of benignancy and malignancy. Eur J Med Res 2001;6:385–90.

[40] Furukawa T, Oohashi K, Yamao K, et al. Intraductal ultrasonography of the pancreas: development and clinical potential. Endoscopy 1997;29:561–9.

[41] Menzel J, Domschke W. Intraductal ultrasonography may localize islet cell tumours negative on endoscopic ultrasound. Scand J Gastroenterol 1998;33:109–12.

[42] Gress FG, Barawi M, Kim D, et al. Preoperative localization of a neuroendocrine tumor of the pancreas with EUS-guided fine needle tattooing. Gastrointest Endosc 2002;55:594–7.

[43] Howell DA, Beveridge RP, Bosco J, et al. Endoscopic needle aspiration biopsy at ERCP in the diagnosis of biliary strictures. Gastrointest Endosc 1992;38:531–5.

[44] Howell DA, Parsons WG, Jones MA, et al. Complete tissue sampling of biliary strictures at ERCP using a new device. Gastrointest Endos 1996;43:498–502.

[45] Jailwala J, Fogel EL, Sherman S, et al. Triple-tissue sampling at ERCP in malignant biliary obstruction. Gastrointest Endosc 2000;51:383–90.

[46] Kurzawinski T, Deery A, Davidson BR. Diagnostic value of cytology for biliary stricture. Br J Surg 1993;80:414–21.

[47] Kosuge T, Yamamoto J, Shimada K, et al. Improved surgical results for hilar cholangiocarcinoma with procedures including major hepatic resection. Ann Surg 1999;230:663–71.

[48] Neuhaus P, Jonas S, Bechstein WO, et al. Extended resections for hilar cholangiocarcinoma. Ann Surg 1999;230:808–18.

[49] Ortner MA, Liebetruth J, Schreiber S, et al. Photodynamic therapy of nonresectable cholangiocarcinoma. Gastroenterology 1998;114:536–42.

[50] Chamberlain RS, Blumgart LH. Hilar cholangiocarcinoma: a review and commentary. Ann Surg Oncol 2000;7:55–66.

[51] Launois B, Reding R, Lebeau G, et al. Surgery for hilar cholangiocarcinoma: French experience in collective survey of 552 extrahepatic bile duct cancers. J Hepato-Biliary-Pancreatic Surg 2000;7:128–34.

[52] Fritscher-Ravens A, Broering DC, Knoefel WT, et al. EUS-guided fine-needle aspiration of suspected hilar cholangiocarcinoma in potentially operable patients with negative brush cytology. Am J Gastroenterol 2004;99:45–51.

[53] Eloubeidi MA, Chen VK, Jhala NC, et al. Endoscopic ultrasound-guided fine needle aspiration biopsy of suspected cholangiocarcinoma. Clin Gastroenterol Hepatol 2004;2:209–13.

[54] Ascher SM, Evans SR, Goldberg JA, et al. Intraoperative bile duct sonography during laparoscopic cholecystectomy: experience with a 12.5 MHz catheter-based US probe. Radiology 1992;185:493–6.

[55] Tamada K, Ueno N, Tomiyama T, et al. Characterization of biliary strictures using intraductal ultrasonography: comparison with percutaneous cholangioscopic biopsy. Gastrointest Endosc 1998;47:341–9.

[56] Menzel J, Poremba C, Dietl KH, et al. Preoperative diagnosis of bile duct strictures comparison of intraductal ultrasonography with conventional endosonography. Scand J Gastroenterol 2000; 35:77–82.

[57] Tamada K, Nagai H, Yasuda Y, et al. Transpapillary intraductal US prior to biliary drainage in the assessment of longitudinal spread of extrahepatic bile duct carcinoma. Gastrointest Endosc 2001;53:300–7.

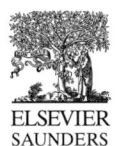

ELSEVIER
SAUNDERS

Gastrointest Endoscopy Clin N Am
15 (2005) 513–531

GASTROINTESTINAL
ENDOSCOPY CLINICS
OF NORTH AMERICA

Endoscopic Palliation of Pancreaticobiliary Malignancies

Janak N. Shah, MD*, V. Raman Muthusamy, MD

*Department of Medicine, Division of Gastroenterology, University of California, San Francisco,
2330 Post Street, Suite 610, San Francisco, CA 94115, USA*

Malignant biliary obstruction is most frequently encountered in the setting of pancreatic adenocarcinoma, but it also occurs with cholangiocarcinoma, ampullary neoplasms, and gallbladder carcinomas. Less commonly, hepatocellular carcinomas and metastatic disease may lead to bile duct obstruction. The incidence of pancreatic adenocarcinoma, the predominant cause of malignant biliary obstruction, seems to be increasing. Recent statistics reveal that more than 31,000 people develop pancreatic cancer in the United States annually [1]. At time of presentation, the disease is often locally advanced or metastatic, and only 18% of patients are candidates for curative resection [2]. Bile duct obstruction develops in over 70% [3]; thus, palliation is an important issue for patients with unresectable pancreatic tumors.

Cholangiocarcinoma is less prevalent than pancreatic cancer, but more than 2000 cases are diagnosed in the United States each year [1]. Similar to pancreatic adenocarcinoma, the tumor is usually advanced at presentation. Only 30% of patients are surgically resectable [4], so adequate palliation is of equal importance for this disease.

Patients with malignant bile duct obstruction usually present with jaundice and associated symptoms of pruritus, anorexia, and malaise. Obstruction may result in other complications, including cholangitis, coagulopathy, malabsorption, and hepatocellular dysfunction [3]. The goal of palliation in these patients is to bypass the site of stricture and thereby improve the associated clinical features of biliary obstruction. Endoscopic stenting has become the favored technique for the

---

* Corresponding author. University of California, San Francisco, VA Medical Center, 4150 Clement Street, Building 203, Suite 2A79, San Francisco, CA 94121.
E-mail address: janak.shah@med.va.gov (J.N. Shah).

1052-5157/05/$ – see front matter © 2005 Elsevier Inc. All rights reserved.
doi:10.1016/j.giec.2005.03.003 *giendo.theclinics.com*

palliation of unresectable malignant biliary obstruction. Not only do stents improve the direct symptoms related to biliary obstruction, but some studies suggest improvement in other areas, such as anorexia, fatigue, insomnia, cognition, and overall quality of life [5,6]. A subset of patients who have normalization of hepatic function may become candidates for palliative chemotherapy [7,8], potentially affecting survival.

Endoscopic stenting

Background

The endoscopic placement of a plastic stent across an obstructed bile duct was first described in 1979 [9]. Self-expanding metallic stents (SEMS) for use in the biliary system were introduced into clinical practice 10 years later. Initial reports of SEMS described percutaneous placement techniques, but endoscopic means of deployment were recognized soon after [10–12]. Commonly used plastic biliary endoprostheses are available in a variety of sizes, lengths, and shapes [13]. The ability to place larger-diameter plastic stents is limited by the size of the endoscope accessory channel. SEMS were developed to overcome this limitation. They have the advantage of larger diameter stenting (up to 10 mm) but are more costly than plastic stents.

Stent choice: plastic versus self-expanding metallic stents

The optimal stent choice for the palliation of malignant biliary obstruction is dependent on multiple factors and varies from patient to patient. The major decision that needs to be made is the type of stent to be placed (ie, plastic or metallic) (Fig. 1). Important measures for this decision include several stent-related factors, such as stent efficacy (relief of jaundice), stent patency, need for

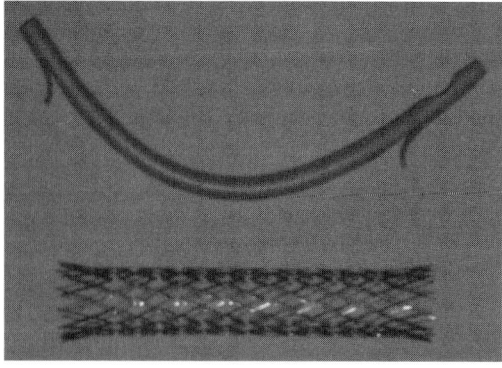

Fig. 1. Photograph of a plastic (*top*) and self-expanding metallic biliary stent (*bottom*). The plastic stent (Cotton-Leung stent; Wilson-Cook) is 11.5 French; the SEMS (Memotherm; Bard) is 30 French.

reinterventions, and cost. Patient-related issues, such as the extent of disease and associated life expectancy, need to be considered because they influence the optimal stent choice.

Several trials directly compare plastic with metal stents for the palliation of malignant biliary obstruction. Plastic stents and SEMS provide palliation of jaundice and improve liver function tests after placement in over 95% of patients and are equivalent in this regard [14–17]. These two stent types significantly differ in duration of patency. Median stent patency ranges from 2 to 5 months for plastic endoprostheses, whereas it is 4 to 10 months or more for SEMS [14–19].

The decreased patency of plastic stents seems to influence the need for additional interventions. In comparative trials, the use of plastic stents led to significantly increased repeat endoscopic interventions to reestablish biliary drainage as compared with SEMS [15–17,19]. In several of these studies, there were significantly increased numbers of hospitalization days associated with plastic stents [15,16,19]. There has been no associated survival benefit based on stent type. Median patient survival ranges from 4 to 6 months after plastic or metallic stenting [14,16].

Cost issues are important and should be considered when making a decision between a plastic and metallic endoprosthetic. Generally, list prices for SEMS are substantially greater than for plastic stents (around $1000 US versus $40 US) [13]. Estimating cost is more complicated than determining the stent price. Given the decreased duration of plastic stent patency, the additional costs of repeat interventions, treatment of occlusion-related complications (eg, cholangitis), and subsequent hospitalizations need to be weighed. Based on two decision analysis models, the placement of SEMS is more economic in patients expected to survive longer than 6 months, whereas plastic stents are cost-saving in patients surviving less than 4 months [20,21]. Cost analysis from a randomized controlled trial was similar: Plastic stents were more economic in patients with a life expectancy of < 3 months, and SEMS were cost-preferred for patients surviving > 6 months [16].

Life expectancy may influence stent choice, but it is difficult to estimate survival in a patient with malignant biliary obstruction. A few clinical factors may help. Patients with hepatic metastases have a decreased median survival (2.7 months) as compared with those without metastatic disease (5.3 months) [19]. The primary tumor size may also reflect life expectancy. Based on multivariate analysis, patients with tumors that are > 3 cm have significantly shorter median survival (3.2 months) than patients with tumors that are < 3 cm (6.6 months) [22]. Thus, plastic stents may be preferred to SEMS in patients with large tumors (> 3 cm) or liver metastases.

There are no strict criteria for selecting between plastic and metallic endoprostheses for the palliation of unresectable malignant biliary obstruction. Balancing life expectancy with stent patency should lead to optimal symptom-free survival at the lowest cost. These decisions must be individualized, and patient factors must be considered. For example, SEMS may be preferred in a patient who is noncompliant or resides in a remote area without medical access, despite a short life expectancy. Patients with difficult endoscopic biliary access

Table 1
Relative strengths of plastic stents versus SEMS for malignant biliary obstruction

	Plastic stent	SEMS
Endoscopic placement success	+++	+++
Large-diameter stenting	+	+++
Relief of obstruction	+++	+++
Decreased stent cost	+++	+
Stent patency	++	+++

Abbreviation: SEMS, self-expanding metallic stents.

from associated duodenal stenosis may benefit from early SEMS placement. Relative strengths and weaknesses of plastic stents and SEMS are summarized in Table 1.

Plastic stents

Once a decision to place a plastic biliary endoprosthetic has been made, additional variables come into consideration. Plastic stents are available in a variety of sizes, designs, and materials [13]. The stent that provides the longest occlusion-free duration should be chosen. Larger-caliber devices (10 French or greater) are preferred to smaller caliber devices (8.5 French or less). This preference is primarily due to the effect on stent patency. In comparative studies, the median occlusion-free life for devices that are 10 French or greater is 21 to 32 weeks, as compared with 10 to 12 weeks for devises that are 8.5 French or less [23,24]. Additionally, there may be a lower associated incidence of cholangitis with larger-gauge endoprosthetics [23]. The superior performance of large-caliber stents is attributed to improved internal flow dynamics [23]. Among the larger sizes, there is no conclusive benefit for using 11.5 French stents compared with 10 French stents [25,26]. Stent length does not seem to affect stent longevity, at least for the large-caliber endoprostheses [26].

Variations of plastic stent design and material composition have been made to improve stent longevity. The concern for the presence of side holes as a contributing factor for stent occlusion on a popular plastic stent model prompted the development of a Teflon stent without side holes [27]. Randomized trials comparing these two designs failed to demonstrate differences in stent patency [28,29]. Materials that allow a lower coefficient of friction may theoretically reduce stent clogging and thereby improve stent life. Such alterations have been of unproven benefit in clinical trials [30,31].

The role of pharmacologic agents to lengthen plastic stent life has been investigated. Choleretic agents may enhance bile flow and thereby reduce stent occlusion. Antibiotics may inhibit stent colonization by bacteria, an important step in occlusion. Both classes of drugs, alone or in combination, have failed to demonstrate improvements in stent longevity [32–36].

Placement of plastic stents above an intact sphincter of Oddi may theoretically prevent stent colonization by bacteria and thereby reduce occlusion rates. This has been observed in a canine study [37]. Such "internally" placed biliary stents demonstrated no patency benefit in a randomized clinical trial and were associated with higher stent migration rates [38]. Moreover, such a technique would be possible in about one third of patients presenting with malignant biliary obstruction and in an even lower proportion when pancreatic tumors are the cause of obstruction [39].

In summary, once a decision to place a plastic stent has been made, the most important variable to consider is stent size. The use of a large-caliber device (10 French or greater) optimizes stent longevity. Data do not support advantages for plastic stent patency based on stent material, design, placement location, or the concurrent use of antibiotics or choleretics. The optimal plastic stent and associated treatment methods in managing malignant biliary obstruction may need to be readdressed with medical and technologic advances.

Self-expanding metallic stents

An assortment of SEMS that vary in design is available. Most SEMS are made of stainless steel or a nickel-titanium alloy (Nitinol) in an open mesh design. They come in several lengths ranging from 40 to 80 mm and have deployed diameters up to 10 mm [13]. Some popular models in the United States include the Wallstent (Boston Scientific, Natick, Massachusetts), the Zilver stent (Wilson-Cook, Winston-Salem, North Carolina), and the Memotherm (Bard Inc., Billerica, Masachusetts) [13,40]. Metallic stents are difficult to remove, so they are generally reserved for patients with established, unresectable, malignant disease.

There are limited published data directly comparing different models of SEMS. One trial comparing the Ultraflex Diamond stent to the Wallstent (both by Boston Scientific) for malignant biliary obstruction revealed similar rates of stent occlusion and patency duration [41]. This study involved a small number of patients—only 23 in each group. A smaller, retrospective comparison ($n = 21$ patients) demonstrated longer patency for the Wallstent [42]. Generally, most biliary endoscopists consider SEMS models to be equivalent. Endoscopist familiarity with the mechanical characteristics of the stent and its delivery system are important to consider when selecting the model.

More recently, polyurethane-covered SEMS were developed to prolong stent patency. The covering provides a physical barrier to prevent tumor ingrowth through the open mesh designs of conventional SEMS and has been associated with low rates of tumor ingrowth in some series [43,44]. Covered SEMS have resulted in less mucosal hyperplasia than uncovered varieties in animal models [45], but early clinical experience with covered SEMS demonstrated similar duration of patency compared with uncovered models [46–48]. In contrast, a recent randomized study revealed significantly decreased occlusion rates (14% versus 38%) and increased mean stent patency (304 versus 166 days) for covered compared with uncovered SEMS [49]. These data may not be generalizable because the investigators used one specific model of SEMS. Radial expansile forces and sizes of mesh interstices differ from model to model [40], and thus the presence of a polyurethane covering may theoretically have less impact on stent patency with other SEMS models. Moreover, covered stents may be prone to migration and may occlude ductal branches, leading to complications such as cholecystitis and cholangitis [3,50]. Both cases of acute cholecystitis that occurred in the recent randomized trial were in patients treated with covered stents [49]. Further clinical data are needed before firm recommendations regarding covered SEMS are made.

Stenting techniques

A detailed cholangiogram is helpful for planning stent placement. Although this is usually obtained during the stent placement procedure at endoscopic retrograde cholangiopancreatography (ERCP), anatomic details can be obtained before ERCP using magnetic resonance cholangiopancreatography (MRCP) or thin-section CT scans with pancreaticobiliary protocols [51]. At least one of these imaging tests has usually been performed during the initial evaluation, and a detailed review of these images may be useful before ERCP and stenting.

Before placement of plastic or metallic biliary stents, selective cannulation of the common bile duct is required. The site of obstruction then needs to be traversed with a guide wire to allow the placement of the stent. Multiple guide wires should be placed if multiple stents are anticipated. Plastic stents are placed directly over a guide wire or smaller "guiding" catheter, using a similar size coaxial "pushing" catheter. SEMS are delivered within an outer, narrower,

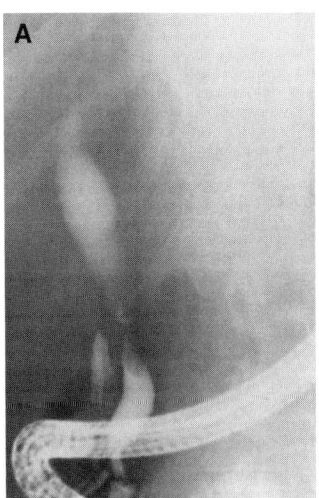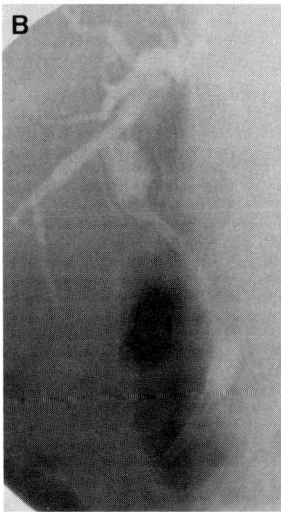

Fig. 2. (*A*) Endoscopic retrograde cholangiogram depicts a mid common bile duct stricture due to a mass in the head of the pancreas. (*B*) A plastic biliary stent (11.5 French, 7 cm) was placed endoscopically and traverses the malignant stricture.

constraining delivery system that is advanced over a stricture-traversing guide wire. When the delivery catheter is in position (confirmed fluoroscopically), the constraining outer catheter is removed to allow SEMS deployment and full expansion. Detailed knowledge of stent mechanical properties and of the delivery system is important because some SEMS models foreshorten during deployment [3]. At experienced centers, the placement of a plastic or metal stent at ERCP is successful in over 90% of patients (Figs. 2 and 3) [16,17,19].

Several technical issues should be considered during stenting. Biliary sphincterotomy may facilitate the introduction of large devices into the common bile duct and is often performed before placing large-caliber or multiple plastic stents and for SEMS that cross the papilla [40]. Biliary sphincterotomy is not

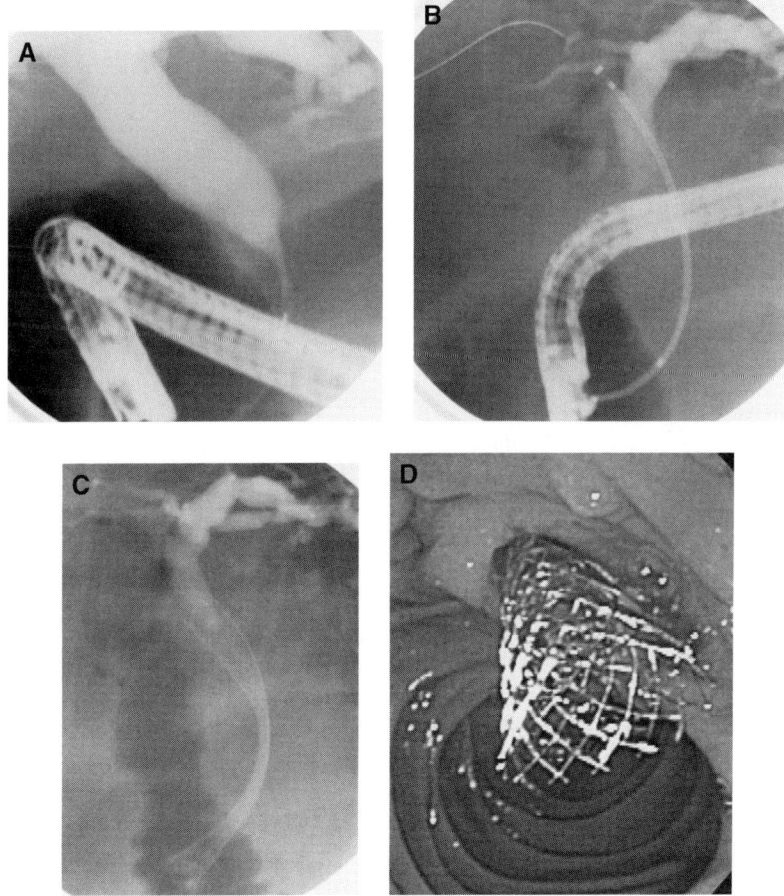

Fig. 3. (*A*) ERCP depicts a distal common bile duct stricture from a pancreatic malignancy. (*B*) A metallic stent (constrained within the delivery catheter) is advanced over a guide wire across the stricture at ERCP. Radiographic (*C*) and endoscopic (*D*) views of a 10 × 60 mm SEMS (Wallstent; Boston Scientific) postdeployment.

mandatory. A recent investigation revealed similar technical success (over 94%) and complication rates (4% to 6%) in patients with and without biliary sphincterotomy undergoing placement of a 10 French plastic stent [52]. Biliary sphincterotomy should be performed in patients with proximal biliary strictures requiring transpapillary stents that extend into the proximal biliary tree. This group has a lower incidence of post-ERCP pancreatitis as compared with those without sphincterotomy [53].

Dilation of strictures may be required to allow stent delivery. This is often performed using mechanical or pneumatic catheters placed over stricture-traversing guide wires [40]. For very high-grade stenoses, the standard endoscopic dilation devices occasionally fail, preventing subsequent access for stent delivery. In this setting, plastic stent retrieval devices (Soehendra Stent Retriever; Wilson-Cook) have been used to traverse strictures to allow subsequent stenting with over 90% success rates at initial ERCP [54,55].

Pancreaticobiliary malignancy may cause duodenal obstruction by direct invasion or extrinsic compression and is encountered in up to 25% of patients with advanced tumors [56]. Luminal stenting should be considered in patients with evidence for duodenal stenosis and can be safely performed during the same endoscopic biliary stenting procedure [57,58].

Endoscopic access to the biliary tree for stent placement may be difficult in patients with duodenal stenosis, tumor invasion of the ampulla of Vater, or large-sized primary tumors [59]. In this setting, a few options exist to facilitate the minimally invasive palliation of biliary obstruction. Using a combined percutaneous and endoscopic approach, a guide wire may be inserted into the biliary system transhepatically, advanced through the ampulla, and retrieved endoscopically in the second portion of the duodenum. A biliary stent can then be placed endoscopically over the retrieved guidewire in standard fashion. Such a "rendezvous" technique allows successful endoscopic stent placement in over 80% of patients with malignant obstruction [60,61]. Subsequent stent exchanges can be performed successfully using only endoscopic methods in over 80% of patients [60].

Plastic and metallic biliary endoprosthetics can be placed by interventional radiologists using solely percutaneous methods with similar outcomes for technical success and stent patency as those placed endoscopically [62,63]. However, an earlier randomized clinical trial comparing endoscopic to percutaneous plastic stent insertion revealed a higher success rate for the relief of jaundice, lower procedural complications, and lower associated mortality for endoscopic stenting [64]. In contrast, a more recent randomized trial comparing the two insertion techniques demonstrated improved clinical success (relief of jaundice) and median survival for the percutaneous approach [65]. These results should be interpreted with caution because the stent types for percutaneous (SEMS) and endoscopic (plastic) delivery were different. Moreover, complication rates were significantly higher for percutaneous stenting (61% versus 35%). Thus, the data favor the endoscopic route for stenting of unresectable pancreaticobiliary malignancies.

Pancreatic duct stenting

Although pancreatic stents are not commonly used for palliation, they have been placed at ERCP to improve pancreatic ductal flow through strictures and to reduce pancreatic ductal pressures, a mechanism believed to decrease pain for patients with pancreatic tumors [66]. Placement techniques mimic those of endoscopic biliary stent insertion, and a few series report substantial reductions of the number of patients in pain (60% to 75%) and analgesia requirements (up to 50% discontinue pain medications) after pancreatic stenting [66,67]. Careful patient selection is important in identifying those who may benefit from such stenting.

Stent dysfunction and complications

The patency of plastic and metal stents is compromised by two different mechanisms. Occlusion of plastic endoprostheses is nearly always the result of the deposition of sludge that is comprised of bacterial biofilm and calcium bilirubinate and palmitate [68]. Sludge deposition within the stent lumen is a complex process that seems to involve bacteria, bacterial proteins, physical stent characteristics, and bile viscosity [69,70]. On the other hand, SEMS occlusion can occur due to a variety of mechanisms. The predominant cause is the ingrowth of tumor through the stent mesh (35% to 55%), followed by overgrowth of tumor at the stent's proximal or distal end (5% to 10%) and combination overgrowth/ingrowth (25%) [71,72]. Less common etiologies include the development of mucosal hyperplasia due to stent induced chronic inflammation and biliary sludge deposition [71,72].

Occluded plastic and metallic biliary stents necessitate intervention to reestablish drainage because patients with occluded stents are at risk to develop cholangitis [16,72]. For patients with plastic stents, treatment options include replacement with another plastic stent or SEMS. Factors involved in deciding between plastic and metallic stents have been previously discussed, but there are a few additional considerations. Patients with prior history of multiple or premature plastic stent occlusions seem to be at risk for future plastic stent dysfunction and may benefit from earlier SEMS placement [73,74]. Patients who are treated with plastic stents should be considered for interval routine stent exchanges. In a randomized trial, routine exchanges every 3 months were associated with longer symptom-free intervals for patients than exchanges at signs of stent occlusion, but there was no difference in overall survival [16].

Occluded SEMS are managed by a variety of methods. The most commonly used techniques include insertion of a plastic stent within the occluded SEMS, insertion of a second SEMS, and mechanical cleaning of the occluded stent lumen (Figs. 4 and 5). Overall success rates for reestablishing biliary drainage are over 80% [72,75]. Mechanical cleaning methods, such as catheter irrigation or the use of stone-extraction balloons, may be less successful and are associated with decreased duration of patency than repeat stenting [72,75]. Given the typical

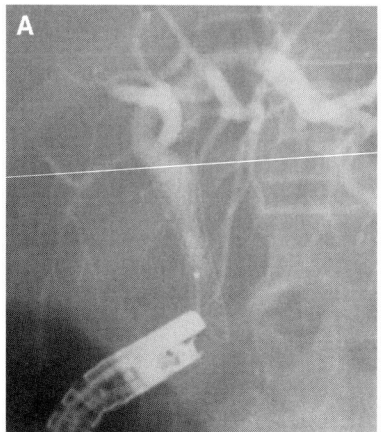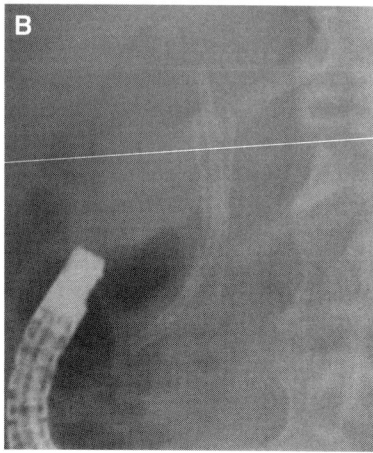

Fig. 4. (*A*) Endoscopic retrograde cholangiogram demonstrates tumor ingrowth compromising the SEMS lumen (10 × 40 mm Wallstent; Boston Scientific) in a patient with advanced pancreatic malignancy and prior Billroth 2 surgery. (*B*) Occlusion was managed with the endoscopic insertion of a plastic biliary stent (10 French, 7 cm) through the SEMS.

short median survival at the time of the first SEMS occlusion, treatment with plastic stents seems to be the most cost-effective method [72]. Other techniques for SEMS recanalization include application of thermal energy and intraductal brachytherapy but are not widely used [76–79].

Additional complications related to biliary stenting include upper gastro-intestinal hemorrhage, duodenal perforation, stent migration, luminal obstruction,

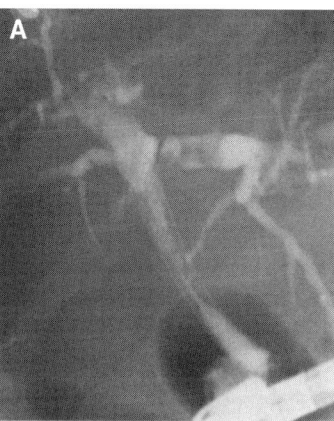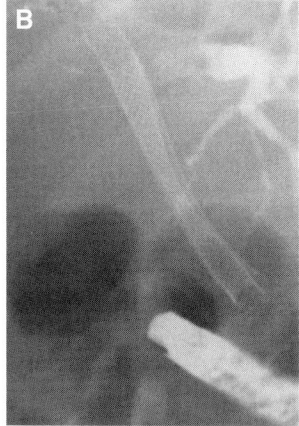

Fig. 5. (*A*) Endoscopic retrograde cholangiogram reveals occlusion at the midportion of the SEMS (Wallstent; Boston Scientific) from tumor ingrowth. (*B*) Occlusion was treated endoscopically with a second SEMS (Wallstent; Boston Scientific).

cholangitis, and cholecystitis [80–85]. These types of complications seem to be infrequent.

Stenting considerations for hilar obstruction

Patients with cholangiocarcinoma, gallbladder carcinoma, and periportal lymph node metastases may develop complex hilar strictures that involve the common hepatic duct, right hepatic duct, left hepatic duct, intrahepatic ducts, or combination thereof. Two or more stents may be required to anatomically drain all obstructed segments. To technically perform such bilateral biliary drainage is more difficult [86], and its clinical utility over a single stent providing unilateral drainage is debated. Although a retrospective evaluation revealed optimal survival in patients receiving bilateral drainage for hilar tumors [87], a more recent randomized trial demonstrated similar rates of jaundice relief, complications, and mortality in patients receiving unilateral biliary drainage [86].

The root of controversy around unilateral versus bilateral drainage is likely related to a procedural issue. The failure of draining opacified, obstructed ductal segments at ERCP raises the risk of postprocedural cholangitis. The reported survival benefit of bilateral drainage in one study seems to be related to a lower incidence of cholangitis [87]. Therefore, many biliary endoscopists decide to place unilateral versus bilateral stents based on contrast opacification during ERCP, ideally placing stents in all opacified, nondrained segments. Minimizing contrast opacification is of utmost importance during ERCP and enables unilateral stenting with good clinical outcomes. To that end, a detailed preprocedural MRI, MRCP, or CT may be helpful. This may allow the biliary endoscopist to plan image-targeted stent placement, minimize contrast injection during ERCP, reduce the risk of cholangitis, and increase the chance for a successful unilateral drainage procedure [88,89].

Endoscopic stenting versus surgical bypass

Before minimally invasive therapy, surgical bypass was the only palliative option for unresectable pancreaticobiliary malignancy. Several randomized trials have compared endoscopic to surgical palliation. Two initial studies showed no difference in survival or overall complications, with effective relief of jaundice (>90%) in both groups [90,91]. Despite increased readmissions in one study among the endoscopically stented group, the overall hospitalization time of patients receiving endoscopic palliation was significantly shorter compared with surgically treated patients [90]. A larger randomized trial of 201 patients demonstrated equivalent technical success and overall survival [92]. The endoscopically stented group had lower procedure-related mortality (3% versus 14%), major complication rates (11% versus 29%), and median total hospital stay (20 versus 26 days) compared with the surgical group. Jaundice recurred in over one third of the stented group, compared with 2% of surgically palliated patients. A recent meta-analysis including these randomized trials revealed no mortality benefit with either palliative therapy, but there were more treatment sessions in the endoscopically stented patients [93]. These studies involved plastic biliary stents, and there are no large randomized trials comparing SEMS to surgery. Given the similar mortality rates with endoscopic stenting compared with surgical bypass in these randomized trials [90–92], the less invasive endoscopic route of palliation seems preferable for patients with unresectable tumors.

Additional analyses have been performed to compare endoscopic stenting with surgical bypass from a cost-effectiveness standpoint. A retrospective evaluation of over 60 patients found a nearly 50% reduction in initial hospital charges between the endoscopic and surgical groups (United States $9663 versus $18,325) [94]. Although more endoscopically treated patients required read-missions, the associated average medical costs remained lower than for patients treated surgically (United States $4029 versus $6776). Similarly, a retrospective case control study involving patients with unresectable cholangiocarcinoma found the median lifetime cost of surgical therapy to be United States $60,986, compared with $24,251 for endoscopic therapy [95]. Thus, available data support the use of endoscopic stenting over surgical bypass from a cost perspective.

Role of endoscopic ultrasound in palliation

Endoscopic ultrasound (EUS) has a variety of roles in the treatment of patients with advanced pancreaticobiliary malignancies. In patients with inaccessible ductal systems at ERCP, EUS may be used to access the biliary or pancreatic ducts. Earlier reports described the ability of EUS to obtain a cholangiogram (EUS-guided cholangiopancreatography) after unsuccessful ERCP [96]. Subsequent reports have described ductal drainage via EUS-guided rendezvous procedures, in which a guide wire is advanced into the duodenal lumen after intraductal puncture, allowing ERCP-guided stent placement [97–99]. These types of procedures may gain increased prominence with the convergence of EUS and ERCP techniques in the management of pancreaticobiliary disease. Others have described EUS-guided hepaticogastrostomy in a porcine model, supporting the feasibility of EUS-guided biliary drainage in patients with inaccessible ducts due to malignant gastric outlet obstruction [100].

EUS may have a therapeutic role in the palliation of pain arising from pancreatic malignancy. Using EUS-guided fine-needle injection (EUS FNI) techniques, a combination of bupivacaine and alcohol can be injected into the celiac plexus under EUS guidance to provide pain control [101,102]. An early report of EUS-guided celiac plexus neurolysis involving 30 patients revealed a reduction in pain medication use and improved pain scores in almost 90% of patients at a median follow-up of 10 weeks [101]. Patients with advanced metastatic disease seemed to have the best responses. A more recent study of 58 patients revealed improved pain scores in 78% at 6 months without major procedural complications [102]. EUS-guided celiac plexus neurolysis may be performed in patients with evidence of unresectable disease at initial endosonographic evaluation and should be considered in patients with substantial pain symptoms.

More recently, new EUS-guided interventions have been developed with the aim of directly treating pancreatic tumors. EUS-targeted radiofrequency ablation of the pancreas in a porcine model has been described [103]. Ablations produced well-demarcated spheres of coagulation necrosis. A pilot study of EUS-guided photodynamic therapy of intraabdominal organs in a porcine model has also been reported [104]. Others have focused on delivery of biologically active agents via EUS-FNI into the pancreas. Delivered agents have included an allogeneic mixed lymphocyte culture (cytoimplant), a gene-deleted, replication-selective adenovirus that selectively targets malignant cells (ONYX-015), and a replication deficient adenovector containing the human tumor necrosis factor-α gene [105–107]. Initial data from these studies suggest that these procedures are technically feasible and safe. Given the relative ease of targeted access to the pancreas at EUS, these types of EUS-guided interventions hold promise for future palliative and nonpalliative treatments.

Recent advances in endoscopic technology

Photodynamic therapy

Photodynamic therapy (PDT) has shown promise in the treatment of cholangiocarcinoma. PDT for cholangiocarcinoma is a two-step process that involves (1) the intravenous administration of a photosensitizing agent that is preferentially retained in dysplastic tissue and (2) tissue exposure to light using an intraductal catheter at ERCP, generating oxygen free radicals and causing tissue injury/cell death. An initial study of nine patients with unresectable Bismuth type III and IV cholangiocarcinomas revealed improvements in jaundice and quality of life indices over a 2-month follow-up period [108]. Subsequently, a study of 24 patients suggested a small survival benefit in patients with PDT and SEMS compared with those with biliary drainage alone [109]. More recently, a randomized trial comparing PDT with plastic stents to stenting alone demonstrated a significant median survival benefit (493 days versus 98 days) in the PDT group [110]. This study was terminated early due to the magnitude of the treatment effect. Given the promising results, PDT may play a more important role in the treatment of advanced biliary tumors in the future.

New stent technology

Technologic advances with respect to stent design and material are expected. Stents that elute chemotherapy have been developed. One group described the use of a carboplatin-coated biliary tube to provide a partial response in three of five patients with advanced cholangiocarcinoma [111]. Others have advocated paclitaxel-eluting stents for improved stent patency in the setting of malignant biliary strictures based on preliminary results from cell cultures [112]. Additionally, bioabsorbable biliary stents have been developed [113]. These may offer advantages of nonpermanent large-diameter stenting, a reduction in biofilm accumulation and cellular proliferation, and prospects for drug impregnation for local delivery.

Summary

   Endoscopic techniques have advanced dramatically over the past two decades and maintain a central role in the palliation of pancreaticobiliary malignancy. Endoscopic stents remain the preferred method for treating malignant biliary obstruction. Advances in stent design are anticipated and should improve outcomes for palliative stenting. Additionally, with progress in interventional EUS techniques and increased abilities to deliver therapy via the endoscope, these methods and others will likely expand the applications for endoscopic palliation of pancreaticobiliary malignancies.

References

[1] Jemal A, Tiwari RC, Murray T, et al. Cancer statistics, 2004. CA Cancer J Clin 2004;54:8–29.
[2] Geer RJ, Brennen MF. Prognostic indicator of survival after resection of pancreatic adeno-carcinoma. Am J Surg 1993;165:68–72.
[3] Levy MJ, Baron TH, Gostout CJ, et al. Palliation of malignant extrahepatic biliary obstruction with plastic versus expandable metal stents: an evidence-based approach. Clin Gastroenterol Hepatol 2004;2:273–85.
[4] Burke EC, Jarnagin WR, Hochwald SN, et al. Hilar cholangiocarcinoma: patterns of spread, the importance of hepatic resection for curative operation, and a presurgical clinical staging system. Ann Surg 1998;228:385–94.
[5] Ballinger AB, McHugh M, Catnach SM, et al. Symptom relief and quality of life after stenting for malignant bile duct obstruction. Gut 1994;35:467–70.
[6] Luman W, Cull A, Palmer KR. Quality of life in patients stented for malignant biliary obstruction. Eur J Gastroenterol Hepatol 1997;9:481–4.
[7] Martin JA, Slivka A, Rabiovitz M, et al. ERCP and stent therapy for progressive jaundice in hepatocellular carcinoma: which patients benefit, which patients don't? Dig Dis Sci 1999;44: 1298–302.
[8] Van Laethem JL, De Broux S, Eisendrath P, et al. Clinical impact of biliary drainage and jaundice resolution in patients with obstructive metastases at the hilum. Am J Gastroenterol 2003;98:1271–7.
[9] Soehendra N, Reynders-Frederix V. [Palliative biliary duct drainage: a new method for endoscopic introduction of a new stent.] Dtsch Med Wochenschr 1979;104:206–7.
[10] Irving JD, Adam A, Dick R, et al. Gianturco expandable metallic biliary stents: results of a European clinical trial. Radiology 1989;172:321–6.
[11] Neuhaus H, Hagenmuller F, Classen M. Self-expanding biliary stents: preliminary clinical experience. Endoscopy 1989;21:225–8.
[12] Deviere J, Cremer M. Endoscopic approach to malignant biliary obstruction. Cardiovasc Intervent Radiol 1990;13:223–30.
[13] Nelson DB, Bosco JJ, Curtis WD, et al. Biliary stents. Gastrointest Endosc 1999;50:938–42.

[14] Davids PH, Groen AK, Rauws EA, et al. Randomized trial of self-expanding metal stents versus polyethylene stents for distal malignant biliary obstruction. Lancet 1992;340:1488–92.

[15] Knyrim K, Wagner HJ, Pausch J, et al. A prospective, randomized, controlled trial of metal stents for malignant obstruction of the common bile duct. Endoscopy 1993;25:207–12.

[16] Prat F, Chapat O, Ducot B, et al. A randomized trial of endoscopic drainage methods for inoperable malignant strictures of the common bile duct. Gastrointest Endosc 1998;47:1–7.

[17] Schmassmann A, von Gunten E, Knuchel J, et al. Wallstents versus plastic stents in malignant biliary obstruction: effects of stent patency of the first and second stent on patient compliance and survival. Am J Gastroenterol 1996;91:654–9.

[18] Carr-Locke DL, Ball TJ, Connors PJ, et al. Multicenter, randomized, controlled trial of metal stents for malignant obstruction of the common bile duct [abstract]. Gastrointest Endosc 1993; 39:310A.

[19] Kaassis M, Boyer J, Dumas R, et al. Plastic or metal stents for malignant stricture of the common bile duct? Results of a randomized prospective study. Gastrointest Endosc 2003;57: 178–82.

[20] Yeoh KG, Zimmerman MJ, Cunningham JT, et al. Comparative costs of metal versus plastic biliary stent strategies for malignant obstructive jaundice by decision analysis. Gastrointest Endosc 1999;49:466–71.

[21] Arguedas MR, Heudebert GH, Stinnett AA, et al. Biliary stents in malignant obstructive jaundice due to pancreatic carcinoma: a cost effectiveness analysis. Am J Gastroenterol 2002; 97:898–904.

[22] Prat F, Chapat O, Ducot B, et al. Predictive factors for survival of patients with inoperable malignant distal biliary strictures: a practical management guideline. Gut 1998;42:76–80.

[23] Speer AG, Cotton PB, MacRae KD. Endoscopic management of malignant biliary obstruction: stents of 10 French gauge are preferable to stents of 8 French gauge. Gastrointest Endosc 1988;34:412–7.

[24] Pederson FM. Endoscopic management of malignant biliary obstruction; is stent size of 10 French gauge better than 7 French gauge? Scand J Gastroenterol 1993;28:185–9.

[25] Kadakia SC, Starnes E. Comparison of 10 French gauge stent with 11.5 French gauge stent in patients with biliary tract disease. Gastrointest Endosc 1992;38:454–9.

[26] Pereira-Lima JC, Jakobs R, Maier M, et al. Endoscopic biliary stenting for the palliation of pancreatic cancer: results, survival predictive factors, and comparison of 10-French with 11.5 French gauge stents. Am J Gastroenterol 1996;91:2179–84.

[27] Binmoeller KF, Seitz U, Seifert H, et al. The Tannenbaum stent: a new plastic biliary stent without sideholes. Am J Gastroenterol 1995;90:1738–40.

[28] Catalano MF, Geenen JE, Lehman GA, et al. "Tannenbaum" Teflon stents versus traditional polyethylene stents for the treatment of malignant biliary stricture. Gastrointest Endosc 2002; 55:354–8.

[29] Terruzzi V, Comin U, De Grazia F, et al. Prospective randomized trial comparing Tannenbaum Teflon and standard polyethylene stents in distal malignant biliary stenosis. Gastrointest Endosc 2000;51:23–7.

[30] Van Berkel AM, Huibregtse IL, Bergman JJ, et al. A prospective randomized trial of Tannenbaum-type Teflon-coated stents versus polyethylene stents for distal malignant biliary obstruction. Eur J Gastroenterol Hepatol 2004;16:213–7.

[31] Costamagna G, Mutignani M, Rotondano G, et al. Hydrophilic hydromer-coated polyurethane stents versus uncoated stents in malignant biliary obstruction: a randomized trial. Gastrointest Endosc 2000;51:8–11.

[32] Halm U, Schiefke I, Fleig WE, et al. Ofloxacin and ursodeoxycholic acid versus ursode-oxycholic acid alone to prevent occlusion of biliary stents: a prospective, randomized trial. Endoscopy 2001;33:491–4.

[33] Ghosh S, Palmer KR. Prevention of biliary stent occlusion using cyclical antibiotics and ursodeoxycholic acid. Gut 1994;35:1757–9.

[34] Luman W, Ghosh S, Palmer KR. A combination of ciprofloxacin and Rowachol does not prevent biliary stent occlusion. Gastrointest Endosc 1999;49:316–21.

[35] De Ledinghen V, Person B, Legoux JL, et al. Prevention of biliary stent occlusion by ur-sodeoxycholic acid plus norfloxacin: a multicenter randomized trial. Dig Dis Sci 2000;45: 145–50.

[36] Sung JJ, Sollano JD, Lai CW, et al. Long-term ciprofloxacin treatment for the prevention of biliary stent blockage: a prospective randomized study. Am J Gastroenterol 1999;94:3197–201.

[37] Geoghegan JG, Branch MS, Costerton JW, et al. Placement of biliary stents above the sphincter of Oddi prolongs stent patency in dogs. [abstract] Gut 1991;32:A1232.

[38] Pedersen FM, Lassen AT, Schaffalitzky de Muckadell OB. Randomized trial of stent placed above and across the sphincter of Oddi in malignant bile duct obstruction. Gastrointest Endosc 2000;51:116–7.

[39] Liu Q, Khay G, Cotton PB. Feasibility of stent placement above the sphincter of Oddi ("inside-stent") for patients with malignant biliary obstruction. Endoscopy 1998;30:687–90.

[40] Costamagna G, Pandolfi M. Endoscopic stenting for biliary and pancreatic malignancies. J Clin Gastroenterol 2004;38:59–67.

[41] Dumonceau JM, Cremer M, Auroux J, et al. A comparison of Ultraflex Diamond stents and Wallstents for palliation of distal malignant biliary strictures. Am J Gastroenterol 2000;95: 670–6.

[42] Ahmad J, Siqueira E, Martin J, et al. Effectiveness of the Ultraflex Diamond stent for the palliation of malignant biliary obstruction. Endoscopy 2002;34:793–6.

[43] Shim CS, Lee YH, Cho YD, et al. Preliminary results of a new covered biliary metal stent for malignant biliary obstruction. Endoscopy 1998;30:345–50.

[44] Isayama H, Komatsu Y, Tsujino T, et al. Polyurethane-covered metal stent for management of distal malignant biliary obstruction. Gastrointest Endosc 2002;55:366–70.

[45] Silvis SE, Sievert Jr CE, Vennes JA, et al. Comparison of covered versus uncovered wire mesh stents in the canine biliary tract. Gastrointest Endosc 1994;40:17–21.

[46] Rossi P, Bezzi M, Salvatori FM, et al. Clinical experience with covered Wallstents for biliary malignancies: 23-month follow-up. Cardiovasc Intervent Radiol 1997;20:441–7.

[47] Hausegger KA, Thurnher S, Bodendorfer G, et al. Treatment of malignant biliary obstruction with polyurethane-covered Wallstents. Am J Roentgenol 1998;170:403–8.

[48] Born P, Neuhas H, Rosch T, et al. Initial experience with a new, partially covered Wallstent for malignant biliary obstruction. Endoscopy 1996;28:699–702.

[49] Isayama H, Komatsu Y, Tsujino T, et al. A prospective, randomized study of "covered" versus "uncovered" diamond stents for the management of distal malignant biliary obstruction. Gut 2004;53:729–34.

[50] Wamsteker EJ, Elta GH. Migration of covered biliary self-expanding metallic stents in two patients with malignant biliary obstruction. Gastrointest Endosc 2003;58:792–3.

[51] Hawes RH, Xiong Q, Waxman I, et al. A multispecialty approach to the diagnosis and management of pancreatic cancer. Am J Gastroenterol 2000;95:17–31.

[52] Giorgio PD, Luca LD. Comparison of treatment outcomes between biliary plastic stent placements with and without endoscopic sphincterotomy for inoperable malignant common bile duct obstruction. World J Gastroenterol 2004;15:1212–4.

[53] Tarnasky PR, Cunningham JC, Hawes RH, et al. Transpapillary stenting of proximal biliary strictures: does biliary sphincterotomy reduce the risk of post-procedure pancreatitis? Gastrointest Endosc 1997;45:46–51.

[54] Van Someren RN, Benson MJ, Glynn MJ, et al. A novel technique for dilating difficult malignant biliary strictures during therapeutic ERCP. Gastrointest Endosc 1996;43:495–8.

[55] Brand B, Thonke F, Obytz S, et al. Stent retriever for dilation of pancreatic and bile duct strictures. Endoscopy 1999;31:142–5.

[56] Schiefke I, Zabel-Langhennig A, Wiedmann M, et al. Self-expandable metallic stents for malignant duodenal obstruction caused by biliary tract cancer. Gastrointest Endosc 2003;58: 213–9.

[57] Profili S, Feo CF, Meloni GB, et al. Combined biliary and duodenal stenting for palliation of pancreatic cancer. Scand J Gastroenterol 2003;38:1099–102.

[58] Kaw W, Singh S, Gagneja H. Clinical outcome of simultaneous self-expandable metal stents for palliation of malignant biliary and duodenal obstruction. Surg Endosc 2003;17:457–61.

[59] Boender J, Nix GA, Schutte HE, et al. Malignant common bile duct obstruction: factors influencing the success rate of endoscopic drainage. Endoscopy 1990;22:259–62.

[60] Dowsett JF, Vaira D, Hatfield AR, et al. Endoscopic biliary therapy using the combined percutaneous and endoscopic technique. Gastroenterol 1989;96:1180–6.

[61] Robertson DA, Ayres R, Hacking CN, et al. Experience with a combined percutaneous and endoscopic approach to stent insertion in malignant obstructive jaundice. Lancet 1987;2: 1449–52.

[62] Kaskarelis IS, Papadaki MG, Papageorgiou GN, et al. Long-term follow-up in patients with malignant biliary obstruction after percutaneous placement of uncovered Wallstent endoprostheses. Acta Radiol 1999;40:528–33.

[63] Nakamura T, Hirai R, Kitagawa M, et al. Treatment of common bile duct obstruction by pancreatic cancer using various stents: single-center experience. Cardiovasc Intervent Radiol 2002;25:373–80.

[64] Speer AG, Cotton PB, Russell RC, et al. Randomized trial of endoscopic versus percutaneous stent insertion in malignant obstructive jaundice. Lancet 1987;2:57–62.

[65] Pinol V, Castells A, Bordas JM, et al. Percutaneous self-expanding metal stents versus endoscopic polyethylene endoprostheses for treating malignant biliary obstruction: randomized clinical trial. Radiology 2002;225:27–34.

[66] Costamagna G, Alveras P, Palladino F, et al. Endoscopic pancreatic stenting in pancreatic cancer. Can J Gastroenterol 1999;13:481–7.

[67] Tham TC, Lichtenstein DR, Vandervoort J, et al. Pancreatic duct stents for "obstructive type" pain in pancreatic malignancy. Am J Gastroenterol 2000;95:956–60.

[68] Prat F, Cosson C, Domingo N, et al. Study of the mechanisms of biliary stent occlusion: an analysis of occluded and nonoccluded stents, with emphasis on the role of antinucleating biliary anionic peptide factor. Endoscopy 2004;36:322–8.

[69] Leung JW, Liu YL, Desta T, et al. Is there a synergistic effect between mixed bacterial infection and in biofilm formation on biliary stents? Gastrointest Endosc 1998;48:250–7.

[70] Dowidar N, Kolmos HJ, Matzen P. Experimental clogging of biliary endoprostheses: role of bacteria, endoprosthesis material, and design. Scand J Gastroenterol 1992;27:77–80.

[71] Kim HS, Lee DK, Kim HG, et al. Features of malignant biliary obstruction affecting the patency of metallic stents: a multicenter study. Gastrointest Endosc 2002;55:359–65.

[72] Tham TCK, Carr-Locke DL, Vandervoort J, et al. Management of occluded biliary Wallstents. Gut 1998;42:703–7.

[73] Matsuda Y, Shimakura K, Akamatsu T. Factors affecting the patency of stents in malignant biliary obstructive disease: univariate and multivariate analysis. Am J Gastroenterol 1991;86: 843–9.

[74] Menon K, Romagnuolo J, Barkun AN. Expandable metal biliary stenting in patients with recurrent premature polyethylene stent occlusion. Am J Gastroenterol 2001;96:1435–40.

[75] Bueno JT, Gerdes H, Kurtz RC. Endoscopic management of occluded biliary Wallstents: a cancer center experience. Gastrointest Endosc 2003;58:879–84.

[76] Lossef SV, Druy E, Jelinger E, et al. Use of hot-tip laser probes to recanalize occluded expandable metallic biliary endoprostheses. Am J Roentgenol 1992;158:199–201.

[77] Maetani I, Ukita T, Inoue H, et al. Micorwave coagulation versus insertion of a second stent for occluded biliary metal stent. Hepatogastroenterology 2001;48:1279–83.

[78] Cremer M, Deviere J, Sugai B, et al. Expandable biliary metal stents for malignancies: endoscopic insertion and diathermic cleaning for tumor ingrowth. Gastrointest Endosc 1990;36: 451–7.

[79] Glasser M, Laurence BH, Cameron FG. Relief of tumorous obstruction of a metal biliary stent with palliative intraluminal iridium-192 therapy. Gastrointest Endosc 1992;38:496–8.

[80] Smilanich RP, Hafner GH. Complications of biliary stents in obstructive pancreatic malignancies: a case report and review. Dig Dis Sci 1994;39:2645–9.

[81] Gardiner MF, Long WB, Haskal ZJ, et al. Upper gastrointestinal hemorrhage secondary to erosion of a biliary Wallstent in a woman with pancreatic cancer. Endoscopy 2000;32:661–3.

[82] Roebuck DJ, Stanley P, Katz MD, et al. Gastrointestinal hemorrhage due to duodenal erosion by a biliary Wallstent. Cardiovasc Intervent Radiol 1998;21:63–5.

[83] Marano BJ, Bonanno CA. Metallic biliary endoprosthesis causing duodenal perforation and acute upper gastrointestinal bleeding. Gastrointest Endosc 1994;40:257–8.

[84] Pescatore P, Meier-Willersen HJ, Manegold BC. A severe complication of the new self-expanding spiral nitinol biliary stent. Endoscopy 1997;29:413–5.

[85] Ainley CC, Williams SJ, Smith AC, et al. Gallbladder sepsis after stent insertion for bile duct obstruction: management by percutaneous cholecystostomy. Br J Surg 1991;78:961–3.

[86] De Palma GD, Galloro G, Siciliano S, et al. Unilateral versus bilateral endoscopic hepatic duct drainage in patients with malignant biliary obstruction: results of a prospective, randomized, and controlled study. Gastrointest Endosc 2001;53:681–4.

[87] Chang WH, Kortan P, Haber GB. Outcome in patients with bifurcation tumors who undergo unilateral versus bilateral hepatic duct drainage. Gastrointest Endosc 1998;47:354–62.

[88] Freeman ML, Overby C. Selective MRCP and CT-targeted drainage of malignant hilar biliary obstruction with self-expanding metallic stents. Gastrointest Endosc 2003;58:41–9.

[89] Hintze RE, Abou-Rebyeh H, Adler A, et al. Magnetic resonance cholangiopancreatography-guided unilateral endoscopic stent placement for Klatskin tumors. Gastrointest Endosc 2001;53:40–6.

[90] Shepherd HA, Royle G, Ross APR, et al. Endoscopic biliary endoprosthesis in the palliation of malignant obstruction of the distal common bile duct: a randomized trial. Br J Surg 1988;75:1166–8.

[91] Andersen JR, Sorensen SM, Kruse A, et al. Randomised trial of endoscopic endoprosthesis versus operative bypass in malignant obstructive jaundice. Gut 1989;30:1132–5.

[92] Smith AC, Dowsett JF, Russell RCG, et al. Randomised trial of endoscopic stenting versus surgical bypass in malignant low bile duct obstruction. Lancet 1994;344:1655–60.

[93] Taylor MC, McLeod RS, Langer B. Biliary stenting versus bypass surgery for the palliation of malignant distal bile duct obstruction: a meta-analysis. Liver Transpl 2000;6:302–8.

[94] Raikar GV, Melin MM, Ress A, et al. Cost-effective analysis of surgical palliation versus endoscopic stenting in the management of unresectable pancreatic cancer. Ann Surg Oncol 1996;3:470–5.

[95] Martin Jr RC, Vitale GC, Reed DN, et al. Cost comparison of endoscopic stenting vs surgical treatment for unresectable cholangiocarcinoma. Surg Endosc 2002;16:667–70.

[96] Wiersema MJ, Sandusky D, Carr R, et al. Endosonography-guided cholangiopancreatography. Gastrointest Endosc 1996;43:102–6.

[97] Bataille L, Deprez P. A new application for therapeutic EUS: main pancreatic duct drainage with a "pancreatic rendezvous technique." Gastrointest Endosc 2002;55:740–3.

[98] Burmester E, Niehaus J, Lieneweber T, et al. EUS-cholangio-drainage of the bile duct: report of 4 cases. Gastrointest Endosc 2003;57:246–51.

[99] Mallery S, Matlock J, Freeman ML. EUS-guided rendezvous drainage of obstructed biliary and pancreatic ducts: report of 6 cases. Gastrointest Endosc 2004;59:100–7.

[100] Sahai AV, Hoffman BJ, Hawes RH. Endoscopic ultrasound-guided hepaticogastrostomy to palliate obstructive jaundice: preliminary results in pigs [abstract]. Gastrointest Endosc 1998;47:AB37.

[101] Wiersema MJ, Wiersema LM. Endosonography-guided celiac plexus neurolysis. Gastrointest Endosc 1996;44:56–62.

[102] Gunaratnam NT, Sarma AV, Norton ID, et al. A prospective study of EUS-guided celiac plexus neurolysis for pancreatic cancer pain. Gastrointest Endosc 2001;54:316–24.

[103] Goldberg SN, Mallery S, Gazelle GS, et al. EUS-guided radiofrequency ablation in the pancreas: results in a porcine model. Gastrointest Endosc 1999;50:392–401.

[104] Chan HH, Nishioka NS, Mino M, et al. EUS-guided photodynamic therapy of the pancreas: a pilot study. Gastrointest Endosc 2004;59:95–9.

[105] Chang KJ, Nguyen PT, Thompson JA, et al. Phase I clinical trial of allogeneic mixed lymphocyte culture (cytoimplant) delivered by endoscopic ultrasound-guided fine-needle injection in patients with advanced pancreatic carcinoma. Cancer 2000;88:1325–35.

[106] Hecht JR, Bedford R, Abbruzzese JL, et al. A phase I/II trial of intratumoral endoscopic ultrasound injection of ONYX-015 with intravenous gemcitabine in unresectable pancreatic carcinoma. Clin Cancer Res 2003;9:555–61.

[107] Chang KJ, Senzer N, Chung T, et al. A novel gene transfer therapy against pancreatic cancer (TNFerade) delivered by endoscopic ultrasound (EUS) and percutaneous guided fine needle injection (FNI) [abstract]. Gastrointest Endosc 2004;59:AB92.

[108] Ortner MA, Liebetruth J, Schreiber S, et al. Photodynamic therapy of nonresectable cholangiocarcinoma. Gastroenterology 1998;114:536–42.

[109] Dumoulin FL, Gerhardt T, Fuchs S, et al. Phase II study of photodynamic therapy and metal stent as palliative treatment for nonresectable hilar cholangiocarcinoma. Gastrointest Endosc 2003;57:860–7.

[110] Ortner MA, Caca K, Berr F, et al. Successful photodynamic therapy for nonresectable cholangiocarcinoma: a randomized prospective study. Gastroenterology 2003;125:1355–63.

[111] Mezawa S, Homma H, Sato T, et al. A study of carboplatin-coated tube for the unresectable cholangiocarcinoma. Hepatology 2000;32:916–23.

[112] Kalinowski M, Alfke H, Kleb B, et al. Paclitaxel inhibits proliferation of cell lines responsible for metal stent obstruction: possible topical application in malignant bile duct obstructions. Invest Radiol 2002;37:399–404.

[113] Ginsberg G, Cope C, Shah J, et al. In vivo evaluation of a new bioabsorbable self-expanding biliary stent. Gastrointest Endosc 2003;58:777–84.

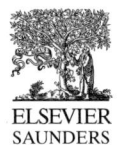

ELSEVIER
SAUNDERS

Gastrointest Endoscopy Clin N Am
15 (2005) 533–547

GASTROINTESTINAL
ENDOSCOPY CLINICS
OF NORTH AMERICA

Screening and Surveillance of Colorectal Cancer

Charles J. Kahi, MD, MSc[a], Douglas K. Rex, MD[b],*

[a]Indiana University School of Medicine, Roudebush VA Medical Center, C-7055, 1481 W 10th Street,
Indianapolis, IN 46202, USA
[b]Indiana University School of Medicine, Indiana University Medical Center, UH 4100,
550 N University Boulevard, Indianapolis, IN 46202, USA

Colorectal cancer (CRC) remains the second leading cause of cancer deaths in the United States [1]. The cumulative lifetime risk is about 5%, and the majority of cases occur after the age of 50 [2]. CRC has several characteristics that make it an attractive target for population-based screening and surveillance. The disease is common and lethal if not detected early, effective treatments are available for early CRC, identification and removal of precursor adenomatous polyps prevent cancer occurrence, and screening modalities are widely disseminated in clinical practice and are available to most patients [3].

Estimating the magnitude of risk for developing CRC is a crucial aspect in deciding on a screening and surveillance strategy. Average-risk persons have no risk factors for CRC other than age. High-risk screening encompasses patients with inflammatory bowel disease, a personal history of CRC or adenomatous polyps, a family history of hereditary nonpolyposis colorectal cancer or familial adenomatous polyposis, and those with a family history of CRC that does not meet the diagnostic criteria for the latter inherited syndromes [4].

This article presents the various modalities available for CRC screening and discusses screening strategies in average-risk persons and surveillance after polypectomy and cancer resection.

* Corresponding author.
E-mail address: drex@iupui.edu (D.K. Rex).

Screening modalities

Fecal occult blood test

Testing stool samples for occult blood is commonly used for CRC screening in the United States [5] and is the only modality that has been shown to decrease CRC incidence and mortality in randomized controlled clinical trials [6–10]. The most commonly used assays use cards that are impregnated with guaiac, which turns blue in the presence of peroxidase-like substances such as heme [11]. Three large, randomized trials conducted in Minnesota [8], Nottingham, England [6], and Denmark [7,10] have shown mortality reductions from CRC ranging from 15% to 33% when positive results were followed by colonoscopy. Mortality reductions are higher in persons who comply with testing. Fecal occult blood test (FOBT) screening has been shown to reduce the incidence of CRC [9].

Several issues affect the performance characteristics and efficacy of the FOBT, particularly screening frequency and rehydration of samples. The two European studies used biennial screening, whereas the Minnesota study randomized patients to annual or biennial screening. The greatest reduction in mortality was observed in the annual arm of the Minnesota study (5.88 versus 8.83 deaths per 1000 in the control group, 33% reduction), and the 13-year follow-up of the Danish study showed a 30% reduction in risk of death for patients who participated in all seven biennial screening rounds [10,12]. Rehydration of stool samples before testing increases the sensitivity of FOBT but at the expense of specificity, thus increasing the number of workups done for false-positive tests. For example, in the Minnesota trial, rehydration increased the rate of positive tests from 2.4% to 9.8%, and this may have increased the number of colonoscopies done for false-positive tests with possible chance detection of CRCs [13,14].

Screening with FOBT has several advantages, including wide availability, ease of performance and lack of invasiveness, ability to perform in the primary care setting, and low cost [5]. Its disadvantages include relatively modest efficacy and high false-positive rates when compared with endoscopic modalities. The sensitivity for CRC detection is 33% to 50% for one-time testing, but this improves with repeat testing at regular intervals [3,15].

The most widely used FOBT is Hemoccult II (SmithKline Diagnostics, Palo Alto, California). Other more sensitive guaiac tests and immunochemical assays for human hemoglobin are available for clinical use [16] and have been endorsed for use in CRC screening.

United States societies' CRC screening guidelines recommend annual FOBT without rehydration or with rehydration at the discretion of the practitioner performing the test [3,17–19]. The appropriate workup of positive tests is critical for effectiveness: Regardless of the assay used, the frequency of screening, or whether the sample was rehydrated, a patient with a positive FOBT should be referred for colonoscopy.

Flexible sigmoidoscopy

Sigmoidoscopic examination of the distal colon with polypectomy reduces rectal cancer mortality by about two thirds, as shown in well-designed case-control studies [20,21]. Sigmoidoscopy is an attractive modality because it is relatively inexpensive, does not require routine sedation, and may be performed in the primary care setting. In addition, it requires less intensive bowel preparation than complete colonoscopy and has a lower risk of perforation [3,5,22]. The major limitation of sigmoidoscopy is its lack of sensitivity for lesions that are beyond the reach of the instrument, which is an important consideration because nearly half of colonic neoplasms occur in the proximal colon [23,24]. The addition of FOBT to sigmoidoscopy to enhance detection of proximal lesions is not an effective solution because FOBT has marginal sensitivity for lesions that bleed intermittently [4]. In a study of one-time screening using colonoscopy and FOBT, sigmoidoscopy alone detected 70.3% of all advanced neoplasms, compared with 75.8% with the addition of FOBT to sigmoidoscopy [25].

The benefit of sigmoidoscopy is not only due to the removal of adenomatous polyps found within the range of the instrument, but also as a result of colonoscopies obtained after a "positive" sigmoidoscopy to examine the proximal colon. There is convincing evidence to support complete colonoscopy in patients with distal advanced adenomas (Box 1) [23,26,27]. The data are less clear for patients with single distal adenomas that are 5 mm or less in size, although in current practice these patients generally undergo complete colonoscopy [3,23,25,28,29].

The optimal interval for screening flexible sigmoidoscopy is uncertain. Several studies have shown low recurrence rates of adenomas up to 3 years after a negative screening examination [30–32]. The Prostate, Lung, Colorectal, and Ovarian trial found a 0.8% incidence rate of advanced adenomas 3 years after a negative screening by flexible sigmoidoscopy [33]; the study by Selby and colleagues [21] suggested that sigmoidoscopy may be protective for up to 10 years after the initial examination. Balancing these facts, societal guidelines state that a 5-year interval between sigmoidoscopies is adequate (Table 1). A recent direct observational study from the Northern California Kaiser Permanente database supported an interval of at least 5 years between examinations [34].

Flexible sigmoidoscopy has several other limitations. The lack of sedation may render it less acceptable to patients and decrease compliance with follow-up

---

Box 1. The advanced adenoma

- Diameter 1 cm or more, or
- High-grade dysplasia, or
- >20% villous elements, or
- Carcinoma

Table 1
Colorectal cancer screening guidelines in average-risk persons

Screening modality	ACG	AGA	ACS
FOBT	Annual	Annual	Annual
Sigmoidoscopy	Every 5 y	Every 5 y	Every 5 y
FOBT + sigmoidoscopy	Annual/every 5 y	Annual/every 5 y	Annual/every 5 y
Colonoscopy	Every 10 y (preferred strategy)	Every 10 y	Every 10 y

Abbreviations: ACG, American College of Gastroenterology; ACS, American Cancer Society; AGA, American Gastroenterological Association; FOBT, fecal occult blood test.
Data from Refs. [3,17–19].

recommendations. In addition, primary care physicians may be more likely to report false-negative examinations than gastroenterologists [35]. For these reasons, complete colonoscopy performed by a specialist is emerging as a preferred screening test for CRC. The American College of Gastroenterology has endorsed colonoscopy every 10 years as the preferred screening strategy for CRC but accepts flexible sigmoidoscopy every 5 years with annual FOBT as an alternative [3]. Other multidisciplinary groups consider these approaches to be equivalent (Table 1) [17–19].

Colonoscopy

Colonoscopy is becoming the dominant CRC screening and surveillance modality for several reasons. First, colonoscopy allows visualization and removal of lesions from the entire colon in one session. The need to adequately examine the proximal colon is supported by the observed shift of CRCs toward the right colon [36,37] and by recent evidence that many advanced proximal lesions can be missed by limiting screening to sigmoidoscopic examination of the distal colon. In a study on 1994 average-risk persons undergoing screening colonoscopy, Imperiale and colleagues [23] found that 46% of patients with proximal advanced lesions had no distal pathology. Another report found that 34.5% of 116 average-risk patients with proximal CRC had neoplasia distal to the splenic flexure [26]. Second, colonoscopy is effective in preventing CRC. The National Polyp Study showed a 76% to 90% reduction in CRC incidence among screened individuals compared with reference populations [38]. Other prospective studies from Europe have confirmed these findings [39,40], although some evidence suggests lower rates of protection [41–43]. Third, colonoscopy every 10 years is cost effective when compared with other CRC screening strategies [44–46]. Finally, the procedure is usually done under sedation, thereby minimizing patient discomfort and improving patient satisfaction and public acceptance of colonoscopy in general [47,48].

The optimal interval between screening colonoscopic examinations has not been determined in large, prospective observational studies. A single, small, observational study indicated a low incidence of advanced adenomas when colonoscopy was repeated 5 years after a negative examination in asymptomatic average-risk persons [49]. The 10-year protective effect of sigmoidoscopy on the distal colon can be extrapolated to the remainder of the colon, given that the two procedures rely on fundamentally the same principles and technology [21]. This approach is consistent with the known natural history of adenomas and the estimated time it would take for an adenoma to become a carcinoma [50].

An attractive feature of colonoscopy is the fact that the procedure is constantly evolving, and new methods are being devised to improve its effectiveness and tolerability. For example, sedation with propofol has been shown to provide better analgesia and more rapid neuropsychologic recovery after colonoscopy, compared with conventional benzodiazepine/narcotic combinations [51]. Cap-fitted colonoscopy [52–54], wide-angle colonoscopy [55], and chromoendoscopy with or without magnification [56–60] are new techniques that may improve polyp detection rates. Bowel preparations that are better tolerated are also becoming available [61,62]. Improvements in effectiveness and cost-effectiveness (by allowing expansion of surveillance intervals) will render colonoscopy even more attractive as the mainstay of CRC screening.

Colonoscopy has its disadvantages. First, although it is the gold standard for examination of the colon, some lesions are missed even by experienced endoscopists. Tandem colonoscopy studies have attempted to quantify this risk. In one report, 27% of adenomas 5 mm or less, 13% of adenomas 6 to 9 mm, and 6% of adenomas 1 cm or larger were missed [63]. Another study used CT colonography as a gold standard and found a 12% miss rate for adenomas 1 cm or larger for complete colonoscopy [64]. A recent study of CT colonography compared with colonoscopy in high-risk patients. Among 31 patients with large polyps, eight were missed by initial colonoscopy, detected by CT colonography, and then confirmed by second-look colonoscopy [65]. The adequacy of a colonoscopic examination also depends on endoscopist skill and technique [66], and the United States Multi-Society Task Force on Colorectal Cancer has developed a set of Continuous Quality Improvement guidelines aimed at defining and implementing high quality standards for the performance of colonoscopy [67]. Second, colonoscopy carries a risk of perforation, although the rate seems to be lower than 0.1% to 0.2% [22]. Finally, there are the inconveniences of bowel preparation and the need to take a day off work for the patient and a designated driver after recovery from sedation [4]. These factors need to be kept in mind when counseling patients about their options in screening for CRC.

Double-contrast barium enema

The use of double-contrast barium enema (DCBE) for CRC screening is declining for several reasons. First, colonoscopy is superior to DCBE. In one study, the sensitivity of DCBE for the detection of CRC was 83% compared with 95% for colonoscopy, and DCBE was four times more likely to miss a malignancy

[35]. The National Polyp Study Workgroup reported that DCBE missed about half of polyps larger than 6 mm and half of those larger than 10 mm, and the overall detection rate for all adenomas was 39% [68]. Second, DCBE is a diagnostic modality, and patients with positive findings have to undergo colonoscopy on another day and with a repeat bowel preparation [4]. Finally, sedation is usually not used, and patients may experience significant discomfort as a result of air insufflation into the colon.

DCBE may have a role in instances where colonoscopy is incomplete or in combination with flexible sigmoidoscopy; however, the latter is often cumbersome to arrange and perform and has not been shown to be more effective than either modality alone.

CT and MR colonography

CT and MR colonography, also known as "virtual colonoscopy," are discussed in detail elsewhere in this issue. Virtual colonoscopy is emerging as a promising technology for CRC screening, but it is not ready for general use as a screening modality in lieu of established strategies. The main problem is the highly variable sensitivity of virtual colonoscopy for the detection of adenomas, which has ranged from 43% to 94% in published studies [69–78]. A recent study on 1233 asymptomatic average-risk adults using novel three-dimensional reconstruction techniques reported sensitivity rates of 94% for polyps 8 mm or larger and 88.7% for polyps 6 mm or larger [74]. These results await confirmation from studies conducted at other centers. Other impediments to virtual colonoscopy include cost, discomfort due to air insufflation, uncertain patient acceptance rates [79,80], and the clinical and medico-legal implications of incidentally detected extracolonic lesions [81].

Fecal DNA tests

Testing for DNA shed from CRC in stool became commercially available in 2003. The assay tests for chromosomal instability genes (APC, K-ras, p53), a microsatellite instability marker (BAT-26), and a marker of cells not undergoing apoptosis called "long DNA" [82] or the DNA integrity assay. Multicenter trials using this assay are in progress. Results of the first of these multicenter trials were reported by Imperiale [23] at an industry symposium at the 2003 ACG National Meeting. The sensitivity of the multi-target DNA assay in 2507 fully evaluated patients was 52% and 15% for CRC and advanced adenomas, respectively. The main issue with this new test is its high cost (about $800), but it is an attractive modality because it is simpler to collect than standard FOBTs (ie, no dietary restrictions, single sample, convenient collection device) and is noninvasive. The test should probably be repeated every 3 to 5 years. This strategy requires further data for validation.

Screening strategies

The relative efficacy of various modalities used to screen for CRC is only one dimension that expert groups have to consider when developing screening guidelines. These guidelines are generally consistent in their recommendations, and all recommend initiating CRC screening in average-risk individuals starting at 50 years of age. The yield of screening in younger patients is sufficiently low to justify starting at this age [2]. The ACG recommends colonoscopy every 10 years as the preferred screening strategy for the reasons outlined previously. Several alternative screening strategies deserve further consideration. For example, it would be reasonable to start screening with flexible sigmoidoscopy and FOBT at 50 years of age and then to continue with colonoscopy at 60 years of age because this would take into account the increased incidence and the proximal shift of CRCs with advancing age [3,83]. A cost-effectiveness analysis reported that single colonoscopy at 65 years of age was a cost-effective alternative to screening colonoscopy every 10 years if the latter option was hampered by high costs or poor patient compliance [84]. Conversely, a cost-utility analysis found that a single screening colonoscopy between 50 and 54 years of age was the most cost-effective strategy [85].

More studies are needed to define the optimal time to begin screening colonoscopy; however, in light of its impressive efficacy and safety record, it is likely that colonoscopy will remain the cornerstone of CRC screening. The use of flexible sigmoidoscopy and FOBT is expected to decline unless available resources do not permit the use of screening colonoscopy. The future role of virtual colonoscopy and fecal DNA tests awaits further data from studies showing effective and cost-effective prevention of CRC.

Postpolypectomy surveillance

About 17% of the colonoscopies performed each year in the United States are done for postpolypectomy surveillance, and this number may increase as the use of screening colonoscopy grows [86,87]. The most important consideration in determining postpolypectomy surveillance intervals is accurately estimating patients' risk of recurrent polyps. Effective and cost-effective surveillance requires balancing the protective effect of clearing the colon of polyps while maximizing intervals between examinations so that patients receive the best care and resources are appropriately used. Recent evidence indicates that colonoscopy is overused for surveillance by some gastroenterologists and surgeons [88].

Risk of recurrence after polypectomy

The overall per procedure yield of colonoscopy for postpolypectomy surveillance is low (about 317 colonoscopies for each CRC detected) [83]; therefore, attention over the past decade has shifted toward stratifying patients according to

---

Box 2. Predictors of recurrent adenomas and advanced adenomas

- Adenoma ≥ 1 cm
- Multiple adenomas
- Advanced adenoma histology
- Older age
- Family history of CRC in parent
- Proximal location of index adenoma

Data from References [2,38,89–100].

---

their risk of developing a metachronous advanced adenoma. These patients should be followed with more intensive surveillance than patients who have a low risk of recurrence. Data from several studies have defined the factors that are known to predict the development of advanced adenomas (Box 2) [27,38,41, 43,89–100]. Although not all studies report the same risk factors, large polyps, histologically advanced adenomas, and multiple (three or more) adenomas are the strongest predictors of recurrent lesions.

Other predictive variables include older patient age, family history of CRC, and proximal location of index polyps. Family history seems to be a significant predictor, particularly when considered along with older age. For example, in the National Polyp Study, the odds ratio for recurrence was 4.3 (95% confidence interval 1.7–10.8) for patients older than 60 years of age with one parent with CRC, compared with younger patients with no family history [38,100].

Surveillance guidelines

To maintain simplicity, current guidelines consider large adenomas (≥ 1 cm), multiple adenomas (three or more), and histologically advanced adenomas (villous features, high-grade dysplasia) as high-risk lesions that warrant intensive follow-up (Table 2). Other factors that are accounted for may be important, such as family history, which is considered only in the American College of Gastroenterology (ACG) guidelines [101].

Current guidelines are fairly consistent regarding the follow-up of large sessile polyps with advanced histology; these should be reassessed endoscopically after 1 to 6 months [17–19,101]. There is disagreement regarding the surveillance of patients with smaller, less advanced lesions. The ACG and the American Gastroenterological Association (AGA) recommend that patients with one or two small (<1 cm) adenomas undergo their first follow-up colonoscopy after 5 years, then at 5-year intervals if this examination is negative [18,19,101]. On the other hand, the American Cancer Society (ACS) states that a patient with one tubular adenoma <1 cm should undergo surveillance in 3 to 6 years and should return to average-risk screening if this examination is negative [17]. The ACG, AGA, and ACS recommend that patients with advanced adenomas at the

Table 2
Postpolypectomy surveillance guidelines

Society	Interval
ACG	
1 or 2 tubular adenomas <1 cm and negative family history of colorectal cancer	5 y
>2 adenomas, adenoma >1 cm, villous histology, high-grade dysplasia, or family history of colorectal cancer	3 y
Negative follow-up	5 y
AGA Consortium	
1–2 tubular adenomas <1 cm	5 y
>2 adenomas, adenoma >1 cm, villous histology, or high-grade dysplasia	3 y
Negative follow-up	5 y
ACS	
1 tubular adenoma <1 cm	3–6 y
Negative follow-up	Average-risk guidelines
1 tubular adenoma >1 cm, ≥2 adenomas, villous histology, or high-grade dysplasia	Within 3 y
Negative follow-up	3 y
Negative follow-up	Average-risk guidelines

Abbreviations: ACG, American College of Gastroenterology; ACS, American Cancer Society; AGA, American Gastroenterological Association.
Data from Refs. [17–19,101].

index colonoscopy have their first follow-up after 3 years. There is disparity regarding the intensity of subsequent surveillance. The ACG and AGA consider that patients with adenomas are at life-long risk for recurrence, and therefore colonoscopies should be repeated every 5 years unless the results of the most recent examination warrant more frequent surveillance. The ACS considers that polypectomy reduces the risk of CRC to or below general population levels, and therefore a patient with an advanced adenoma can return to general screening guidelines if two consecutive 3-year colonoscopies are negative (Table 2).

Postcancer resection surveillance

Patients with a history of CRC who have undergone surgical resection with curative intent represent a special high-risk population that should be discussed separately. The initial role of colonoscopy is to clear the colon of synchronous neoplasms; this examination can be performed preoperatively or up to 6 months postoperatively if malignant obstruction precluded a complete colonoscopy before surgery [102–104]. After resection, the focus of colonoscopy is to detect metachronous lesions. Randomized trials comparing various surveillance regimens have concluded that the majority of CRC recurrences are extraluminal and are likely best detected using imaging with CT and carcinoembryonic antigen measurements [105–110]. A recent meta-analysis of these trials reported a low rate of intraluminal anastomotic recurrences detected by colonoscopy (3.2%) [111]. The ACG, AGA, and American Society of Colon and Rectal Surgeons recommend that the first colonoscopy be performed 3 years after resection, provided perioperative clearing was satisfactory [18,19,101,102]. The ACS states that the first colonoscopy should be performed 1 year postoperatively. Recent studies have identified a substantial yield of colonoscopy for metachronous lesions in the first 2 years after CRC resection [112,113]. This approach can be justified if there are concerns about the early occurrence of a second primary cancer [114]; however, available data suggest that annual colonoscopy does not influence survival from the original CRC [111], and recurrent cancers detected at the anastomosis are usually not resectable for cure.

Rectal cancer represents a special case in post-CRC resection surveillance because of its higher propensity for local recurrence. This is largely dependent on the type of surgical technique used. Blunt dissection is associated with local recurrence rates of up to 45%, compared with less than 10% with total mesorectal excision and local recurrence rates as low as 2.4% when neoadjuvant chemoradiation is given followed by total mesorectal excision [115]. In cases where the rate of recurrence is expected to be high, such as after low anterior resection using traditional blunt dissection technique, there is a rationale to perform flexible sigmoidoscopy every 6 months for the first 2 years after surgery [116,117]. The role of endorectal ultrasonography (EUS) for the routine evaluation of the surgical anastomosis is evolving. Some studies have suggested that the earlier detection of locally recurrent rectal cancers by EUS imparts a survival advantage [118,119], and one multidisciplinary group has suggested combining EUS with flexible sigmoidoscopy during postoperative surveillance [116]. No randomized controlled clinical trials have evaluated the value of EUS in surveillance for recurrent rectal cancer. The rationale for flexible sigmoidoscopy and EUS decreases in patients who are appropriately treated up front for locally advanced rectal cancer using neoadjuvant chemoradiation followed by total mesorectal excision [120] because local recurrence rates are as low as those with colon cancer.

References

[1] Jemal A, Tiwari RC, Murray T, et al. Cancer statistics, 2004. CA Cancer J Clin 2004;54:8–29.
[2] Imperiale TF, Wagner DR, Lin CY, et al. Results of screening colonoscopy among persons 40 to 49 years of age. N Engl J Med 2002;346:1781–5.
[3] Rex DK, Johnson DA, Lieberman DA, et al. Colorectal cancer prevention 2000: screening recommendations of the American College of Gastroenterology. Am J Gastroenterol 2000;95: 868–77.
[4] Kahi CJ, Rex DK. Current and future trends in colorectal cancer screening. Cancer Metastasis Rev 2004;23:137–44.
[5] Ransohoff DF, Sandler RS. Clinical practice: screening for colorectal cancer. N Engl J Med 2002;346:40–4.
[6] Hardcastle JD, Chamberlain JO, Robinson MH, et al. Randomised controlled trial of faecal-occult-blood screening for colorectal cancer. Lancet 1996;348:1472–7.

[7] Kronborg O, Fenger C, Olsen J, et al. Randomised study of screening for colorectal cancer with faecal-occult-blood test. Lancet 1996;348:1467–71.

[8] Mandel JS, Bond JH, Church TR, et al. Reducing mortality from colorectal cancer by screening for fecal occult blood. Minnesota Colon Cancer Control Study. N Engl J Med 1993;328: 1365–71.

[9] Mandel JS, Church TR, Bond JH, et al. The effect of fecal occult-blood screening on the incidence of colorectal cancer. N Engl J Med 2000;343:1603–7.

[10] Jorgensen OD, Kronborg O, Fenger C. A randomised study of screening for colorectal cancer using faecal occult blood testing: results after 13 years and seven biennial screening rounds. Gut 2002;50:29–32.

[11] Rockey DC. Occult gastrointestinal bleeding. N Engl J Med 1999;341:38–46.

[12] Sawhney MS, Nelson DB. The winner after 7 rounds–fecal occult blood testing! Gastroenterology 2002;122:2081–2 [discussion: 2082].

[13] Ederer F, Church TR, Mandel JS. Fecal occult blood screening in the Minnesota study: role of chance detection of lesions. J Natl Cancer Inst 1997;89:1423–8.

[14] Lang CA, Ransohoff DF. Fecal occult blood screening for colorectal cancer: is mortality reduced by chance selection for screening colonoscopy? JAMA 1994;271:1011–3.

[15] Ahlquist DA, Wieand HS, Moertel CG, et al. Accuracy of fecal occult blood screening for colorectal neoplasia: a prospective study using Hemoccult and HemoQuant tests. JAMA 1993;269:1262–7.

[16] Allison JE, Tekawa IS, Ransom LJ, et al. A comparison of fecal occult-blood tests for colorectal-cancer screening. N Engl J Med 1996;334:155–9.

[17] Smith RA, von Eschenbach AC, Wender R, et al. American Cancer Society guidelines for the early detection of cancer: update of early detection guidelines for prostate, colorectal, and endometrial cancers. Also: update 2001–for testing early lung cancer detection. CA Cancer J Clin 2001;51:38–75 [quiz: 77–80].

[18] Winawer S, Fletcher R, Rex D, et al. Colorectal cancer screening and surveillance: clinical guidelines and rationale-Update based on new evidence. Gastroenterology 2003;124:544–60.

[19] Winawer SJ, Fletcher RH, Miller L, et al. Colorectal cancer screening: clinical guidelines and rationale. Gastroenterology 1997;112:594–642.

[20] Newcomb PA, Norfleet RG, Storer BE, et al. Screening sigmoidoscopy and colorectal cancer mortality. J Natl Cancer Inst 1992;84:1572–5.

[21] Selby JV, Friedman GD, Quesenberry Jr CP, et al. A case-control study of screening sigmoidoscopy and mortality from colorectal cancer. N Engl J Med 1992;326:653–7.

[22] Gatto NM, Frucht H, Sundararajan V, et al. Risk of perforation after colonoscopy and sigmoidoscopy: a population-based study. J Natl Cancer Inst 2003;95:230–6.

[23] Imperiale TF, Wagner DR, Lin CY, et al. Risk of advanced proximal neoplasms in asymptomatic adults according to the distal colorectal findings. N Engl J Med 2000;343: 169–74.

[24] Lieberman DA, Weiss DG, Bond JH, et al. Use of colonoscopy to screen asymptomatic adults for colorectal cancer. Veterans Affairs Cooperative Study Group 380. N Engl J Med 2000;343: 162–8.

[25] Lieberman DA, Weiss DG. One-time screening for colorectal cancer with combined fecal occult-blood testing and examination of the distal colon. N Engl J Med 2001;345:555–60.

[26] Rex DK, Chak A, Vasudeva R, et al. Prospective determination of distal colon findings in average-risk patients with proximal colon cancer. Gastrointest Endosc 1999;49:727–30.

[27] Atkin WS, Morson BC, Cuzick J. Long-term risk of colorectal cancer after excision of rectosigmoid adenomas. N Engl J Med 1992;326:658–62.

[28] Opelka FG, Timmcke AE, Gathright Jr JB, et al. Diminutive colonic polyps: an indication for colonoscopy. Dis Colon Rectum 1992;35:178–81.

[29] Read TE, Read JD, Butterly LF. Importance of adenomas 5 mm or less in diameter that are detected by sigmoidoscopy. N Engl J Med 1997;336:8–12.

[30] Brint SL, DiPalma JA, Herrera JL. Colorectal cancer screening: is one-year surveillance sigmoidoscopy necessary? Am J Gastroenterol 1993;88:2019–21.

[31] Rex DK, Lehman GA, Ulbright TM, et al. The yield of a second screening flexible sigmoidoscopy in average-risk persons after one negative examination. Gastroenterology 1994; 106:593–5.

[32] Riff ER, Dehaan K, Garewal GS. The role of sigmoidoscopy for asymptomatic patients: results of three annual screening sigmoidoscopies, polypectomy, and subsequent surveillance colonoscopy in a primary-care setting. Cleve Clin J Med 1990;57:131–6.

[33] Schoen RE, Pinsky PF, Weissfeld JL, et al. Results of repeat sigmoidoscopy 3 years after a negative examination. JAMA 2003;290:41–8.

[34] Doria-Rose VP, Levin TR, Selby JV, et al. The incidence of colorectal cancer following a negative screening sigmoidoscopy: implications for screening interval. Gastroenterology 2004; 127:714–22.

[35] Rex DK, Rahmani EY, Haseman JH, et al. Relative sensitivity of colonoscopy and barium enema for detection of colorectal cancer in clinical practice. Gastroenterology 1997;112:17–23.

[36] Kee F, Wilson RH, Gilliland R, et al. Changing site distribution of colorectal cancer. BMJ 1992;305:158.

[37] Mamazza J, Gordon PH. The changing distribution of large intestinal cancer. Dis Colon Rectum 1982;25:558–62.

[38] Winawer SJ, Zauber AG, Ho MN, et al. Prevention of colorectal cancer by colonoscopic polypectomy. The National Polyp Study Workgroup. N Engl J Med 1993;329:1977–81.

[39] Citarda F, Tomaselli G, Capocaccia R, et al. Efficacy in standard clinical practice of colonoscopic polypectomy in reducing colorectal cancer incidence. Gut 2001;48:812–5.

[40] Thiis-Evensen E, Hoff GS, Sauar J, et al. Population-based surveillance by colonoscopy: effect on the incidence of colorectal cancer. Telemark Polyp Study I. Scand J Gastroenterol 1999;34:414–20.

[41] Alberts DS, Martinez ME, Roe DJ, et al. Lack of effect of a high-fiber cereal supplement on the recurrence of colorectal adenomas. Phoenix Colon Cancer Prevention Physicians' Network. N Engl J Med 2000;342:1156–62.

[42] Muller AD, Sonnenberg A. Prevention of colorectal cancer by flexible endoscopy and polypectomy: a case-control study of 32,702 veterans. Ann Intern Med 1995;123:904–10.

[43] Schatzkin A, Lanza E, Corle D, et al. Lack of effect of a low-fat, high-fiber diet on the recurrence of colorectal adenomas. Polyp Prevention Trial Study Group. N Engl J Med 2000; 342:1149–55.

[44] Frazier AL, Colditz GA, Fuchs CS, et al. Cost-effectiveness of screening for colorectal cancer in the general population. JAMA 2000;284:1954–61.

[45] Lieberman DA. Cost-effectiveness model for colon cancer screening. Gastroenterology 1995; 109:1781–90.

[46] Sonnenberg A, Delco F, Inadomi JM. Cost-effectiveness of colonoscopy in screening for colorectal cancer. Ann Intern Med 2000;133:573–4.

[47] Rex DK. Barium studies/virtual colonoscopy: the gastroenterologist's perspective. Gastrointest Endosc 2002;55(Suppl):S33–6 [discussion: S36].

[48] Kim LS, Koch J, Yee J, et al. Comparison of patients' experiences during imaging tests of the colon. Gastrointest Endosc 2001;54:67–74.

[49] Rex DK, Cummings OW, Helper DJ, et al. 5-year incidence of adenomas after negative colonoscopy in asymptomatic average-risk persons [see comment]. Gastroenterology 1996; 111:1178–81.

[50] Zauber AG, Winawer SJ. Initial management and follow-up surveillance of patients with colorectal adenomas. Gastroenterol Clin North Am 1997;26:85–101.

[51] Sipe BW, Rex DK, Latinovich D, et al. Propofol versus midazolam/meperidine for outpatient colonoscopy: administration by nurses supervised by endoscopists. Gastrointest Endosc 2002;55:815–25.

[52] Dafnis GM. Technical considerations and patient comfort in total colonoscopy with and without a transparent cap: initial experiences from a pilot study. Endoscopy 2000;32:381–4.

[53] Inoue H, Takeshita K, Hori H, et al. Endoscopic mucosal resection with a cap-fitted panendoscope for esophagus, stomach, and colon mucosal lesions. Gastrointest Endosc 1993;39:58–62.

[54] Tada M, Inoue H, Yabata E, et al. Colonic mucosal resection using a transparent cap-fitted endoscope. Gastrointest Endosc 1996;44:63–5.

[55] Rex DK, Chadalawada V, Helper DJ. Wide angle colonoscopy with a prototype instrument: impact on miss rates and efficiency as determined by back-to-back colonoscopies. Am J Gastroenterol 2003;98:2000–5.

[56] Brooker JC, Saunders BP, Shah SG, et al. Total colonic dye-spray increases the detection of diminutive adenomas during routine colonoscopy: a randomized controlled trial. Gastrointest Endosc 2002;56:333–8.

[57] Fujii T, Rembacken BJ, Dixon MF, et al. Flat adenomas in the United Kingdom: are treatable cancers being missed? Endoscopy 1998;30:437–43.

[58] Hurlstone DP, Cross SS, Adam I, et al. A prospective clinicopathological and endoscopic evaluation of flat and depressed colorectal lesions in the United Kingdom. Am J Gastroenterol 2003;98:2543–9.

[59] Hurlstone DP, Cross SS, Slater R, et al. Detecting diminutive colorectal lesions at colonoscopy: a randomised controlled trial of pan-colonic versus targeted chromoscopy. Gut 2004;53:376–80.

[60] Saitoh Y, Waxman I, West AB, et al. Prevalence and distinctive biologic features of flat colorectal adenomas in a North American population. Gastroenterology 2001;120:1657–65.

[61] Berkelhammer C, Ekambaram A, Silva RG. Low-volume oral colonoscopy bowel preparation: sodium phosphate and magnesium citrate. Gastrointest Endosc 2002;56:89–94.

[62] Rex DK, Chasen R, Pochapin MB. Safety and efficacy of two reduced dosing regimens of sodium phosphate tablets for preparation prior to colonoscopy. Aliment Pharmacol Ther 2002; 16:937–44.

[63] Rex DK, Cutler CS, Lemmel GT, et al. Colonoscopic miss rates of adenomas determined by back-to-back colonoscopies. Gastroenterology 1997;112:24–8.

[64] Pickhardt PJ, Nugent PA, Mysliwiec PA, et al. Location of adenomas missed by optical colonoscopy. Ann Intern Med 2004;141:352–9.

[65] Van Gelder RE, Nio CY, Florie J, et al. Computed tomographic colonography compared with colonoscopy in patients at increased risk for colorectal cancer. Gastroenterology 2004;127: 41–8.

[66] Rex DK. Colonoscopic withdrawal technique is associated with adenoma miss rates. Gastrointest Endosc 2000;51:33–6.

[67] Rex DK, Bond JH, Winawer S, et al. Quality in the technical performance of colonoscopy and the continuous quality improvement process for colonoscopy: recommendations of the US Multi-Society Task Force on Colorectal Cancer. Am J Gastroenterol 2002;97:1296–308.

[68] Winawer SJ, Stewart ET, Zauber AG, et al. A comparison of colonoscopy and double-contrast barium enema for surveillance after polypectomy. National Polyp Study Work Group. N Engl J Med 2000;342:1766–72.

[69] Fenlon HM, Nunes DP, Schroy III PC, et al. A comparison of virtual and conventional colonoscopy for the detection of colorectal polyps. N Engl J Med 1999;341:1496–503.

[70] Macari M, Bini EJ, Xue X, et al. Colorectal neoplasms: prospective comparison of thin-section low-dose multi-detector row CT colonography and conventional colonoscopy for detection. Radiology 2002;224:383–92.

[71] Mendelson RM, Foster NM, Edwards JT, et al. Virtual colonoscopy compared with conventional colonoscopy: a developing technology. Med J Aust 2000;173:472–5.

[72] Miao YM, Amin Z, Healy J, et al. A prospective single centre study comparing computed tomography pneumocolon against colonoscopy in the detection of colorectal neoplasms. Gut 2000;47:832–7.

[73] Pescatore P, Glucker T, Delarive J, et al. Diagnostic accuracy and interobserver agreement of CT colonography (virtual colonoscopy). Gut 2000;47:126–30.

[74] Pickhardt PJ, Choi JR, Hwang I, et al. Computed tomographic virtual colonoscopy to screen for colorectal neoplasia in asymptomatic adults. N Engl J Med 2003;349:2191–200.

[75] Rex DK, Vining D, Kopecky KK. An initial experience with screening for colon polyps using spiral CT with and without CT colography (virtual colonoscopy). Gastrointest Endosc 1999;50:309–13.

[76] Spinzi G, Belloni G, Martegani A, et al. Computed tomographic colonography and conventional colonoscopy for colon diseases: a prospective, blinded study. Am J Gastroenterol 2001; 96:394–400.

[77] Yee J, Akerkar GA, Hung RK, et al. Colorectal neoplasia: performance characteristics of CT colonography for detection in 300 patients. Radiology 2001;219:685–92.

[78] Cotton PB, Durkalski VL, Pineau BC, et al. Computed tomographic colonography (virtual colonoscopy): a multicenter comparison with standard colonoscopy for detection of colorectal neoplasia. JAMA 2004;291:1713–9.

[79] Akerkar GA, Yee J, Hung R, et al. Patient experience and preferences toward colon cancer screening: a comparison of virtual colonoscopy and conventional colonoscopy. Gastrointest Endosc 2001;54:310–5.

[80] Taylor SA, Halligan S, Saunders BP, et al. Acceptance by patients of multidetector CT colonography compared with barium enema examinations, flexible sigmoidoscopy, and colonoscopy. AJR Am J Roentgenol 2003;181:913–21.

[81] Hara AK, Johnson CD, MacCarty RL, et al. Incidental extracolonic findings at CT colonography. Radiology 2000;215:353–7.

[82] Ahlquist DA, Skoletsky JE, Boynton KA, et al. Colorectal cancer screening by detection of altered human DNA in stool: feasibility of a multitarget assay panel. Gastroenterology 2000; 119:1219–27.

[83] Rex DK. Colonoscopy: a review of its yield for cancers and adenomas by indication. Am J Gastroenterol 1995;90:353–65.

[84] Sonnenberg A, Delco F. Cost-effectiveness of a single colonoscopy in screening for colorectal cancer. Arch Intern Med 2002;162:163–8.

[85] Ness RM, Holmes AM, Klein R, et al. Cost-utility of one-time colonoscopic screening for colorectal cancer at various ages. Am J Gastroenterol 2000;95:1800–11.

[86] Lieberman DA, De Garmo PL, Fleischer DE, et al. Patterns of endoscopy use in the United States. Gastroenterology 2000;118:619–24.

[87] Rex DK, Lieberman DA. Feasibility of colonoscopy screening: discussion of issues and recommendations regarding implementation. Gastrointest Endosc 2001;54:662–7.

[88] Mysliwiec PA, Brown ML, Klabunde CN, et al. Are physicians doing too much colonoscopy? A national survey of colorectal surveillance after polypectomy. Ann Intern Med 2004;141:264–71.

[89] Baron JA, Beach M, Mandel JS, et al. Calcium supplements for the prevention of colorectal adenomas. Calcium Polyp Prevention Study Group. N Engl J Med 1999;340:101–7.

[90] Baron JA, Cole BF, Sandler RS, et al. A randomized trial of aspirin to prevent colorectal adenomas. N Engl J Med 2003;348:891–9.

[91] Bertario L, Russo A, Sala P, et al. Risk of colorectal cancer following colonoscopic polypectomy. Tumori 1999;85:157–62.

[92] Grossman S, Milos ML, Tekawa IS, et al. Colonoscopic screening of persons with suspected risk factors for colon cancer: II. Past history of colorectal neoplasms. Gastroenterology 1989; 96:299–306.

[93] Jorgensen OD, Kronborg O, Fenger C. A randomized surveillance study of patients with pedunculated and small sessile tubular and tubulovillous adenomas. The Funen Adenoma Follow-up Study. Scand J Gastroenterol 1995;30:686–92.

[94] Lotfi AM, Spencer RJ, Ilstrup DM, et al. Colorectal polyps and the risk of subsequent carcinoma. Mayo Clin Proc 1986;61:337–43.

[95] Martinez ME, Sampliner R, Marshall JR, et al. Adenoma characteristics as risk factors for recurrence of advanced adenomas. Gastroenterology 2001;120:1077–83.

[96] Noshirwani KC, van Stolk RU, Rybicki LA, et al. Adenoma size and number are predictive of adenoma recurrence: implications for surveillance colonoscopy. Gastrointest Endosc 2000; 51:433–7.

[97] Otchy DP, Ransohoff DF, Wolff BG, et al. Metachronous colon cancer in persons who have had a large adenomatous polyp. Am J Gastroenterol 1996;91:448–54.

[98] Spencer RJ, Melton III LJ, Ready RL, et al. Treatment of small colorectal polyps: a population-based study of the risk of subsequent carcinoma. Mayo Clin Proc 1984;59:305–10.

[99] van Stolk RU, Beck GJ, Baron JA, et al. Adenoma characteristics at first colonoscopy as predictors of adenoma recurrence and characteristics at follow-up. The Polyp Prevention Study Group. Gastroenterology 1998;115:13–8.

[100] Winawer SJ, Zauber AG, O'Brien MJ, et al. Randomized comparison of surveillance intervals after colonoscopic removal of newly diagnosed adenomatous polyps. The National Polyp Study Workgroup. N Engl J Med 1993;328:901–6.

[101] Bond JH. Polyp guideline: diagnosis, treatment, and surveillance for patients with colorectal polyps. Practice Parameters Committee of the American College of Gastroenterology. Am J Gastroenterol 2000;95:3053–63.

[102] Anthony T, Simmang C, Hyman N, et al. Practice parameters for the surveillance and follow-up of patients with colon and rectal cancer. Dis Colon Rectum 2004;47:807–17.

[103] Desch CE, Benson III AB, Smith TJ, et al. Recommended colorectal cancer surveillance guidelines by the American Society of Clinical Oncology. J Clin Oncol 1999;17:1312.

[104] Tate JJ, Rawlinson J, Royle GT, et al. Pre-operative or postoperative colonic examination for synchronous lesions in colorectal cancer. Br J Surg 1988;75:1016–8.

[105] Kjeldsen BJ, Kronborg O, Fenger C, et al. A prospective randomized study of follow-up after radical surgery for colorectal cancer. Br J Surg 1997;84:666–9.

[106] Makela JT, Laitinen SO, Kairaluoma MI. Five-year follow-up after radical surgery for colorectal cancer: results of a prospective randomized trial. Arch Surg 1995;130:1062–7.

[107] Ohlsson B, Breland U, Ekberg H, et al. Follow-up after curative surgery for colorectal carcinoma: randomized comparison with no follow-up. Dis Colon Rectum 1995;38:619–26.

[108] Pietra N, Sarli L, Costi R, et al. Role of follow-up in management of local recurrences of colorectal cancer: a prospective, randomized study. Dis Colon Rectum 1998;41:1127–33.

[109] Schoemaker D, Black R, Giles L, et al. Yearly colonoscopy, liver CT, and chest radiography do not influence 5-year survival of colorectal cancer patients. Gastroenterology 1998;114: 7–14.

[110] Secco GB, Fardelli R, Gianquinto D, et al. Efficacy and cost of risk-adapted follow-up in patients after colorectal cancer surgery: a prospective, randomized and controlled trial. Eur J Surg Oncol 2002;28:418–23.

[111] Renehan AG, Egger M, Saunders MP, et al. Impact on survival of intensive follow up after curative resection for colorectal cancer: systematic review and meta-analysis of randomised trials. BMJ 2002;324:813.

[112] Barillari P, Ramacciato G, Manetti G, et al. Surveillance of colorectal cancer: effectiveness of early detection of intraluminal recurrences on prognosis and survival of patients treated for cure. Dis Colon Rectum 1996;39:388–93.

[113] Brady PG, Straker RJ, Goldschmid S. Surveillance colonoscopy after resection for colon carcinoma. South Med J 1990;83:765–8.

[114] Green RJ, Metlay JP, Propert K, et al. Surveillance for second primary colorectal cancer after adjuvant chemotherapy: an analysis of Intergroup 0089. Ann Intern Med 2002;136:261–9.

[115] Kapiteijn E, Marijnen CA, Nagtegaal ID, et al. Preoperative radiotherapy combined with total mesorectal excision for resectable rectal cancer. N Engl J Med 2001;345:638–46.

[116] ESMO minimum clinical recommendations for diagnosis, adjuvant treatment and follow-up of colon cancer. Ann Oncol 2003;1:400–5.

[117] Berman JM, Cheung RJ, Weinberg DS. Surveillance after colorectal cancer resection. Lancet 2000;355:395–9.

[118] Lohnert MS, Doniec JM, Henne-Bruns D. Effectiveness of endoluminal sonography in the identification of occult local rectal cancer recurrences. Dis Colon Rectum 2000;43:483–91.

[119] Rotondano G, Esposito P, Pellecchia L, et al. Early detection of locally recurrent rectal cancer by endosonography. Br J Radiol 1997;70:567–71.

[120] Rex DK. Postpolypectomy and post-cancer resection surveillance. Rev Gastroenterol Disord 2003;3:202–9.

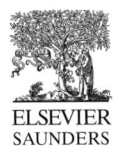

ELSEVIER
SAUNDERS

Gastrointest Endoscopy Clin N Am
15 (2005) 549–580

GASTROINTESTINAL
ENDOSCOPY CLINICS
OF NORTH AMERICA

Endoscopic Management of Familial Colonic Neoplasia

Yuki Young, MD, Jonathan P. Terdiman, MD*

Division of Gastroenterology, Department of Medicine, University of California, 2330 Post Street, Suite 610, San Francisco, CA 94115, USA

Although the major risk factors for sporadic colorectal cancer (CRC) are advancing age and environmental exposures, approximately 20% to 25% of cases occur in younger individuals or in those with a personal or family history of cancer, suggesting a heritable susceptibility [1]. The genetic predisposition to colorectal cancer falls into two major groups: (1) common familial colorectal cancer (15% to 20% of CRC) and (2) hereditary colorectal cancer (5% of CRC) [2]. In common familial CRC, first-degree relatives of persons with CRC or adenomatous polyps have an approximately twofold risk of developing colorectal cancer, and the risk increases with the number of relatives affected and the earlier the age of onset in the family [3]. A family history of extracolonic cancers (eg, uterine) or the presence in individual family members of multiple colorectal or other cancers also increases the risk. Increased risk for CRC in common familial CRC is conveyed by the inheritance of one or more of likely many possible low-penetrance susceptibility alleles, most of which have yet to be identified [4]. Carriage of these susceptibility alleles increases the risk of acquiring CRC, but the development of CRC is not certain. In the large majority of allele carriers, CRC does not occur. Common familial CRC are discussed in greater detail in a subsequent part of this article.

Nearly 5% of colorectal cancers are hereditary in etiology, meaning that they are caused by carriage of a highly penetrant, dominantly inherited, susceptibility allele. Hereditary colorectal cancer is conventionally divided between the polyposis syndromes and hereditary nonpolyposis colorectal cancer (Box 1) [2]. The polyposis syndromes are defined by the presence of multiple polyps in

---

* Corresponding author.
  E-mail address: jonathan.terdiman@ucsf.edu (J.P. Terdiman).

1052-5157/05/$ – see front matter © 2005 Elsevier Inc. All rights reserved.
doi:10.1016/j.giec.2005.03.007

giendo.theclinics.com

Box 1. Classification of hereditary colorectal cancer syndromes

Polyposis syndromes (< 1% of all colorectal cancers)
Adenomatous polyposis syndromes

• Familial adenomatous polyposis
    Gardner syndrome
    Turcot syndrome
    Attenuated adenomatous polyposis coli

Hamartomatous polyposis syndromes

• Peutz-Jeghers syndrome
• Juvenile polyposis
    Hereditary mixed polyposis syndrome
• Cowden syndrome
    Bannayan-Riley-Ruvalcaba syndrome
    Ruvulcaba-Myhre syndrome
    Bannayan-Zonana syndrome
    Soto syndrome
    Lhermitte-Duclos disease
• Gorlin syndrome

Hereditary nonpolyposis colorectal cancer (3% to 5% of all colorectal cancers)

• Lynch syndrome
• Muir-Torre syndrome
• Turcot syndrome

---

the gut lumen and have conventionally been categorized by polyp histology. The most common and important of the polyposis syndromes is familial adenomatous polyposis (FAP). The other major category of hereditary polyposes are the hamartomatous polyposis syndromes, most importantly Peutz-Jeghers syndrome, hereditary juvenile polyposis, Cowden syndrome, and a number of other rare hereditary polyposis syndromes.

Hereditary nonpolyposis rectal cancer (HNPCC) is much more common than any of the polyposis syndromes. At least 2% to 3% of all CRC is secondary to HNPCC [5,6]. In HNPCC, the lifetime risk of CRC approaches 70% to 80% but not as a consequence of an increased number of colorectal adenomas [7].

The primary importance of familial and hereditary colorectal cancer is the increased risk of CRC and, often, other cancer, for individuals with these conditions. Failure to recognize common familial CRC, or more importantly, one of the hereditary syndromes, leads to inadequate cancer screening and surveillance in individuals at risk, with subsequent premature loss of life. Recently, the elucidation of the genes responsible for many of these syndromes has revolutionized the care of at-risk individuals and families. Genetic testing has the potential to greatly improve the efficiency and reduce the costs and morbidity of cancer screening and surveillance. Genetic testing is commercially available and is the standard of care for individuals and families with or suspected of having FAP or HNPCC [8,9]. Genetic testing will ultimately make an impact on the management of individuals at risk for common familial colorectal cancer. However, genetic testing raises a number of vexing clinical, ethical, legal, and psychosocial questions.

This article discusses the clinical features, genetics, and management of common familial and hereditary colorectal cancer, specifically the polyposis syndromes and HNPCC.

Polyposis syndromes

Familial adenomatous polyposis

Clinical features: intestinal

FAP is an autosomal dominant disorder that affects about 1 in 10,000 to 15,000 individuals and accounts for probably <0.1% of colorectal cancers [10]. The diagnosis is made on the basis of the presence of >100 adenomatous colorectal polyps. In classic FAP, affected individuals develop hundreds to thousands of colonic adenomas by the mid to late teens, with over 95% of affected individuals demonstrating polyposis by 35 years of age. Colorectal cancer is inevitable in untreated patients, with the majority of cancers appearing by age 40 and over 90% by age 45 [11,12]. Variants of FAP are recognized in which polyps are greatly reduced in number, are predominantly or exclusively located in the right colon, and occur approximately a decade later than in classic FAP. This latter condition has been termed attenuated adenomatous polyposis coli (AAPC) or attenuated FAP and can have a lower cancer penetrance [13,14].

In addition to colonic polyps, up to 90% of individuals with FAP develop small bowel adenomas, most commonly at or near the ampulla of Vater [15–18]. These polyps are usually multiple and sessile, often forming carpet-like lesions. Because the ampulla of Vater is almost invariably involved, duodenoscopy, in addition to routine upper endoscopy, is required to assess the full extent of duodenal polyposis [19]. The lifetime risk for small bowel carcinoma is approximately 5%, and duodenal cancer is the leading cause of cancer death in patients with FAP who have undergone a colectomy [12,20–22]. Individuals with stage III or IV polyposis by the Spigelman classification, based on size and number of polyps and degree of dysplasia, are at greatest risk for periampullary/duodenal carcinoma [23].

Most patients with FAP develop gastric polyposis. Gastric polyps are usually of the fundic-gland histologic type, but adenomas rarely do occur [18]. Gastric carcinoma risk is not much increased in Western families but is reported to be increased three- to fourfold in Japanese and Korean families with FAP. Overall, the lifetime risk of gastric cancer in individuals with FAP has been reported at 0.5% [18]. The gastric adenoma is felt to be the precursor lesion for gastric cancer because fundic gland polyps are considered to have almost no malignant potential. There has been a case reported of gastric cancer arising in an area of fundic gland polyposis [24].

Clinical features: extra-intestinal

Approximately two thirds of FAP patients develop congenital hypertrophy of the retinal pigment epithelium (CHRPE). CHRPE lesions typically are flat, oval, and pigmented and are best detected by opthalmoscopy after pupillary dilation. In FAP, the lesions are usually multiple (≥ 4), bilateral, or large [25,26]. Although CHRPE does not affect vision and has no malignant potential, it is important as an early marker to identify susceptible individuals because it can be detected at birth. In CHRPE-positive families, nearly all individuals with FAP in the family have CHRPE. Thus, an examination of the fundus can identify susceptible family members at a young age [26].

Individuals with FAP are at increased risk for cancer at sites other than the colon and rectum and small bowel. Malignancies associated with FAP include hepatoblastoma in young children, medulloblastoma, papillary carcinoma of the thyroid, and pancreatic cancer [11,27,28]. The association of FAP and central nervous systems tumors, primarily medulloblastoma, has been termed Turcot syndrome [29,30]. The association of FAP and extra-intestinal lesions, such as desmoid tumors, sebaceous or epidermoid cysts, lipomas, osteomas, supernumerary teeth, and juvenile nasopharyngeal angiofibromas, has been termed Gardner syndrome.

Genetics

The great majority of cases of FAP are caused by a germ-line mutation of the tumor supressor *APC* gene located on chromosome 5q21 [31–33]. Normally, each individual has two functional copies of *APC*. Loss of *APC* function in a colonic epithelial cell by mutation of one gene copy and loss of the other is an early and critical genetic step in the development of most sporadic colorectal neoplasms. Owing to a germ-line mutation of *APC*, which usually is inherited from a parent but can occur spontaneously in about one third of cases, individuals with FAP have only one functional copy of the *APC* per cell, and initiation of colonic neoplasia is far more likely to occur, resulting in a dramatic increase in the number of colorectal adenomas and cancers. In some circumstances, mutation of one gene copy may be enough to eliminate *APC* function in a cell because the mutant *APC* gene product can interfere with the function of the wild-type gene product [34,35].

The APC protein is involved in the control of cellular proliferation, apoptosis, and cellular adhesion. APC mutations most commonly result in a truncated protein that cannot participate in the regulation of cytoplasmic β-catenin levels via APC-mediated degradation (in coordination with axin/conductin and glycogen synthase kinase 3β) [36–38]. Degradation of β-catenin prevents its translocation into the nucleus where it binds one of the T-cell factors to initiate transcription of genes that promote cellular proliferation and prevent cell death, such as *cyclin D* and *c-myc* [39,40].

Recently, a small number of cases of FAP have been attributed to inherited defects of the base excision repair gene *MYH* [41,42]. Germline *MYH* mutations must be biallelic to cause polyposis, so in this circumstance the adenomatous polyposis is the consequence of recessive rather than dominant inheritance, as it is with germline *APC* mutations. Mutations in *MYH* may account for some of the cases of FAP that occur without a family history that had previously been felt to be secondary to spontaneous germline mutations of *APC* [43].

Screening and surveillance

Colonic and extra-colonic screening and surveillance recommendations for FAP are summarized in Box 2 [2,44]. Endoscopic surveillance reduces the rates of colorectal cancer and mortality in FAP patients [45]. Individuals at risk for FAP should undergo annual flexible sigmoidoscopy beginning at age 10 to 12 years. Once adenomas have been identified, yearly colonscopy is required. Colectomy should be undertaken once any of the polyps is ≥5 mm or if any polyp biopsies demonstrate villous features or high-grade dysplasia. In families with suspected AAPC, surveillance should be undertaken with complete colonoscopy rather than sigmoidoscopy because of the proximal location of the polyps. Due to the later onset of polyposis in these families, some experts recommend that surveillance can sometimes be safely deferred until approximately 20 years of age. In our opinion, delaying the onset of surveillance in AAPC families can be problematic because of the phenotypic variability in such families.

All patients with FAP develop cancer of the colon or rectum. Three factors have led to a significant improvement in the prognosis of these patients: (1) The earlier identification of at-risk family members, (2) endoscopic screening of colonic polyps in the premalignant stage, and (3) definitive surgical treatment to eradicate the progression of colorectal polyposis to cancer. A total proctocolectomy with ileal pouch-anal anastomosis (IPAA) has increasingly become the operation of choice for FAP. This operation theorectically removes almost all of the mucosa at risk and obviates the need for a proctectomy in the future. Because the absolute risk estimate of developing polyps or cancer in the ileal pouch, ileoanal anastomosis, or anal transition zone is not known even when mucosectomy is performed, patients should undergo routine pouch surveillance [46,47]. After colectomy, ongoing surveillance is required. If the rectum is re-

Box 2. Options for cancer prevention in FAP for known or suspected gene mutation carriers

Primary recommendations

- Annual flexible sigmoidoscopy beginning by 10 to 12 years of age
- Annual colonoscopy, beginning by 20 years of age when attenuated FAP suspected
- Prophylactic colectomy in teen years or when polyps detected at colonoscopy
- Endoscopic surveillance every 4 to 6 months after ileorectal anastomosis and annually after ileoanal anastomosis
- Upper endoscopy, including duodenoscopy, every 6 months to 3 years starting by 20 to 25 years of age

Secondary recommendations

- Annual thyroid examination beginning by 10 to 12 years of age
- Annual palpation of liver during first decade of life (consider annual hepatic ultrasound and measure of alpha feto-protein)
- Consider serial MRI of brain in families with Turcot syndrome.
- Consider serial MRCP or endoscopic ultrasound in families with with multiple pancreatic cancers.
- Consider the use of sulindac or celecoxib chemoprevention in individuals with colorectal adenomas.

tained, endoscopic examination should be performed approximately every 6 to 12 months to remove or ablate any adenomas found. The risk of rectal cancer in individuals with FAP with an ileorectal anastomosis exceeds 10%, and nearly 20% of patients who undergo a colectomy with ileorectal anastomosis require completion proctectomy [48]. Even after IPAA, a substantial risk of the development of pouch adenomas exists, although the risk of developing invasive cancer seems to be low [47,49]. Therefore, endoscopic examination of the ileal pouch is recommended every 1 to 2 years.

The American Society for Gastrointestinal Endoscopy recommends surveillance for upper tract adenomas in patients with FAP. [19] Upper GI endoscopy and duodenoscopy, with biopsy of the ampulla of Vater, should be initiated once colonic adenomas have been identified or no later than 25 years of age [44]. Enteroscopy or enteroclysis are advocated by some experts to exclude small bowel adenoms distal to the duodenum, but significant lesions in the middle or distal small bowel are rare. The upper GI surveillance interval remains empirical, but generally screening should be undertaken every 1 to 3 years depending on the polyp burden. Once detected, upper tract adenomas can be removed or ablated by a variety of methods, although there are no data to show that this improves long-term outcomes [50–52]. If invasive cancer or high-risk adenomas are encountered (Spigelman stage IV), then operative resection is indicated. Surgical treatment of duodenal cancers results in high mortality from metastatic disease (46%), and even patients with severe adenomatosis are susceptible to death from metastatic disease (9%). Recurrence rates are high unless pancreas-sparing duodenectomy is performed. It is therefore important to treat these lesions before the detection of invasive cancer and to follow carefully for recurrences [53].

In addition to endoscopic screening, cancer prevention efforts in FAP may be augmented by chemoprevention with use of nonsteroidal anti-inflammatory drugs (NSAIDs) or cyclooxygenase 2 (COX-2) selective inhibitors. The NSAID sulindac and the COX-2 inhibitor celecoxib have been demonstrated to reduce the size and number of adenomas in individuals with FAP [54,55]. In a recent study, sulindac did not prevent the development of adenomas [56], but sulindac, celecoxib, and similar drugs may slow polyp progression [57]. They are unlikely to obviate the need for surgery.

Gene testing

Genetic testing for FAP is commercially available and is the standard of care for families suspected of having the syndrome [8,9]. Genetic counseling should be offered before genetic testing. The indications and strategy for FAP testing have been suggested by the American Gastroenterological Assocation based upon concensus expert opinion and are summarized in Fig. 1. Testing starts with a family member suspected of having FAP based on clinical presentation. If the disease-causing mutation can be identified, nonaffected family members can then be tested to determine if they carry the mutation. Family members proven not to have inherited the family mutation are spared burdensome screening and surveillance. If the mutation is not found in an affected person, it does not mean that FAP is not present but that the test is noninformative [58]. Because up to one third of individuals with FAP have a spontaneous germ-line *APC* mutation, testing should not be limited to members of classic FAP kindred. Individuals with the FAP phenotype but without a family history are also eligible for testing. Beause children can develop polyposis and therefore require cancer screening, predisposition testing of is appropriate, although this is best deferred until early adolescence [59,60]. Opthalmologic examinations of families with CHRPE can be used as a surrogate for genetic testing, but the validity of this approach to FAP screening has not been demonstrated. It may be difficult to determine whether an individual has the FAP phenotype and therefore merits testing, especially if the diagnosis of attenuated FAP is being considered. A finding of multiple polyps in an individual over 45 to 50 years of age, especially in the absence of a family history, is far more likely to be part of the spectrum of sporadic colonic neoplasms rather than FAP, but this remains an area of controversy. Some experts would test patients with 20 or more cumulative colorectal adenomas [2,9].

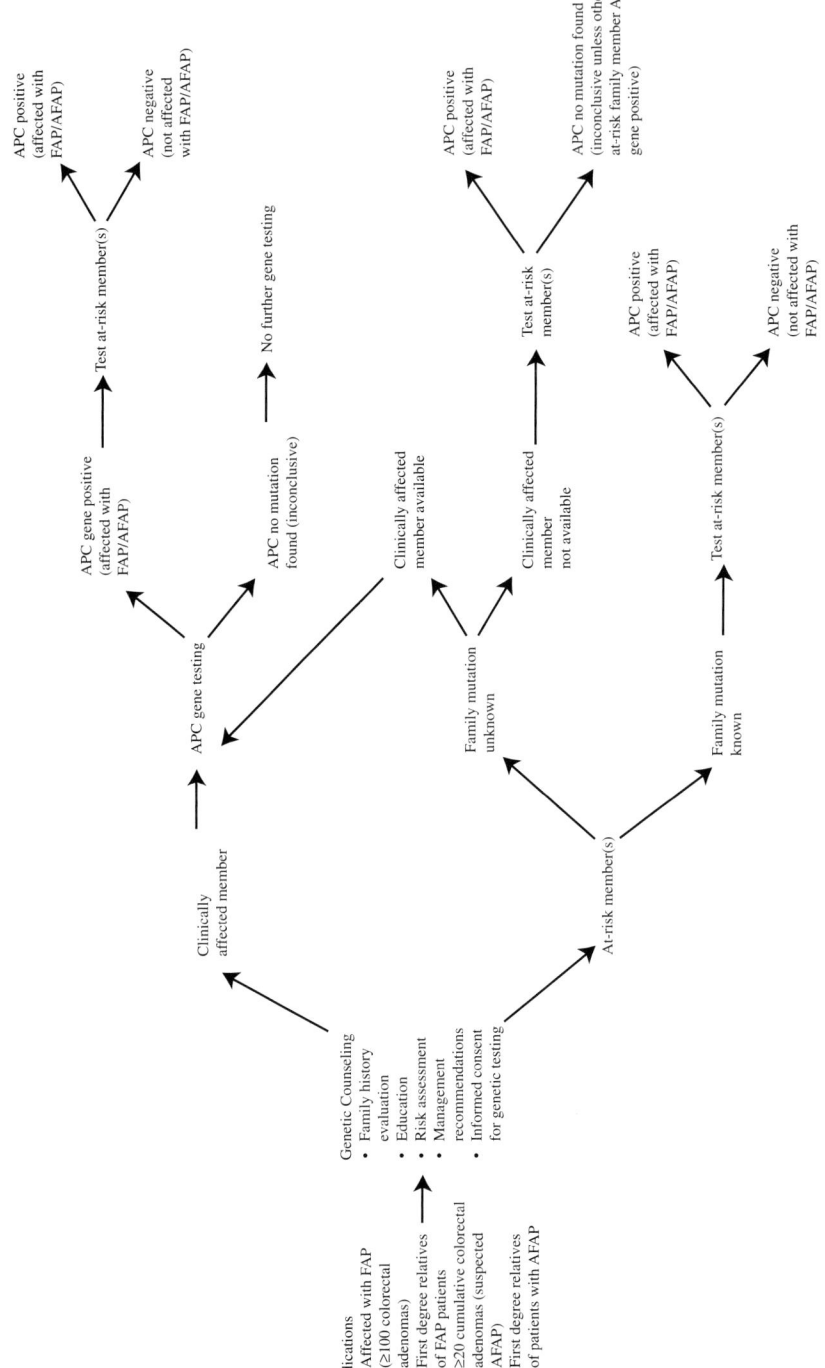

Hereditary hamartomatous polyp syndromes

Peutz-Jeghers syndrome

Clinical features

Peutz-Jeghers syndrome (PJS) is an autosomal dominantly inherited cancer predisposition syndrome characterized by the presence of numerous hamartomatous polyps in the GI tract and mucocutaneous pigmentation [61]. The syndrome is rare, occurring in approximately 1 in 200,000 births [11]. The classic mucocutaneous melanin pigment spots occur on the lips and buccal mucosa but can also be found on other areas of the skin, such as the dorsal and volar aspects of the hands and feet [62]. Pigment spots can be identified in 95% of patients with PJS, often from birth or early infancy. The spots can fade with age, and therefore the absence of typical pigmentation does not exclude the diagnosis. No malignant potential has been ascribed to the hyperpigmentation of PJS.

The predominant clinical feature of PJS is the presence of numerous GI harmartomatous polyps. The polyps have a distinctive histology with an arborizing pattern of smooth muscle in the lamina propria that distinguishes them from the hamartomas seen in juvenile polyposis or Cowden syndrome [63]. The polyps can be pedunculated or sessile, and they range in size from several millimeters to 3 to 4 cm. Polyps are seen in the stomach in approximately 40% of cases, in the small bowel in 80% (especially in the jejunum), and in the colon and rectum in 40% [62,63]. The polyps occur at a young age, and the typical age of diagnosis of PJS secondary to polyp complications is in the mid 20s. One third of PJS patients experience polyp-related symptoms by 10 years of age, and 50% to 60% have symptoms before 20 years of age [64].

Although the major complications related to PJS polyps are recurrent GI bleeding and obstruction, often secondary to intussusception, PJS is associated with high rates of intestinal and extra-intestinal cancer [65,66]. The majority of PJS-related deaths after 30 years of age are secondary to malignancy, and the lifetime risk of cancer in PJS approaches 90% [66]. Intestinal cancers may be secondary to the malignant degeneration of the hamartomatous polyps, and foci of dysplasia can sometimes be found in large PJS polyps [67]. The majority of intestinal cancers are adenocarcinomas, although an increased risk for malignant GI stromal tumors, such as leiomyosarcoma, exists. Extra-intestinal cancers are more common than intestinal cancers in PJS. The most common extra-intestinal cancer is cancer of the pancreas. Increased risk for cancer of the breast, ovary, lung, cervix, uterus, testes, and other organs has been documented [62,66]. In addition to the more common intestinal and extra-intestinal cancers, PJS is associated with an increased frequency of unusual neoplastic and non-neoplastic tumors of the genital tract. Most of these lesions occur in women, and

Fig. 1. FAP gene testing recommendations and strategy. (*From* American Gastroenterological Association Medical Position Statement. Hereditary colorectal cancer and genetic testing. Gastroenterology 2001;121:195–7; with permission.)

they are often small, bilateral, multifocal, and benign. The lesions include ovarian sex cord tumors with annular tubules, mucinous neoplasms of the ovary, mucinous metaplasia of the fallopian tube, and extremely well differentiated adenocarcinoma (adenoma malignum) of the cervix [11]. Men can develop rare Sertoli cell or testicular tumors of the seminiferous tubules.

Genetics

PJS is caused by a germline mutation in the tumor-supressor *STK11* gene (also called *LKB1*) located on 19p. The *STK11* gene product is a serine threonine kinase involved in the transduction of intracellular growth signals [68,69]. Mutations in *STK11* can be documented in about one half of PJS families. Some mutations may not be readily detectable by the methods generally used, but it is possible that some PJ families may be the consequence of germline mutations in other genes, possibly one or more of those in the STK11 molecular pathway [70]. As with FAP testing, if a pathogenic gene alteration can be detected in an affected family member, nonaffected family members can then be tested with essentially 100% accuracy.

Screening and surveillance

Genetic testing for PJS is not commercially available. At-risk first-degree relatives should be screened with an upper GI series and small bowel follow-through or upper endoscopy and push enteroscopy at least once during the second decade of life.

Box 3. Cancer prevention options in Peutz-Jeghers syndrome

- Upper endoscopy every 2 years starting at 10 to 15 years of age
- Enteroscopy/small bowel x-ray (small bowel follow-through or enteroclysis) every 2 years starting at 10 to 15 years of age
- Colonoscopy every 3 years starting at 15 to 20 years of age
- Removal of all polyps found >1 to 1.5 cm (by endoscopy methods or at laparatomy with intra-operative endoscopy)
- Endoscopic ultrasound or MRCP every 1 to 2 years starting at 30 years of age
- Annual breast examination and mammography starting at 25 years of age
- Annual pelvic examination, pap smear, transvaginal ultrasound, and CA-125 levels starting at 20 to 25 years of age
- Annual testicular examination starting at 10 years of age, with testicular ultrasound for onset of feminizing features

Although the lifetime risk of cancer in PJS is extremely high, the ability to reduce cancer incidence and cancer-related mortality in patients with PJS through intensive surveillance remains unproved. Surveillance guidelines for PJS remain empirical and have not been formally adopted by any of the major professional organizations (Box 3) [44,62,71]. Most experts recommend surveillance, and they further recommend that any intestinal polyps encountered, especially those >1 to 1.5 cm in size, be removed, even if that requires exploratory laparotomy and intraoperative endoscopy [72].

Juvenile polyposis

Clinical features

Juvenile polyps occur in about 2% of children. Typically, the polyps are few in number, with juvenile polyposis defined as the presence of 10 or more juvenile polyps. Approximately one third of cases of juvenile polyposis have a hereditary etiology, whereas the remainder is sporadic. Hereditary juvenile polyposis is rare, occurring in roughly 1 in 100, 000 individuals [71]. Histologically, juvenile polyps are hamartomas with a characteristic hyperplastic appearance of the surface epithelium, expansion of the lamina propria, and frequent cyst formation with mucus engorgement. The characteristic cystically dilated glands have led these polyps to be termed juvenile retention polyps [73]. The polyps can range in size from several millimeters to several centimeters, and they may be sessile or pedunculated (more often the latter). Juvenile polyps are most commonly found in the colon and rectum, but in hereditary juvenile polyposis, the polyps can be found throughout the GI tract and in the colon and rectum [74]. In contrast to individuals with sporadic juvenile polyps, those with hereditary juvenile polyposis continue to form polyps throughout their lifetime.

The primary clinical manifestation of juvenile polyposis is colorectal bleeding, but, as with the other hereditary hamartomatous polyp syndromes, juvenile polyposis is associated with an increased risk for colorectal cancer [75,76]. Increased cancer risk is not seen among individuals with sporadic juvenile polyps. The exact magnitude of the risk in hereditary juvenile polyposis remains uncertain but may approach that seen in FAP. Cancer risk is increased many-fold [77]. Colorectal cancer occurs in juvenile polyposis patients at a young age, often in the mid 30s [74,75]. Cancer arises from a juvenile polyp that has developed dysplastic/adenomatous features, and therefore increased cancer risk can extend to other segments of the bowel involved with polyps. Individuals with many polyps with mixed histologic features of juvenile polyps and adenomas are termed as having hereditary mixed polyposis sydrome. Colorectal cancer can occur in individuals with no prior evidence of dysplastic polyps [71]. It is not clear if there is an increased risk for extracolonic cancer in the absence of polyps in that segment of bowel or if there is an increased risk of extraintestinal (eg, pancreatic) cancer.

Genetics

Hereditary juvenile polyposis is an autosomal dominant disorder, and disease-causing germline mutations can be found in about 50% of patients. The majority of mutations are found in *SMAD4*, located on 18q, and commercial genetic testing is available [74,78–80]. *SMAD4* is a tumor suppressor gene of importance in the development of sporadic pancreatic, colorectal, and other cancers [81]. *SMAD4* is a critical component of the growth inhibitory TGF β signaling pathway [82]. Some juvenile polyposis families are found to have disease-causing mutations in the *PTEN* gene (see below) [83] or in the bone morpho-genetic protein receptor 1A (*BMPR1A*) gene [84]. *BMPR1A* is a serine-threonine kinase type receptor belonging to the superfamily of TGF β receptors involved in growth inhibitory signaling.

Screening and surveillance

Genetic testing for juvenile polyposis is not commercially available. No formal screening or surveillance recommendations exist for hereditary juvenile polyposis. In asymptomatic children from families with the syndrome, complete colonoscopy should commence in the early teen years and should be repeated every 1 to 3 years depending on the size and number of polyps found [44,71]. Polyps should be removed. In hereditary juvenile polyposis, as with all the hereditary polyposis syndromes, polyps continue to recur throughout the patient's lifetime, and intensive surveillance should continue until 70 years of age [44]. If the number of polyps is great, colectomy is indicated, especially if polyps with dysplastic features are encountered. At the time that colonic polyps are detected, upper endoscopy and small bowel contrast x-rays should be performed to look for extracolonic polyps. If none is found, repeat upper GI screening examinations may be performed approximately every 1 to 3 years [44,71].

Cowden syndrome

Clinical features

Cowden syndrome, also termed the gingival multiple hamartoma syndrome, is a rare syndrome (occurring 1 in 200,000 individuals) characterized by skin lesions, intestinal hamartomas, and an increased risk of cancer [11]. The syndrome is inheredited in an autosomal dominant fashion. It is most widely recognized on the basis of characteristic mucocutaneous lesions that include facial trichilem-momas, acral keratoses, café au lait spots, and verrucous papules of the oral mucosa, gingiva, and tongue. Subcutaneous lipomas and fibromas are common, as are benign thyroid nodules, uterine leiomyomas, and fibrocystic disease of the breast. The characteristic cutaneous lesions are found in approximately 85% of patients with Cowden syndrome. Sixty percent of patients with Cowden syndrome develop hamartomatous polyps of the GI tract [71,85]. The GI polyps most often resemble juvenile polyps, but other benign GI tract polyps can occur, including lipomas, ganglioneuromas, inflammatory polyps, and lymphoid hyperplasia [73]. Juvenile-type polyps that contain some neural elements are particularly characteristic of the syndrome.

The syndrome is often associated with congenital abnomalities (50% of the time) that include craniomegaly and mental retardation. Families with macrocephaly, lipomas, and pigmentation of the glans penis belong to the Bannayan-Ruvalcaba-Riley syndrome (syndrome variations have been termed Soto syndrome, Ruvalcaba-Myhre syndrome, Ruvalcaba-Myrhe-Smith syndrome, and Bannyan-Zonana syndrome), whereas families with glial mass in the cerebellum leading to altered gait and seizures belong to the subsyndrome called Lhermitte-Duclos disease [11].

Cowden syndrome is a cancer susceptibility syndrome, and cancer is the primary source of morbidity and mortality among affected individuals. The lifetime incidence of breast cancer among women with Cowden syndrome is 25% to 50%. The cancer often is bilateral and often has an early age of onset (median age 41 years) [11]. Individuals with Cowden syndrome also have a lifetime risk of follicular carcinoma of the thyroid that approaches 10%. Although many affected individuals have GI tract hamartomas, an excess of GI cancer risk has not been clearly described [71,85]. There is probably a modest increased risk for colorectal cancer among individuals with colorectal hamartomas. Increased risk of other cancers, including cancer of the skin, ovary, uterus, lung, or kidney, is likely present.

Genetics

Cowden syndrome and its associated subsyndromes are caused by a germline mutation in the tumor supressor gene *PTEN* on 10q [86,87]. *PTEN* is an intracellular tyrosine phosphatase that has been shown to be mutated in a significant percentage of sporadic tumors, including glioblastomas, prostate, thyroid, and kidney cancers. *PTEN* mutation testing is commercially available, and mutations can be detected in about 90% of affected individuals [11]. Principles of clinical genetic testing would mirror those in FAP, PJ, and hereditary juvenile polyposis.

Screening and surveillance

The major cancer morbidity from Cowden syndrome is secondary to breast cancer. Breast cancer surveillance should begin at age 20 years of age and should include monthly self-examination and yearly physician examination and mammography [11]. Annual thyroid examinations are recommended to start in the teens. No guidelines regarding GI screening or surveillance have been established [85]. Upon diagnosis, it makes sense to perform upper and lower GI endoscopy to look for GI polyps. Among individuals with GI polyps, regular surveillance and polypectomy should be perormed. Paients without polyps initially might undergo screening colonoscopy starting at 40 years of age, with repeat examinations every 3 to 5 years.

Hereditary nonpolyposis colorectal cancer

Clinical features

HNPCC, like FAP, is an autosomal dominant disorder characterized by the occurrence of multiple colorectal cancers in a family. HNPCC, also called the Lynch syndrome, accounts for approximately 1% to 5% of all CRC cases [6,7,88–91]. It is a misnomer because adenomatous polyps are the precursor of CRC in the syndrome. Unlike FAP, the number of polyps seems to be not much greater than in the general population, but the polyps are far more likely to be flat, to have villous features or high-grade dysplasia, and, more importantly, to grow rapidly and progress to invasive cancer [92–97]. Population-based data on HNPCC gene carriers are few, but individuals with HNPCC seem to have a lifetime risk of CRC of about 80% [98–101]. The mean age of onset of colorectal cancer in HNPCC is approximately 45 years, but colorectal cancer may appear in patients in their teens [93,102]. Furthermore, synchronous and metachronous colorectal cancer is far more common in HNPCC than in sporadic CRC. Synchronous cancers present in 5% to 20% of patients, and the rate of metachronous cancers approaches 1% to 3% per year, depending on the length of the colon remaining after initial resection [103]. This represents a many-fold increase in the rate of metachronous cancers compared with the sporadic colorectal cancer [104]. Compared with sporadic colorectal cancer, HNPCC cancers occur more commonly on the right side of the colon, are more poorly differentiated, and have other unusual histologic characteristics (most importantly, the presence of tumor-infiltrating lymphocytes) [105–107]. Nonetheless, several studies have found that survival is better than in sporadic cancer when matched for stage [108–110].

The risk for other cancers in HNPCC is greatly increased. For example, endometrial cancer occurs in 20% to 60% of women with HNPCC, as compared with 3% in the general population [98]. Individuals with HNPCC are at an increased risk of gastric, ovarian, small bowel, transitional cell (renal pelvis, ureter), sebaceous, central nervous system, and possibly other cancers (Table 1) [98,99, 101,111]. When HNPCC was first described in the 1920s, gastric cancer was the primary malignancy. The decreasing frequency of gastric cancers and increasing frequency of colorectal cancers in HNPCC kindred has mirrored this change in the general population in Western Europe and the United States [93,112]. Gastric cancer is still an important part of HNPCC in regions in which that cancer is endemic, such as Korea [113,114]. The occurrence of sebaceous adenomas, carcinomas, and keratoacanthomas in conjunction with HNPCC-related visceral malignancies define the Muir-Torre syndrome, a variant of HNPCC [115,116].

Table 1
Lifetime risk for cancer among HNPCC gene carriers

Cancer type	Lifetime risk (%)
Colorectal	70–80
Endometrial	20–60
Ovarian	10–12
Gastric	5–13
Renal pelvis/ureter/kidney	4–10
Biliary tract/gallbladder/pancreas	2–18
Small bowel	1–4
CNS (usually glioblastoma)	1–4

Some cases of Turcot syndrome are also variants of HNPCC, with glioblastoma as the associated central nervous system cancer [29,30].

Diagnostic criteria

Obtaining a personal and family cancer history from all patients is critical, and a high index of suspicion needs to be maintained if individuals with HNPCC are to be detected. Many diagnostic criteria have been proposed for HNPCC, the best known of which are the Amsterdam criteria [117]: (1) histologically verified colorectal cancer in three or more relatives, one of whom is a first-degree relative of the other two, having excluded familial adenomatous polyposis; (2) CRC involving at least two generations; and (3) one or more of the colorectal cancers diagnosed before 50 years of age. The criteria were designed specifically to facilitate research on HNPCC before the mutations responsible for the syndrome had been identified but are felt to be overly restrictive and insensitive [118–121]. In response to this problem, a number of other less stringent diagnostic criteria and guidelines for HNPCC have been promulgated, including the Amsterdam II criteria and the original and revised Bethesda guidelines (Table 2) [122–124]. At the heart of all of these criteria are certain basic features that are typical of HNPCC: early age of onset of colorectal or endometrial cancer (<50 years of age); multiple family member with colorectal, endometrial, or another HNPCC-related cancer; and multiple HNPCC-related cancers in the same individual. If one or more of these features is identified, the diagnosis of HNPCC should be considered. The personal and family cancer history need not be striking in cases of HNPCC detected in the general population, so vigilance is required.

Genetics

The genetic basis of HNPCC is a germline mutation in one of a set of genes responsible for DNA mismatch repair (MMR). The growing number of mismatch repair MMR genes includes *MSH2*, *MLH1*, *PMS1*, *PMS2*, *MSH3*, *MSH6*, and others [125–130]. Over 90% of the identified mutations are in two genes, *MSH2* and *MLH1*, located on chromosome 2p and 3p, respectively [131]. Nearly 5% to

Table 2
Clinical criteria for HNPCC

Name	Criteria
Amsterdam	There should be at least three relatives with CRC; all the following criteria should be present. One should be the first-degree relative of the other two. At least two successive generations should be affected. At least one CRC should be diagnosed before 50 years of age. Familial adenomatous polyposis should be excluded.
Amsterdam II	There should be at least three relatives with an HNPCC-associated cancer (CRC, cancer of the endometrium, small bowel, ureter, or renal pelvis); all the following criteria should be present. One should be the first-degree relative of the other two. At least two successive generations should be affected. At least one CRC should be diagnosed before 50 years of age. Familial adenomatous polyposis should be excluded.
Bethesda 1997	Individuals with cancer in families that meet the Amsterdam criteria [*Note: Three affected relatives with histologically verified colorectal cancer with one of them a first-degree relative of the other two and two affected generations and one member diagnosed with colorectal cancer before 50 years of age; FAP should be excluded*] Individuals with two HNPCC-related cancers, including synchronous and metachronous colorectal cancers or associated extracolonic cancers [*Note: Endometrial, ovarian, gastric, hepatobiliary or small bowel cancer or transitional cell carcinoma of the renal pelvis or ureter*] Individuals with colorectal cancer and a first-degree relative with colorectal cancer or HNPCC-related extracolonic cancer or a colorectal adenoma; one of the cancers diagnosed at >45 years of age, and the adenoma diagnosed at age >40 years of age Individuals with colorectal cancer or endometrial cancer diagnosed at >45 years of age Individuals with right-sided colorectal cancer with an undifferentiated pattern (solid/cribiform) on histopathology diagnosed at >45 years of age [*Note: Solid/cribiform defined as poorly differentiated or undifferentiated carcinoma composed of irregular, solid sheets of large eosinophilic cells and containing small gland-like spaces*] Individuals with signet-ring-cell-type colorectal cancer diagnosed at >45 years of age [*Note: Composed of 50% signet-ring cells*] Individuals with adenomas diagnosed at >40 years of age
Bethesda (revised 2004)	Colorectal cancer diagnosed in a patient >50 years of age Presence of synchronous, metachronous colorectal cancer or other HNPCC associated tumor, regardless of age [*Note: Stomach, ovarian, pancreas, ureter and renal pelvis, biliary tract, and brain, sebaceous gland adenomas and keratoacanthomas, and small bowel*] Colorectal cancer with MSI-high histology diagnosed in a patient >60 years of age. [*Note: Tumor infiltrating lymphocytes, Crohn's–like lymphocytic reaction, mucinous/signet ring differentiation, or medullary growth pattern*] Colorectal cancer diagnosed in at least one first-degree relative with an HNPCC-related tumor diagnosed at >50 years of age Colorectal cancer diagnosed in two or more first- or second-degree relatives with HNPCC related tumors, regardless of age

10% of HNPCC families, often with some atypical or attenuated features, are accounted for by a germline mutation in *MSH6* [130,132–137]. Persons with HNPCC have a nonfunctioning copy of the gene in the germline, usually through an inherited, or occasionally spontaneous, germline mutation. When the remaining working copy of the gene is inactivated by mutation, loss, or other mechanisms, the cell loses the ability to repair the inevitable mismatches of DNA base pairs during DNA replication and short insertion and deletion loops [138,139].

Particularly vulnerable to mutation during replication are DNA regions in which nucleotide bases are repeated several or many times. Called microsatellites, such DNA repeat sequences are distributed throughout the genome. More than 90% of colorectal cancers in HNPCC demonstrate multiple change-of-length mutations of these microsatellites, termed microsatellite instability (MSI) [140–142]. MSI is classified as being absent, low, or high, depending on the frequency of microsatellite mutation. The instability of HNPCC tumors is almost always high frequency [143,144]. Microsatellites are found in the coding regions of genes involved in growth regulation, such as the gene for the transforming growth factor β receptor type II and *BAX* [145–149]. A simple laboratory assay can detect the presence or absence and degree of MSI in tumor tissue using a standard set of microsatellite markers. In addition, tumors that have lost the function of one of the mismatch repair genes show negative staining for the protein product of that gene by immunohistochemistry. Staining tumors for MSH2 or mLH1 also may aide in the diagnosis of HNPCC [150–153].

Surveillance and treatment

Recommendations for surveillance in individuals with known or suspected HNPCC are summarized in Box 4. Colonoscopy is recommended every 1 to 2 years staring at 20 to 25 years of age, or at least 10 years before the earliest age of cancer in the family [154]. Complete colonoscopy is essential because of the preponderance of right-sided tumors in HNPCC. Colonoscopy needs to be repeated frequently because of the accelerated rate at which adenomas transform into invasive cancer in HNPCC. Colonoscopic surveillance is of demonstrated efficacy in HNPCC. Individuals who undergo regular total colonic surveillance have a markedly lower incidence of CRC, CRC-related mortality, and all cause mortality than those not undergoing regular surveillance [155], and surveillance is cost-effective [156,157]. With respect to treatment for colon cancers associated with HNPCC, many experts advocate total abdominal colectomy with ileorectal anastomosis (IRA) at the time of the initial cancer resection because of the high rate of metachronous tumors [44,158]. What seems to be most important is adequate postoperative surveillance, rather than the extent of the initial resection [157]. Unless patients are diagnosed with synchronous cancers or if they cannot be relied upon to follow-up for colonoscopic surveillance, a partial colectomy can be offered. As with FAP, the rate of rectal cancer in HNPCC can exceed 10% over an extended follow-up period, so ongoing surveillance is essential, even if an IRA is performed [159]. When adenomas are encountered during surveillance

---

Box 4. Options for cancer prevention in HNPCC for known or suspected gene mutation carriers

Primary recommendations

- Colonoscopy every 1 to 2 years beginning at 20 to 25 years of age (or 10 years before the earliest diagnosis of colorectal cancer in the family, whichever comes first) until 40 years of age and then annual colonoscopy
- Annual transvaginal ultrasound with color Doppler or endometrial aspirate beginning at 25 to 35 years of age

Secondary recommendations

- Consider total abdominal colectomy with ileorectal anastomosis at diagnosis of colorectal cancer.
- Consider prophylactic hysterectomy and oopherectomy in known gene carriers at time of colonic operation or after child bearing is complete.
- Consider annual measure of CA-125 level.
- Consider serial upper endoscopy among families with gastric cancer.
- Consider annual urine cytology or CT urogram among families with urinary tract cancers.

---

colonoscopy, they are removed endoscopically using standard techniques, and in general, colonoscopic surveillance is continued. HNPCC-related polyps are often sessile, so adequate endoscopic resection can be difficult to perform. If there is any doubt, one should proceed with operative resection.

In addition to colorectal cancer surveillance, surveillance for endometrial cancer is recommended for individuals at risk for HNPCC [160]. There is no consensus on the optimal method of surveillance, but choices include yearly endometrial biopsy or yearly transvaginal ultrasound, which also serves as a surveillance test for ovarian cancer, especially if coupled with regular (every 6 to 12 months) determination of CA-125 levels. Surveillance for other HNPCC-related cancers is not recommended generally. Recommendations should be tailored to the tumors appearing in the family being treated. For example, genitourinary cancers may be screened by periodic urine cytology and gastric cancer by upper GI endoscopy. The need for and efficacy of surveillance for extracolonic cancer in HNPCC remains unproved [161,162].

Because of the high risk of endometrial and ovarian cancer, some experts have advocated prophylactic hysterectomy and oophorectomy for women beyond the age of child bearing, especially if they are undergoing a colonic resection

Table 3
Likelihood of detecting a germline *MSH2* or *MLH1* mutatation depending on family history and tumor MSI status

Clinical criteria met	Likelihood of detecting a mutation (%)
Amsterdam criteria met	40–70
Amsterdam criteria met and MSI-H tumor	80
Near Amsterdam criteria met[a]	20–50
Near Amsterdam and MSI-H tumor	50–60
Bethesda guidelines met	30
Bethesda guidelines met and MSI-H tumor	50
Early onset CRC w/o family history	0–30
Early onset CRC and MSI-H tumor	30
Sporadic CRC	<1
Sporadic CRC with MSI-H tumor	10

[a] Meeting all except one of the Amsterdam criteria.

for colorectal cancer. A recent panel of experts, however, found insufficient evidence to recommend for or against prophylactic hysterectomy and oophorectomy [163].

Genetic testing

As with FAP, genetic testing is a standard part of the care of individuals and families at risk for HNPCC [8,59]. However, determining when genetic testing is indicated for HNPCC is a far more difficult problem than in FAP because individuals with HNPCC do not have a unique phenotype to help establish the clinical diagnosis. Some investigators have suggested direct germline *MSH2* and *MLH1* testing of colorectal cancer patients who meet appropriate and fairly stringent clinical criteria, such as Amsterdam criteria, Amsterdam II criteria, or the first three Bethesda guidelines [118,119]. The likelihood of detecting a germline *MSH2* or *MLH1* mutation based on clinical criteria met is summarized in Table 3. Other investigators have suggested that tumor MSI testing or MSH2/MLH1 protein inmmunohistochemistry should be performed first and that germline testing be reserved for those found to have MSI-H tumors or those with loss of mismatch repair protein expression [121,123,153,164]. The

Table 4
Appropriate interpretation of genetic test results

Proband result	Family member result	Interpretation
Positive	Positive	Positive
Positive	Negative	Negative
Negative	Do not test	Not informative[a]
Ambiguous	Do not test	Not informative[a]

[a] Must assume that family member carries the deleterious gene given the inability to prove otherwise because of the negative test in the proband. Proceed with cancer screening appropriate for a gene carrier in the family member.

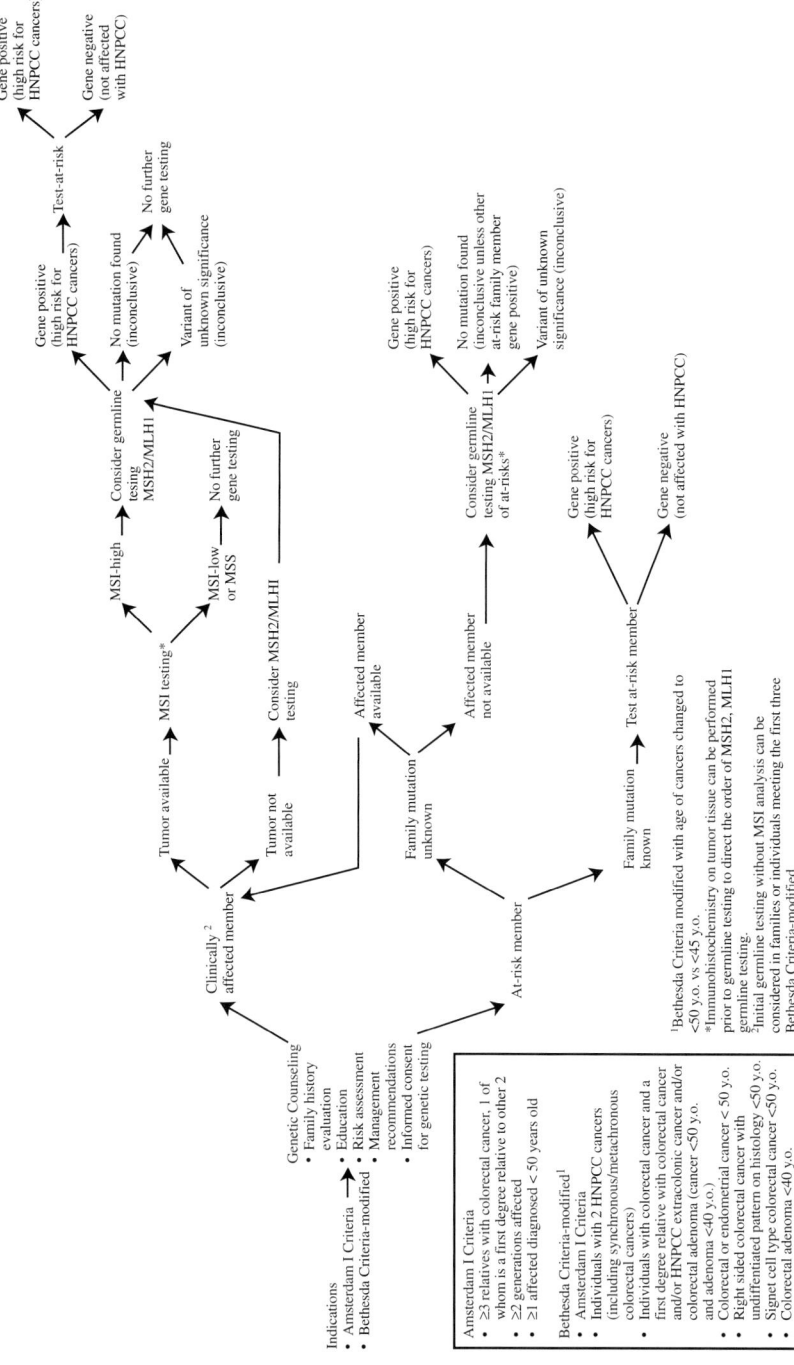

Indications
• Amsterdam I Criteria
• Bethesda Criteria-modified

Genetic Counseling
• Family history
  evaluation
• Education
• Risk assessment
• Management
  recommendations
• Informed consent
  for genetic testing

Amsterdam I Criteria
• ≥3 relatives with colorectal cancer, 1 of
  whom is a first degree relative to other 2
• ≥2 generations affected
• ≥1 affected diagnosed < 50 years old

Bethesda Criteria-modified[1]
• Amsterdam I Criteria
• Individuals with 2 HNPCC cancers
  (including synchronous/metachronous
  colorectal cancers)
• Individuals with colorectal cancer and a
  first degree relative with colorectal cancer
  and/or HNPCC extracolonic cancer and/or
  colorectal adenoma (cancer <50 y.o.
  and adenoma <40 y.o.)
• Colorectal or endometrial cancer < 50 y.o.
• Right sided colorectal cancer with
  undiffentiated pattern on histology <50 y.o.
• Signet cell type colorectal cancer <50 y.o.
• Colorectal adenoma <40 y.o.

[1]Bethesda Criteria modified with age of cancers changed to
<50 y.o. vs <45 y.o.
*Immunohistochemistry on tumor tissue can be performed
prior to germline testing to direct the order of MSH2, MLH1
germline testing.
[2]Initial germline testing without MSI analysis can be
considered in families or individuals meeting the first three
Bethesda Criteria-modified

decision to perform tumor MSI or immunohistochemistry testing is based on clinical criteria, although these criteria are often less stringent than those used to decide for germline testing, such as modified Bethesda guidelines [9]. The likelihood of detecting a germline mutation after a positive tumor MSI test also is summarized in Table 3.

Once a germline mutation is detected in the affected proband, germline testing can be performed in other family members. In this situation, if family members are found not to carry the family mutation, their result is considered a true negative, and their risk for cancer is that of the general population. As with FAP, if a mutation is not detected in a family suspected of having HNPCC, the test result is not informative. Failure to detect a mutation in a family without a known mutation does not mean that the family does not have HNPCC (Table 4).

The indications and strategy for HNPCC gene testing are summarized in Fig. 2 [8].

Common familial colorectal cancer

Clinical features

The rare hereditary syndromes, such as FAP and HNPCC, confer the highest risks of colon cancer; however, these entities account for no more than 5% of all colorectal cancers. Nevertheless, familial history is an important risk factor in the development of CRC, suggesting a critical hereditary component in upward of 25% of cases [2,165]. The magnitude of the risk depends on the number of first-degree relatives affected and the age at diagnosis (Table 5) [3]. In a recent meta-analysis, individuals with a single first-degree relative with colorectal cancer have a risk about 2.25 times that in the general population. Individuals with more than one first-degree relative with colorectal cancer have a risk about 4.25 times that in the general population, and individuals with a relative diagnosed with colorectal cancer before the age of 45 have a risk about 4 times higher than the general population [4]. Individuals with a first-degree relative with colorectal adenoma also have a risk of colon cancer about twice that in the general population [166]. Colon cancer in a second- or third-degree relative increases colon cancer risk, but only about 50% above average risk [154]. Individuals with a first-degree relative with a family history of colon cancer have a colon cancer risk at age 40, which is similar to the general population risk at age 50 [154,167]. Although family history of CRC increases an individual's risk for the disease, especially at a younger age than seen in pure sporadic cancer, there is no convincing evidence that the clinical presentation

Fig. 2. HNPCC gene testing recommendations and strategy. (*From* American Gastroenterological Association Medical Position Statement. Hereditary colorectal cancer and genetic testing. Gastroenterology 2001;121:195–7; with permission.)

Table 5
Risk for colorectal cancer based on family history

Family history	Lifetime risk for colorectal cancer
No family history	3–6%
One first degree relative with CRC	2- to 3-fold increased risk
One first degree relative with CRC <50 years of age	3- to 5-fold increased risk
Two first degree relatives with CRC	3- to 5-fold increased risk
One second or third degree relative with CRC	1.5-fold increased risk
Two second or third degree relative with CRC	2- to 3-fold increased risk
One first degree relative with adenoma	1.5- to 2-fold increased risk

of these common familial colorectal cancers differs in important ways from sporadic CRC with respect to features such as tumor location or aggressiveness.

Genetics

The gene alterations responsible for common familial colorectal cancer are being discovered in increasingly greater numbers, although for the most part these cancer susceptibility alleles remain unknown [1,4]. Kindred studies suggest that these genes are dominantly inherited, but unlike in true hereditary colorectal cancer, the altered genes that cause familial colorectal cancer are generally low penetrance [168]. Thus, inheriting a disease susceptibility gene increases one's risk for colorectal cancer but does not guarantee that the disease will occur. Candidate susceptibility alleles are many and include minor mutations in the same genes that cause hereditary colorectal cancer. An example of this is the *I1307K* allele of *APC* found in Ashkenazi Jews [169]. The protein product of the allele is full length and functional but is 30 times more likely to mutate than the wild-type allele, most commonly through an insertion that leads to APC protein truncation [170,171]. Inheritance of this unstable *APC* allele increases the chance of developing colorectal cancer by approximately 1.5- to 2-fold, rather than the near 100% risk of colorectal cancer that occurs in classic FAP [172]. A recent, large, community-based study of Ashkenazi Jews estimated that by 70 years of age, 5.1% of allele carriers develop CRC, compared with 3.1% of noncarriers [172]. It seems that the magnitude of increased risk conferred by carriage of *APC I1307K* is low to modest, and there is little evidence that the adenomas or CRC in those with *I1307K* appears at an earlier age or differs in presentation or prognosis from sporadic forms [173–179]. Nevertheless, even a small increase in CRC risk conferred by a gene that is common in a particular population has important implications for that population.

The *I1307K APC* allele is one example of the minor colorectal cancer susceptibility genes that will be identified with increasing frequency in the future. Other colorectal cancer predisposition alleles likely include one of a number of variants of genes involved in carcinogen metabolism or certain inherited alleles of many of the oncogenes and tumor suppressor genes involved in the molecular progression of sporadic colorectal cancer [1,4,180]. Colorectal cancer resistance genes will likely be described as well. The particular combination of minor susceptibility and resistance genes a person inherits will prove to be a major determinant of the differing risk of CRC between individuals.

Surveillance and treatment

Several screening recommendations for individuals with familial risk have been published. A recent task force, comprising several different professional organizations, recommended that colorectal cancer screening in individuals with a family history of CRC or adenomatous polyps start with a colonoscopy at 40 years of age or 10 years younger than the earliest familial diagnosis, whichever comes first [154]. Colonoscopy screening intervals depend on the age and number of family members involved. Individuals with a single first-degree relative initially diagnosed at age <60 years or two first-degree relatives with adenomas or CRC should have minimum screening intervals of 5 years [154]. Individuals with a first-degree relative diagnosed at age ≥60 years or two second-degree relatives with adenomas or CRC may undergo 10-year screening intervals if colonoscopy is normal. Screening options for the general population include yearly fecal occult blood testing, flexible sigmoidoscopy every 5 years, or both, or air-contrast barium enema every 5 years, or colonoscopy every 10 years [154]. Earlier guidelines from the American College of Gastroenterology were similar, recommending that individuals with a strong family history of colon cancer (eg, those with multiple first-degree relatives with colorectal cancer) or a single first-degree relative with cancer diagnosed age <60 years should undergo screening colonoscopy starting at 40 years of age or 10 years younger than the age at diagnosis of the youngest affected relative. They recommend that colonoscopy be repeated at 3- to 5-year intervals [181]. The United States Preventive Services Task Force does not address familial risk outside of the hereditary syndromes [182]. Treatment of colon and rectal cancer in this setting involves partial colectomy with close surveillance of the residual colon and rectum thereafter.

Summary

Heredity plays an important causative role in a large percentage of colorectal cancers. The clinician must maintain a high index of suspicion for familial colon cancer syndromes when colonic neoplasia is diagnosed in a patient who is unusually young, when multiple tumors develop in a single organ or paired organs, when family history of cancer of the same type is present in one or more first-degree relatives, when a high rate of cancer occurs in the family, or when cancer occurs in an individual or within a family with congenital anomalies or birth defects. Clinical recognition of the hereditary polyposis syndromes, hereditary nonpolyposis colorectal cancer, and common familial colorectal cancer is essential because screening, surveillance, and treatment among affected individuals and their family members differ from that recommended to the general population. More intensive cancer screening and surveillance is required if premature death is to be avoided. Genetic testing is commercially available for most of the hereditary colorectal cancer syndromes and can greatly facilitate the management of patients if properly undertaken.

References

[1] Calvert PM, Frucht H. The genetics of colorectal cancer. Ann Intern Med 2002;137:603–12.
[2] Burt RW. Colon cancer screening. Gastroenterology 2000;119:837–53.
[3] Johns LE, Houlston RS. A systematic review and meta-analysis of familial colorectal cancer risk. Am J Gastroenterol 2001;96:2992–3003.
[4] Houlston RS, Tomlinson IP. Polymorphisms and colorectal tumor risk. Gastroenterology 2001;121:282–301.
[5] Samowitz WS, Curtin K, Lin H, et al. The colon cancer burden of genetically defined hereditary nonpolyposis colon cancer. Gastroenterology 2001;121:830–8.
[6] Salovaara R, Loukola A, Kristo P, et al. Population-based molecular detection of hereditary nonpolyposis colorectal cancer. J Clin Oncol 2000;18:2193–200.
[7] Terdiman JP, Conrad PG, Sleisenger MH. Genetic testing in hereditary colorectal cancer: indications and procedures. Am J Gastroenterol 1999;94:2344–56.
[8] American Gastroenterological Association Medical Position Statement. Hereditary colorectal cancer and genetic testing. Gastroenterology 2001;121:195–7.
[9] Giardiello FM, Brensinger JD, Petersen GM. AGA technical review on hereditary colorectal cancer and genetic testing. Gastroenterology 2001;121:198–213.
[10] Bisgaard ML, Fenger K, Bulow S, et al. Familial adenomatous polyposis (FAP): frequency, penetrance and mutation rate. Hum Mutat 1994;3:121–5.
[11] Lindor NM, Greene MH. The concise handbook of family cancer syndromes. Mayo Familial Cancer Program. J Natl Cancer Inst 1998;90:1039–71.
[12] Galle TS, Juel K, Bulow S. Causes of death in familial adenomatous polyposis. Scand J Gastroenterol 1999;34:808–12.
[13] Spirio L, Olschwang S, Groden J, et al. Alleles of the APC gene: an attenuated form of familial polyposis. Cell 1993;75:951–7.
[14] Lynch HT, Smyrk T, McGinn T, et al. Attenuated familial adenomatous polyposis (AFAP): a phenotypically and genotypically distinctive variant of FAP. Cancer 1995;76:2427–33.
[15] Church JM, McGannon E, Hull-Boiner S, et al. Gastroduodenal polyps in patients with familial adenomatous polyposis. Dis Colon Rectum 1992;35:1170–3.
[16] Campbell WJ, Spence RA, Parks TG. Familial adenomatous polyposis. Br J Surg 1994;81: 1722–33.
[17] Offerhaus GJ, Giardiello FM, Krush AJ, et al. The risk of upper gastrointestinal cancer in familial adenomatous polyposis. Gastroenterology 1992;102:1980–2.
[18] Wallace MH, Phillips RK. Upper gastrointestinal disease in patients with familial adenomatous polyposis. Br J Surg 1998;85:742–50.
[19] Saurin JC, Chayvialle JA, Ponchon T. Management of duodenal adenomas in familial adenomatous polyposis. Endoscopy 1999;31:472–8.
[20] Belchetz LA, Berk T, Bapat BV, et al. Changing causes of mortality om patients with familial adenomatous polyposis. Dis Colon Rectum 1996;39:384–7.
[21] Bjork J, Akerbrant H, Iselius L, et al. Periampullary adenomas and the adenocarcinomas in familial adenomatous polyposis: cumulative risks and APC gene mutations. Gastroenterology 2001;121:1127–35.
[22] Kadmon M, Tandara A, Herfath C. Duodenal adenomatosis in familial adenomatous polyposis coli: a review of the literature and results from the Heidelberg Polyposis Register. Int J Colorectal Dis 2001;16:63–75.

[23] Burke W, Daly M, Garber J, et al. Recommendations for follow-up care of individuals with an inherited predisposition to cancer. II. BRCA1 and BRCA2. Cancer Genetics Studies Consortium. JAMA 1997;277:997–1003.

[24] Hofgartner WT, Thorp M, Ramus MW, et al. Gastric adenocarcinoma associated with fundic gland polyps in a patient with attenuated familial adenomatous polyposis. Am J Gastroenterol 1999;94:2275–81.

[25] Tiret A, Taiel-Sartral M, Tiret E, et al. Diagnostic value of fundus examination in familial adenomatous polyposis. Br J Ophthalmol 1997;81:755–8.

[26] Ruhswurm I, Zehetmayer M, Dejaco C, et al. Ophthalmic and genetic screening in pedigrees with familial adenomatous polyposis. Am J Ophthalmol 1998;125:680–6.

[27] Giardiello FM, Offerhaus GJA, Lee DH, et al. Increased risk of thyroid and pancreatic carcinoma in familial adenomatous polyposis. Gut 1993;34:1394–6.

[28] Cetta F, Montalto G, Gori M, et al. Germline mutations of the APC gene in patients with familial adenomatous polyposis-associated thyroid carcinoma: results for a European cooperative study. J Clin Endocrinol Metab 2000;85:286–92.

[29] Hamilton SR, Liu B, Parsons RE, et al. The molecular basis of Turcot's syndrome. N Engl J Med 1995;332:839–47.

[30] Paraf F, Jothy S, Van Meir EG. Brain tumor-polyposis syndrome: two genetic diseases? J Clin Oncol 1997;15:2744–58.

[31] Kinzler KW, Nilbert MC, Su LK, et al. Identification of FAP locus genes from chromosome 5q21. Science 1991;253:661–5.

[32] Groden J, Thliveris A, Samowitz W, et al. Identification and characterization of the familial adenomatous polyposis coli gene. Cell 1991;66:589–600.

[33] Miyoshi Y, Ando H, Nagase H, et al. Germ-line mutations of the APC gene in 53 familial adenomatous polyposis patients. Proc Natl Acad Sci USA 1992;89:4452–6.

[34] Polakis P. The adenomatous polyposis coli (APC) tumor suppressor. Biochim Biophys Acta 1997;1332:F127–47.

[35] Dihlmann S, Gebert J, Siermann A, et al. Dominant negative effect of the APC 1309 mutation: a possible explanation for genotype-phenotype correlations in familial adenomatous polyposis. Cancer Res 1999;59:1857–60.

[36] Bullions LC, Levine AJ. The role of beta-catenin in cell adhesion, signal transduction, and cancer. Curr Opin Oncol 1998;10:81–7.

[37] Behrens J, Jerchow BA, Wurtele M, et al. Functional interaction of an axin homolog, conductin, with beta- catenin, APC, and GSK3beta. Science 1998;280:596–9.

[38] Kishida S, Yamamoto H, Ikeda S, et al. Axin, a negative regulator of the wnt signaling pathway, directly interacts with adenomatous polyposis coli and regulates the stabilization of beta-catenin. J Biol Chem 1998;273:10823–6.

[39] He TC, Sparks AB, Rago C, et al. Identification of c-MYC as a target of the APC pathway. Science 1998;281:1509–12.

[40] Tetsu O, McCormick F. Beta-catenin regulates expression of cyclin D1 in colon carcinoma cells. Nature 1999;398:422–6.

[41] Jones S, Emmerson P, Maynard J, et al. Biallelic germline mutations in MYH predispose to multiple colorectal adenoma and somatic G:C to T:A mutations. Hum Mol Genet 2002;11:2961–7.

[42] Sieber OM, Lipton L, Crabtree M, et al. Multiple colorectal adenomas, classic adenomatous polyposis, and germ-line mutations in MYH. N Engl J Med 2003;348:791–9.

[43] Venesio T, Molatore S, Cattaneo F, et al. High frequency of MYH gene mutations in a subset of patients with familial adenomatous polyposis. Gastroenterology 2004;126:1681–5.

[44] Dunlop MG. Guidance on gastrointestinal surveillance for hereditary nonpolyposis colorectal cancer, familial adenomatous polyposis, juvenile polyposis, and Peutz-Jeghers syndrome. Gut 2002;51:v21–7.

[45] Heiskanen I, Luostarinen T, Jarvinen HJ. Impact of screening examinations on survival in familial adenomatous polyposis. Scand J Gastroenterol 2000;35:1284–7.

[46] Remzi FH, Church JM, Bast J, et al. Mucosectomy vs. stapled ileal pouch-anal anastomosis in

patients with familial adenomatous polyposis: functional outcome and neoplasia control. Dis Colon Rectum 2001;44:1590–6.

[47] van Duijvendijk P, Vasen HFA, Betario L, et al. Cumulative risk of developing polyps or malignancy at the ileal pouch-anal anastomosis in patients with familial adenomatous polyposis. J Gastrointest Surg 1999;3:325–30.

[48] Betario L, Russo A, Radice P, et al. Genotype and phenotype factors as determinants for rectal stump cancer in patients with familial adenomatous polyposis. Ann Surg 2000;231: 538–43.

[49] Wu JS, McGannon EA, Church JM. Incidence of neoplastic polyps in the ileal pouch of patients with familial adenomatous polyposis after restorative proctocolectomy. Dis Colon Rectum 1998;41:552–6 [discussion 556–7].

[50] Alacorn FJ, Burke CA, Church JM, et al. Familial adenomatous polyposis: efficacy of endoscopic and surgical treatment for advanced duodenal adenomas. Dis Colon Rectum 1999;42: 1533–6.

[51] Heiskanen I, Kellokumpu I, Jarvinen H. Management of duodenal adenomas in 98 patients with familial adenomatous polyposis. Endoscopy 1999;31:412–6.

[52] Norton ID, Geller A, Petersen BT, et al. Endoscopic surveillance and ablative therapy for periampullary adenomas. Am J Gastroenterol 2001;96:101–6.

[53] de Vos tot Nederveen Cappel WH, Jarvinen HJ, Bjork J, et al. Worldwide survey among polyposis registries of surgical management of severe duodenal adenomatosis in familial adenomatous polyposis. Br J Surg 2003;90:705–10.

[54] Giardiello FM, Hamilton SR, Krush AJ, et al. Treatment of colonic and rectal adenomas with sulindac in familial adenomatous polyposis. N Engl J Med 1993;328:1313–6.

[55] Steinbach G, Lynch PM, Phillips RK, et al. The effect of celecoxib, a cyclooxygenase-2 inhibitor, in familial adenomatous polyposis. N Engl J Med 2000;342:1946–52.

[56] Giardiello FM, Yang VW, Hylind LM, et al. Primary chemoprevention of familial adenomatous polyposis with sulindac. N Engl J Med 2002;346:1054–9.

[57] Cruz-Correa M, Hylind LM, Romans KE, et al. Long-term treatment with sulindac in familial adenomatous polyposis: a prospective study. Gastroenterology 2002;122:641–5.

[58] Giardiello FM, Brensinger JD, Petersen GM, et al. The use and interpretation of commercial APC gene testing for familial adenomatous polyposis. N Engl J Med 1997;336:823–7.

[59] Murphy P, Petersen G, Thibodeau S, et al. ACMG/ASHG statement. Genetic testing for colon cancer: joint statement of the American College of Medical Genetics and the American Society of Human Genetics. Genet Med 2000;2:362–6.

[60] Giardiello FM. Genetic testing in hereditary colorectal cancer. JAMA 1997;278:1278–81.

[61] Jeghers H, McKusick VA, Katz KH. Generalized intestinal polyposis and melanin spots of the oral mucosa, lips and digits: a syndrome of diagnostic significance. N Engl J Med 1949; 241:993–1005.

[62] McGarrity TJ, Kulin HE, Zaino RJ. Peutz-Jeghers syndrome. Am J Gastroenterol 2000;95: 596–604.

[63] Bartholomew LG, Dahlin DC, Waugh JM. Intestinal polyposis associated with mucocutaneous melanin pigmentation (Peutz-Jeghers syndrome): review of the literature and report of six cases with special reference to pathologic findings. Gastroenterology 1957;32:434–51.

[64] Foley TR, McGarrity TJ, Abt A. Peutz-Jeghers syndrome: a 38 year follow up of the "Harrisburg Family." Gastroenterology 1988;95:1535–40.

[65] Boardman LA, Thibodeau SN, Schaid DJ, et al. Increased risk for cancer in patients with the Peutz-Jeghers syndrome. Ann Intern Med 1998;128:896–9.

[66] Giardiello FM, Brensinger JD, Tersmette AC, et al. Very high risk of cancer in familial Peutz-Jeghers syndrome. Gastroenterology 2000;119:1447–53.

[67] Perzin KH, Bridge MF. Adenomatous and carcinomatous changes in hamartomatous polyps of the small intestine (Peutz-Jeghers syndrome): report of a case and review of the literature. Cancer 1982;49:971–83.

[68] Jenne DE, Reimann H, Nezu J, et al. Peutz-Jeghers syndrome is caused by mutations in a novel serine threonine kinase. Nat Genet 1998;18:38–43.

[69] Hemminki A, Markie D, Tomlinson I, et al. A serine/threonine kinase gene defective in Peutz-Jeghers syndrome. Nature 1998;391:184–7.

[70] Boardman LA, Couch FJ, Burgart LJ, et al. Genetic heterogeneity in Peutz-Jeghers syndrome. Hum Mutat 2000;16:23–30.

[71] Wirtzfeld DA, Petrelli NJ, Rodriguez-Bigas MA. Hamartomatous polyposis: molecular genetics, neoplastic risk, and surveillance recommendations. Ann Surg Oncol 2001;8:319–27.

[72] Amaro R, Diaz G, Schneider J, et al. Peutz-Jeghers syndrome managed with a complete intraoperative endoscopy and extensive polypectomy. Gastrointest Endosc 2000;52:552–4.

[73] Rubio CA, Jaramillo E, Lindblom A, et al. Classification of colorectal polyps: guidelines for the endoscopist. Endoscopy 2002;34:226–36.

[74] Woodford-Richens K, Bevan S, Churchman M, et al. Analysis of genetic and phenotypic heterogeneity in juvenile polyposis. Gut 2000;46:656–60.

[75] Giardiello FM, Offerhaus JG. Phenotype and cancer risk of the various polyposis syndromes. Eur J Cancer 1995;31a:1085–7.

[76] Jarvinen H, Franssila KO. Famial juvenile polyposis coli; increased risk of colorectal cancer. Gut 1984;25:792–800.

[77] Howe JR, Mitros FA, Summers RW. The risk of gastrointestinal carcinoma in familial juvenile polyposis. Ann Surg Oncol 1998;5:751–6.

[78] Howe JR, Roth S, Ringold JC, et al. Mutations in the SMAD4/DPC4 gene in juvenile polyposis. Science 1998;280:1086–8.

[79] Houlston R, Bevan S, Williams A, et al. Mutations in DPC4 (SMAD4) cause juvenile polyposis syndrome, but only account for a minority of cases. Hum Mol Genet 1998;7:1907–12.

[80] Woodford-Richens KL, Rowan AJ, Poulsom R, et al. Comprehensive analsysi of SMAD4 mutations and protein expression in juvenile polyposis: evidence for a distinct pathway and polyp morphology in SMAD4 mutation carriers. Am J Pathol 2001;159:1293–300.

[81] Takagi Y, Kohmura H, Futamura M, et al. Somatic alterations of the DPC4 gene in human colorectal cancers in vivo. Gastroenterology 1996;111:1369–72.

[82] Riggins GJ, Thiagalingam S, Rozenblum E, et al. Mad-related genes in the human. Nat Genet 1996;13:347–9.

[83] Olschwang S, Serova-Sinilnikova OM, Lenoir GM, et al. PTEN germline mutations in juvenile polyposis. Nat Genet 1998;18:12–3.

[84] Zhou XP, Woodford-Richens K, Lehtonen R, et al. Germline mutations in BMPR1A/ALK3 cause a subset of cases of juvenile polyposis syndrome and of Bannayan-Riley-Ruvalcaba syndromes. Am J Hum Genet 2001;69:704–11.

[85] Burt RW. Polyposis syndromes. Clin Perspec Gastroenterol 2002;1:51–9.

[86] Liaw D, Marsh DJ, Li J, et al. Germline mutations of the PTEN gene in Cowden disease, an inherited breast and thyroid cancer syndrome. Nat Genet 1997;16:64–7.

[87] Zigman AF, Lavine JE, Jones MC. Localization of the Bannayan-Riley-Ruvalcaba syndrome gene to chromosome 10q23. Gastroenterology 1997;113:1433–7.

[88] Ponz de Leon M, Sassatelli R, Benatti P, et al. Identification of hereditary nonpolyposis colorectal cancer in the general population: the 6-year experience of a population-based registry. Cancer 1993;71:3493–501.

[89] Evans DG, Walsh S, Jeacock J, et al. Incidence of hereditary non-polyposis colorectal cancer in a population-based study of 1137 consecutive cases of colorectal cancer. Br J Surg 1997;84:1281–5.

[90] Aaltonen LA, Salovaara R, Kristo P, et al. Incidence of hereditary nonpolyposis colorectal cancer and the feasibility of molecular screening for the disease. N Engl J Med 1998;338:1481–7.

[91] Ravnik-Glavac M, Potocnik U, Glavac D. Incidence of germline hMLH1 and hMSH2 mutations (HNPCC patients) among newly diagnosed colorectal cancers in a Slovenian population. J Med Genet 2000;37:533–6.

[92] Lynch HT, Smyrk TC, Watson P, et al. Genetics, natural history, tumor spectrum, and pathology of hereditary nonpolyposis colorectal cancer: an updated review. Gastroenterology 1993;104:1535–49.

[93] Lynch HT, Smyrk T, Lynch JF. Overview of natural history, pathology, molecular genetics and management of HNPCC Lynch Syndrome. Int J Cancer 1996;69:38–43.

[94] Kinzler KW, Vogelstein B. Lessons from hereditary colorectal cancer. Cell 1996;87:159–70.

[95] Watanabe T, Muto T, Sawada T, et al. Flat adenoma as a precursor of colorectal carcinoma in hereditary nonpolyposis colorectal carcinoma. Cancer 1996;77:627–34.

[96] Rijcken FEM, Hollema H, Kleibeuker JH. Proximal adenomas in hereditary nonpolyposis colorectal cancer are prone to rapid malignant transformation. Gut 2002;50:382–6.

[97] Lindgren G, Liljegren A, Jaramillo E, et al. Adenoma prevalence and cancer risk in familial nonpolyposis colorectal cancer. Gut 2002;50:228–34.

[98] Vasen HF, Wijnen JT, Menko FH, et al. Cancer risk in families with hereditary nonpolyposis colorectal cancer diagnosed by mutation analysis. Gastroenterology 1996;110:1020–7.

[99] Dunlop MG, Farrington SM, Carothers AD, et al. Cancer risk associated with germline DNA mismatch repair gene mutations. Hum Mol Genet 1997;6:105–10.

[100] Aarnio M, Sankila R, Pukkala E, et al. Cancer risk in mutation carriers of DNA mismatch repair genes. Int J Cancer 1999;81:214–8.

[101] Vasen HFA, Stormorken A, Menko FH, et al. MSH2 mutation carriers are at a higher risk of cancer than MLH1 mutation carriers: a study of hereditary nonpolyposis colorectal cancer families. J Clin Oncol 2001;19:4074–80.

[102] Lynch HT, Smyrk TC, Watson P, et al. Genetics, natural history, tumor spectrum and pathology of hereditary nonpolyposis colorectal cancer: an updated review. Gastroenterology 1993;104:1535–49.

[103] Mecklin JP, Järvinen H. Treatment and follow-up strategies in hereditary nonpolyposis colorectal carcinoma. Dis Colon Rectum 1993;36:927–9.

[104] Hemminki K, Li X, Dong C. Second primary cancers after sporadic and familial colorectal cancer. Cancer Epidemiol Biomarkers Prev 2001;10:793–8.

[105] Jass JR, Smyrk TC, Stewart SM, et al. Pathology of hereditary non-polyposis colorectal cancer. Anticancer Res 1994;14:1631–4.

[106] Michael-Robinson JM, Biemere-Huttmann A, Purdie DM, et al. Tumor infiltrating lymphocytes and apoptosis are independent features in colorectal cancer according to microsatellite instability status. Gut 2001;48:360–6.

[107] Young J, Simms LA, Biden KG, et al. Features of colorectal cancers with high-level microsatellite instability occurring in familail and sporadic settings: parallel pathways of tumorigenesis. Am J Pathol 2001;159:2107–16.

[108] Lynch HT, Smyrk T. Colorectal cancer, survival advantage, and hereditary nonpolyposis colorectal carcinoma. Gastroenterology 1996;110:943–7.

[109] Sankila R, Aaltonen LA, Järvinen HJ, et al. Better survival rates in patients with MLH1-associated hereditary colorectal cancer. Gastroenterology 1996;110:682–7.

[110] Myrhøj T, Bisgaard ML, Bernstein I, et al. Hereditary non-polyposis colorectal cancer: clinical features and survival. Results from the Danish HNPCC register. Scand J Gastroenterol 1997;32:572–6.

[111] Watson P, Lynch HT. Extracolonic cancer in hereditary nonpolyposis colorectal cancer. Cancer 1993;71:677–85.

[112] Lynch HT, Smyrk T. Hereditary nonpolyposis colorectal cancer (Lynch syndrome): an updated review. Cancer 1996;78:1149–67.

[113] Park YJ, Shin KH, Park JG. Risk of gastric cancer in hereditary nonpolyposis colorectal cancer in Korea. Clin Cancer Res 2000;6:2994–8.

[114] Kim JC, Kim HC, Roh SA, et al. hMLH1 and hMSH2 mutations in families with familial clustering of gastric cancer and hereditary nonpolyposis colorectal cancer. Cancer Detect Prev 2001;25:503–10.

[115] Suspiro A, Fidalgo P, Cravo M, et al. The Muir-Torre syndrome: a rare variant of hereditary nonpolyposis colorectal cancer associated with hMSH2 mutation. Am J Gastroenterol 1998;93:1572–4.

[116] Kruse R, Rütten A, Lamberti C, et al. Muir-Torre phenotype has a frequency of DNA

mismatch-repair-gene mutations similar to that in hereditary nonpolyposis colorectal cancer families defined by the Amsterdam criteria. Am J Hum Genet 1998;63:63–70.

[117] Vasen HF, Mecklin JP, Khan PM, et al. The International Collaborative Group on Hereditary Non-Polyposis Colorectal Cancer (ICG-HNPCC). Dis Colon Rectum 1991;34:424–5.

[118] Wijnen JT, Vasen HF, Khan PM, et al. Clinical findings with implications for genetic testing in families with clustering of colorectal cancer. N Engl J Med 1998;339:511–8.

[119] Syngal S, Fox EA, Li C, et al. Interpretation of genetic test results for hereditary nonpolyposis colorectal cancer: implications for clinical predisposition testing. JAMA 1999;282:247–53.

[120] Syngal S, Fox EA, Eng C, et al. Sensitivity and specificity of clinical criteria for hereditary non-polyposis colorectal cancer associated mutations in MSH2 and MLH1. J Med Genet 2000; 37:641–5.

[121] Terdiman JP, Gum Jr JR, Conrad PG, et al. Efficient detection of hereditary nonpolyposis colorectal cancer gene carriers by screening for tumor microsatellite instability before germline genetic testing. Gastroenterology 2001;120:21–30.

[122] Vasen HF, Watson P, Mecklin JP, et al. New clinical criteria for hereditary nonpolyposis colorectal cancer (HNPCC, Lynch syndrome) proposed by the International Collaborative group on HNPCC. Gastroenterology 1999;116:1453–6.

[123] Rodriguez-Bigas MA, Boland CR, Hamilton SR, et al. A National Cancer Institute Workshop on Hereditary Nonpolyposis Colorectal Cancer Syndrome: meeting highlights and Bethesda guidelines. J Natl Cancer Inst 1997;89:1758–62.

[124] Umar A, Boland CR, Terdiman JP, et al. Revised Bethesda Guidelines for hereditary non-polyposis colorectal cancer (Lynch syndrome) and microsatellite instability. J Natl Cancer Inst 2004;96:261–8.

[125] Leach FS, Nicolaides NC, Papadopoulos N, et al. Mutations of a mutS homolog in hereditary nonpolyposis colorectal cancer. Cell 1993;75:1215–25.

[126] Papadopoulos N, Nicolaides NC, Wei Y-F, et al. Mutation of a mutL homolog in hereditary colon cancer. Science 1994;263:1625–9.

[127] Bronner CE, Baker SM, Morrison PT, et al. Mutation in the DNA mismatch repair gene homologue hMLH1 is associated with hereditary non-polyposis colon cancer. Nature 1994; 368:258–61.

[128] Nicolaides NC, Papadopoulos N, Liu B, et al. Mutations of two PMS homologues in hereditary nonpolyposis colon cancer. Nature 1994;371:75–80.

[129] Fishel R, Lescoe MK, Rao MR, et al. The human mutator gene homolog MSH2 and its association with hereditary nonpolyposis colon cancer. Cell 1993;75:1027–38.

[130] Miyaki M, Konishi M, Tanaka K, et al. Germline mutation of MSH6 as the cause of hereditary nonpolyposis colorectal cancer [letter]. Nat Genet 1997;17:271–2.

[131] Peltomäki P, Vasen HF. Mutations predisposing to hereditary nonpolyposis colorectal cancer: database and results of a collaborative study. The International Collaborative Group on Hereditary Nonpolyposis Colorectal Cancer. Gastroenterology 1997;113:1146–58.

[132] Kolodner RD, Tytell JD, Schmeits JL, et al. Germ-line msh6 mutations in colorectal cancer families. Cancer Res 1999;59:5068–74.

[133] Wu Y, Berends MJ, Mensink RG, et al. Association of hereditary nonpolyposis colorectal cancer-related tumors displaying low microsatellite instability with MSH6 germline mutations. Am J Hum Genet 1999;65:1291–8.

[134] Wang Q, Lasset C, Desseigne F, et al. Prevalence of germline mutations of hMLH1, hMSH2, hPMS1, hPMS2, and hMSH6 genes in 75 French kindreds with nonpolyposis colorectal cancer. Hum Genet 1999;105:79–85.

[135] Plaschke J, Kruppa C, Tischler R, et al. Sequence analysis of the mismatch repair gene hMSH6 in the germline of patients with familial and sporadic colorectal cancer. Int J Cancer 2000; 85:606–13.

[136] Huang J, Kuismanen SA, Liu T, et al. MSH6 and MSH3 are rarely involved in genetic predisposition to nonpolyotic colon cancer. Cancer Res 2001;61:1619–23.

[137] Wagner A, Hendriks Y, Meijers-Heijboer EJ, et al. Atypical HNPCC owing to MSH6 germline mutations: analysis of a large Dutch pedigree. J Med Genet 2001;38:318–22.

[138] Fishel R. The selection for mismatch repair defects in hereditary nonpolyposis colorectal cancer syndrome (HNPCC): revising the mutator hypothesis. Cancer Res 2001;61:7369–74.

[139] Heinen CD, Schmutte C, Fishel R. DNA repair and tumorigenesis: lessons from hereditary cancer syndromes. Cancer Biol Ther 2002;1:477–85.

[140] Parsons R, Li LGM, Longley MJ, et al. Hypermutability and mismatch repair deficiency in RER + tumor cells. Cell 1993;75:1227–36.

[141] Peltomaki P, Lothe RA, Aaltonen LA, et al. Microsatellite instability is associated with tumors that characterize the hereditary non-polyposis colorectal carcinoma syndrome. Cancer Res 1993;53:5853–5.

[142] Aaltonen LA, Peltomaki P, Mecklin JP, et al. Replication errors in benign and malignant tumors from hereditary nonpolyposis colorectal cancer patients. Cancer Res 1994;54:1645–8.

[143] Dietmaier W, Wallinger S, Bocker T, et al. Diagnostic microsatellite instability: definition and correlation with mismatch repair protein expression. Cancer Res 1997;57:4749–56.

[144] Boland CR, Thibodeau SN, Hamilton SR, et al. A National Cancer Institute Workshop on Microsatellite Instability for cancer detection and familial predisposition: development of international criteria for the determination of microsatellite instability in colorectal cancer. Cancer Res 1998;58:5248–57.

[145] Markowitz S, Wang J, Myeroff L, et al. Inactivation of the type II TGF-beta receptor in colon cancer cells with microsatellite instability. Science 1995;268:1336–8.

[146] Parsons R, Myeroff LL, Liu B, et al. Microsatellite instability and mutations of the transforming growth factor beta type II receptor gene in colorectal cancer. Cancer Res 1995;55:5548–50.

[147] Rampino N, Yamamoto H, Ionov Y, et al. Somatic frameshift mutations in the BAX gene in colon cancers of the microsatellite mutator phenotype. Science 1997;275:967–9.

[148] Yamamoto H, Sawai H, Weber TK, et al. Somatic frameshift mutations in DNA mismatch repair and proapoptosis genes in hereditary nonpolyposis colorectal cancer. Cancer Res 1998;58:997–1003.

[149] Yagi OK, Akiyama Y, Nomizu T, et al. Proapoptotic gene BAX is frequently mutated in hereditary nonpolyposis colorectal cancers but not in adenomas. Gastroenterology 1998;114:268–74.

[150] Cawkwell L, Gray S, Murgatroyd H, et al. Choice of management strategy for colorectal cancer based on a diagnostic immunohistochemical test for defective mismatch repair. Gut 1999;45:409–15.

[151] Salahshor S, Koelble K, Rubio C, et al. Microsatellite instability and hMLH1 and hMSH2 expression analysis in familial and sporadic colorectal cancer. Lab Invest 2001;81:535–41.

[152] Wahlberg SS, Schmeits J, Thomas G, et al. Evaluation of microsatellite instability and immunohistochemistry for the prediction of germline MSH2 and MLH1 mutations in hereditary nonpolyposis colon cancer families. Cancer Res 2002;62:3485–92.

[153] Christensen M, Katballe N, Wikman F, et al. Antibody-based screening for hereditary nonpolyposis colorectal carcinoma compared with microsatellite analysis and sequencing. Cancer 2002;95:2422–30.

[154] Winawer S, Fletcher R, Rex D, et al. Colorectal cancer screening and surviellance: clinical guidelines and rationale–update based on new evidence. Gastroenterology 2003;124:544–60.

[155] Jarvinen HJ, Aarnio M, Mustonen H, et al. Controlled 15-year trial on screening for colorectal cancer in families with hereditary nonpolyposis colorectal cancer. Gastroenterology 2000;118:829–34.

[156] Vasen HF, van Ballegooijen M, Buskens E, et al. A cost-effectiveness analysis of colorectal screening of hereditary nonpolyposis colorectal carcinoma gene carriers. Cancer 1998;82:1632–7.

[157] Syngal S, Weeks JC, Schrag D, et al. Benefits of colonoscopic surveillance and prophylactic colectomy in patients with hereditary nonpolyposis colorectal cancer mutations. Ann Intern Med 1998;129:787–96.

[158] Church JM. Prophylactic colectomy in patients with hereditary nonpolyposis colorectal cancer. Ann Med 1996;28:479–82.

[159] Rodríguez-Bigas MA, Vasen HF, Pekka-Mecklin J, et al. Rectal cancer risk in hereditary nonpolyposis colorectal cancer after abdominal colectomy. International Collaborative Group on HNPCC. Ann Surg 1997;225:202-7.

[160] Brown GJ, St John DJ, Macrae FA, et al. Cancer risk in young women at risk of hereditary nonpolyposis colorectal cancer: implications for gynecologic surveillance. Gynecologic Oncology 2001;80:346-9.

[161] Dove-Edwin I, Boks D, Goff S, et al. The outcome of endometrial carcinoma surveillance by ultrasound scan in women at risk for hereditary nonpolyposis colorectal carcinoma and familial colorectal carcinoma. Cancer 2002;94:1708-12.

[162] Renkonen-Sinisalo L, Sipponen P, Aarnio M, et al. No support for endoscopic surveillance for gastric cancer in hereditary nonpolyposis colorectal cancer. Scan J Gastroenterol 2002; 37:574-7.

[163] Burke W, Petersen G, Lynch P, et al. Recommendations for follow-up care of individuals with an inherited predisposition to cancer: I. Hereditary nonpolyposis colon cancer. Cancer Genetics Studies Consortium. JAMA 1997;277:915-9.

[164] Lamberti C, Kruse R, Ruelfs C, et al. Microsatellite instability-a useful diagnostic tool to select patients at high risk for hereditary non-polyposis colorectal cancer: a study in different groups of patients with colorectal cancer. Gut 1999;44:839-43.

[165] Lichtenstein P, Holm NV, Verkasalo PK, et al. Environmental and heritable factors in the causation of cancer: analyses of cohorts of twins from Sweden, Denmark, and Finland. N Engl J Med 2000;343:78-85.

[166] Winawer SJ, Zauber AG, Gerdes H, et al. Risk of colorectal cancer in the families of patients with adenomatous polyps. National Polyp Study Workgroup. N Engl J Med 1996;334:82-7.

[167] Fuchs CS, Giovannucci EL, Colditz GA, et al. A prospective study of family history and the risk of colorectal cancer. N Engl J Med 1994;331:1669-74.

[168] Sandler RS. Epidemiology and risk factors for colorectal cancer. Gastroenterol Clin N Am 1996;25:717-35.

[169] Laken SJ, Petersen GM, Gruber SB, et al. Familial colorectal cancer in Ashkenazim due to a hypermutable tract in APC. Nat Genet 1997;17:79-83.

[170] Gryfe R, Di Nicola N, Gallinger S, et al. Somatic instability of the APC I1307K allele in colorectal neoplasia. Cancer Res 1998;58:4040-3.

[171] White RL. Excess risk of colon cancer associated with a polymorphism of the APC gene? [editorial] Cancer Res 1998;58:4038-9.

[172] Woodage T, King SM, Wacholder S, et al. The APCI1307K allele and cancer risk in a community-based study of Ashkenazi Jews. Nat Genet 1998;20:62-5.

[173] Frayling IM, Beck NE, Ilyas M, et al. The APC variants I1307K and E1317Q are associated with colorectal tumors, but not always with a family history. Proc Natl Acad Sci USA 1998;95:10722-7.

[174] Rozen P, Shomrat R, Strul H, et al. Prevalence of the I1307K APC gene variant in Israeli Jews of differing ethnic origin and risk for colorectal cancer. Gastroenterology 1999;116:54-7.

[175] Gryfe R, Di Nicola N, Lal G, et al. Inherited colorectal polyposis and cancer risk of the APC I1307K polymorphism. Am J Hum Genet 1999;64:378-84.

[176] Drucker L, Shpilberg O, Neumann A, et al. Adenomatous polyposis coli I1307K mutation in Jewish patients with different ethnicity: prevalence and phenotype. Cancer 2000;88:755-60.

[177] Syngal S, Schrag D, Falchuk M, et al. Phenotypic characteristics associated with the APC gene I1307K mutation in Ashkenazi Jewish patients with colorectal polyps. JAMA 2000;284: 857-60.

[178] Stern HS, Viertelhausen S, Hunter AG, et al. APC I1307K increases risk of transition from polyp to colorectal carcinoma in Ashkenazi Jews. Gastroenterology 2001;120:392-400.

[179] Rozen P, Naiman T, Strul H, et al. Clinical and screening implications of the I1307K adenomatous polyposis coli gene variant in Israeli Ashkenazi Jews with familial colorectal neoplasia. Cancer 2002;94:2561-8.

[180] Potter JD. Colorectal cancer: molecules and populations. J Natl Cancer Inst 1999;91:916-32.

[181] Rex DK, Johnson DA, Lieberman DA, et al. Colorectal cancer prevention 2000: screening recommendations of the American College of Gastroenterology. American College of Gastroenterology. Am J Gastroenterol 2000;95:868–77.

[182] U.S. Preventive Services Task Force. Screening for colorectal cancer: recommendation and rationale. Ann Intern Med 2002;137:129–31.

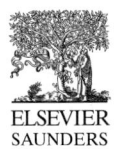

ELSEVIER
SAUNDERS

Gastrointest Endoscopy Clin N Am
15 (2005) 581–614

GASTROINTESTINAL
ENDOSCOPY CLINICS
OF NORTH AMERICA

State-of-the-Art Computed Tomographic and Magnetic Resonance Imaging of the Gastrointestinal System

Sukru Mehmet Erturk, MD, Koenraad J. Mortelé, MD*,
M. Raquel Oliva, MD, Matthew A. Barish, MD

*Division of Abdominal Imaging and Intervention, Department of Radiology,
Brigham and Women's Hospital, Harvard Medical School, 75 Francis Street, Boston, MA 02115, USA*

Among the major innovations in radiology of the gastrointestinal (GI) system are the replacement of classic invasive diagnostic methods with noninvasive ones and the improvement in lesion characterization and staging of pancreatobiliary malignancies. Recent developments in CT and MR technology, such as the introduction of multidetector-row CT (MDCT) and the development of phased-array coils and fast MR sequences, have made GI radiologists essential physicians in these areas. In this article, we discuss the impact of advanced imaging technologies in some selected fields of GI radiology.

Selected developments in GI radiology

Multidetector-row computed tomography for characterization and preoperative staging of pancreatic tumors

With the introduction of MDCT, the visualization of the pancreas has dramatically improved [1]. The fast (subsecond) and thin-section (0.75 mm collimation) scanning ability of MDCT allows for images with high spatial and temporal resolution and thus results in improved detection of minute neoplasms

* Corresponding author.
E-mail address: kmortele@partners.org (K.J. Mortelé).

1052-5157/05/$ – see front matter © 2005 Elsevier Inc. All rights reserved.
doi:10.1016/j.giec.2005.04.002

giendo.theclinics.com

and anatomic structures, such as minor vessels, ducts, and lymph nodes [2,3]. Thin collimation also makes isovolumetric reconstructions that demonstrate pancreas and surrounding vessels in any plane possible. Multi-phasic, contrast-enhanced studies performed with MDCT reveal critical data that are essential evaluating different enhancement characteristics of pancreatic tumors, and, more importantly, detecting vascular invasion. Therefore, MDCT has become a superb tool for detection of small neoplasms with an increasing overall diagnostic accuracy (by means of better differentiating pancreatitis from neoplasm and characterizing the different neoplasms) and an accurate method to assess unresectability [1,2].

Magnetic resonance cholangiopancreatography versus endoscopic retrograde cholangiopancreatography in pancreatobiliary malignancies

At the time of its introduction, MR cholangiopancreatography (MRCP) was considered an interesting technique with potential for detecting pathologies of biliary tract and pancreatic duct [4]. Since that time, MRCP has undergone a number of technical refinements, including new volumetric sequences and breath-hold techniques [5–9]. Today, in the initial diagnostic work-up of biliopancreatic disorders, it has replaced the use of diagnostic endoscopic retrograde cholangiopancreatography (ERCP) in many institutions [10–12]. Compared with ERCP, MRCP offers a number of advantages, such as noninvasiveness and short examination times [13–15]. It avoids a variety of possible complications, including pancreatitis and hemorrhage, which occur in 5% of ERCP attempts. MRCP does not expose patients to ionizing radiation or iodinated contrast material, unlike ERCP [16]. It can be performed in patients in whom it is impossible to perform ERCP due to anatomic alterations from previous surgery [13]. Furthermore, the combination of MRCP with dynamic contrast-enhanced MR imaging and MR angiography optimizes the evaluation of abdominal organs, including the pancreas, liver, gallbladder, and surrounding vascular structures [17]. This so called "all-in-one" imaging approach is presumably the most comprehensive and cost-effective imaging technique in the evaluation of biliopancreatic malignancies. Nevertheless, the major strength of ERCP is the access for therapeutic interventions it offers. Unlike ERCP, MRCP is a purely diagnostic technique.

Computed tomographic colonography (virtual colonoscopy)

Virtual colonoscopy is a promising technique that has been improved dramatically as a result of the recent developments in CT technology. The high-resolution images obtained with MDCT and the noninvasiveness are its main strengths. It is less expensive and less time-consuming than conventional colonoscopy. Virtual colonoscopy is best suited and highly recommended for patients who have undergone a failed or incomplete conventional colonoscopy and for patients who are unable (due to the reasons such as obstructing neoplasms or tortuosity) or unwilling to undergo conventional colonoscopy.

Computed tomographic enteroclysis and computed tomographic enterography

Another benefit of MDCT is the improved ability of CT enteroclysis and CT enterography to examine the small bowel. Combining the advantages of enteral evaluation by cross-sectional imaging and depicting extra-intestinal manifestations of diseases, CT enteroclysis is an efficient diagnostic tool. Many conditions, such as small bowel obstruction, Crohn's disease, and neoplasms, that would traditionally be imaged with other modalities are now routinely examined with CT enteroclysis. The main disadvantage of CT enteroclysis is the need for naso-enteric tube placement, which causes patient discomfort and lengthens examination time. In this context, CT enterography is an efficient alternative for CT enteroclysis. In our experience, the thin collimation ability of MDCT and proper use of enteral contrast material allow CT enterography to obtain images with high diagnostic capacity noninvasively.

Magnetic resonance imaging in preoperative staging of rectal cancer

In the past, MR imaging suffered from technical limitations in the evaluation of rectal cancer because it was unable to accurately determine the depth of tumor invasion or lymph node involvement due to the low signal to noise ratios and poor spatial resolution. Recent technical improvements, including the development of phased-array and endoluminal coils, which yield high signal-to-noise ratios, allow high-resolution imaging of the rectal wall and pelvic organs. With these techniques, higher accuracy in preoperative staging of rectal cancer has become possible.

Multidetector-row computed tomography of pancreatic malignancies

Technique

Accurate CT imaging of the pancreas requires careful attention to technique. First, especially if 3-dimensional (3D) imaging will be performed, low-density or neutral contrast agents (eg, water or milk) should be administered. Water allows excellent visualization of duodenum and does not require editing when performing CT angiography. A fast injection (3 to 5 mL/sec) of contrast material is essential for optimal visualization of the peripancreatic vascular structures and pancreatic parenchyma. Fast data acquisition using thin collimation (1 mm in arterial phase and 2.5 mm in the pancreatic phase) is essential. Modern MDCT scanners allow thin collimation generating thin slices and reconstructions and are, therefore, preferable. A triple-phase imaging protocol, including an arterial phase (with a delay of 20 seconds after the start of injection), a pancreatic parenchymal phase (with a delay of 40 seconds), and a portal venous phase (with a delay of 60 seconds) is optimal to detect pancreatic neoplasms, their local extensions, their possible metastases to the liver and to regional lymph nodes, and involvement of vascular structures.

Pancreatic adenocarcinoma

Ductal pancreatic adenocarcinoma, which is the fourth or fifth leading cause of cancer death in the Western hemisphere, accounts for nearly 90% of all malignant pancreatic neoplasms and is the ninth most common malignancy [18]. It usually occurs in the elderly people presenting with jaundice due to biliary obstruction, pain secondary to involvement of splanchnic or retroperitoneal nerves, or new-onset diabetes. Prognosis is poor, with a 5-year survival rate ranging from 1% to 5%; at the time of clinical presentation, 66% of patients have an advanced tumor stage, with metastatic disease present in 85% of cases [19]. The majority of tumors are located in the pancreatic head and, because of the involvement of the common bile duct, they present earlier than tumors arising in the body or tail of pancreas [3,20].

CT is the imaging modality of choice for the detection and preoperative staging of pancreatic adenocarcinoma [21]. With single-row spiral CT scanners, the accuracy rates for the detection of pancreatic tumors ranged between 80% and 91% [22–24]; however, the obtained images were suboptimal in the detection of small peritoneal implants and small hepatic metastases [3]. The new MDCTs provide radiologists enormous capabilities for fast data acquisition and narrow collimation, resulting in 96% accuracy for detecting pancreatic tumors [25].

On contrast-enhanced MDCT images obtained after bolus injection of nonionic iodinated contrast followed by rapid, thin-section scanning, adenocarcinomas present as hypoattenuating lesions with respect to the surrounding normal pancreatic parenchyma (Fig. 1) [26,27]. There are also some indirect signs

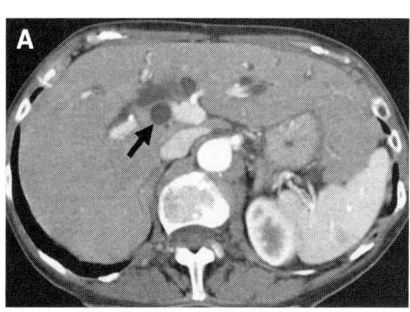 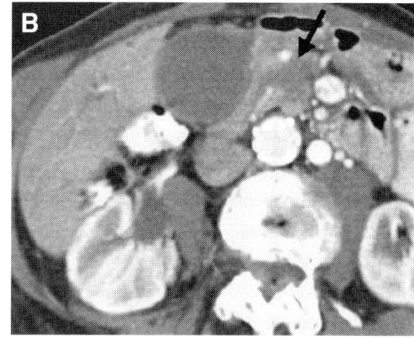

Fig. 1. Pancreatic adenocarcinoma. (*A*) CT image shows dilated intrahepatic bile ducts (*arrow*). (*B*) Pancreatic parenchymal phase CT image demonstrates a hypoattenuating mass located in the pancreatic neck (*arrow*).

for the presence of a tumor on CT without identification of the tumor itself: dilatation of common bile and pancreatic duct without calculi, dilatation of the pancreatic duct in the body and tail but not in the head, a homogenous zone within a heterogeneous atrophic gland, bulging of the uncinate process, and atrophy of the pancreatic tail (Fig. 2) [28,29]. An optimal tumor-to-pancreatic parenchymal contrast difference enables the radiologist to detect even very small lesions. According to a study by McNulty et al [1], maximum tumor conspicuity can be achieved during the pancreatic parenchymal or portal venous phases of a dynamic contrast-enhanced CT examination. The detection of hepatic metastases is critical in the preoperative staging of the patients because the presence of metastatic foci within the liver makes the tumor unresectable. MDCT scanners have the ability to depict very small lesions (< 5 mm), but it may be impossible to characterize them due to their small size. Mostly because of this "characterization" limitation, dynamic CT has a sensitivity around 75% for diagnosing liver metastases [28]. In the study by McNulty et al [1], the pancreatic parenchymal phase exhibited maximum opacification of the celiac and superior mesenteric arteries, whereas the portal venous phase exhibited maximum opacification of the superior mesenteric and portal veins. In the absence of obvious liver metastases, tumor resectability depends on the presence of local invasion or vascular involvement. In a recent prospective study comparing endoscopic ultrasonography, CT, MR imaging, and angiography in preoperative staging and tumor resectability assessment of pancreatic cancer, Soriano et al [30] reported that CT is the mainstay for pancreatic cancer staging, with the best figures in the evaluation of extent of primary tumor, local extension, vascular invasion, and metastatic spread (with accuracies of 73%, 74%, 83%, and 88%, respectively). In this study, endoscopic ultrasound (EUS) was evaluated as essential in assessing tumor size and lymph node involvement. Nevertheless, it can be assumed that the initial enthusiasm for EUS staging of pancreatic cancer has diminished as a result of studies reporting that EUS is not as accurate as it was earlier suggested in locoregional staging, especially in the diagnosis of vascular involvement (Fig. 3) [31,32]. Furthermore, detection of distant metastases, including nonregional

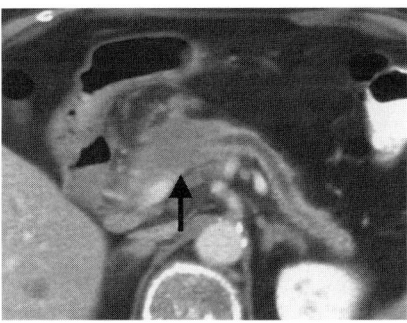

Fig. 2. Pancreatic adenocarcinoma. Portal venous-phase CT image shows a hypoattenuating mass in the pancreatic head (*arrow*), atrophied pancreatic tail, and dilated main pancreatic duct.

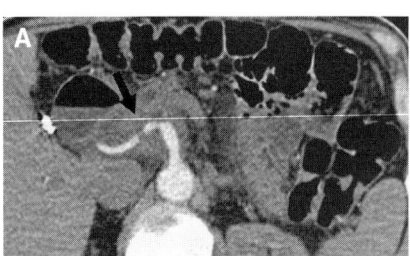
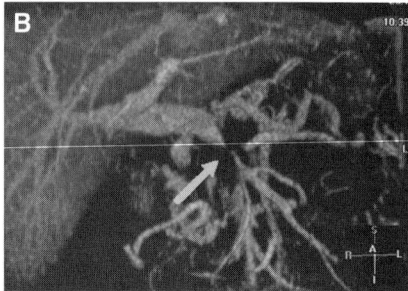

Fig. 3. Pancreatic adenocarcinoma. (*A*) Contrast-enhanced axial CT image shows vascular invasion of the common hepatic artery (*arrow*). (*B*) 3D CT venogram demonstrates an obstruction at the portal venous confluence (*arrow*).

lymph node groups, is beyond the capability of EUS because of restricted field of view, thus favoring MDCT as a single imaging technique for staging pancreatic cancer [33].

Serous cystic tumor

Serous cystic tumor (microcystic adenoma, serous cystadenoma/cystadeno-carcinoma, or glycogen-rich cystadenoma) is considered generally a benign neoplasm. There are only sporadic reports of malignant degeneration [34]. It occurs most frequently in elderly patients with a 1.5:1 female-to-male ratio.

On gross pathology, the tumor is large (mean diameter 10–13 cm) and well circumscribed and contains a central, stellate, and sometimes calcified scar (Fig. 4). It is composed of small cysts (0.2–2.0 cm in diameter) that contain clear fluid and are separated by thin septations (Fig. 5). Serous cystic tumors are typically hypervascular neoplasms due to their rich stromal capillary network and therefore have a tendency for internal bleeding.

On unenhanced MDCT examinations, serous cystic tumors are low-density, solid, or more commonly multicystic lesions with Hounsfield values similar to water [3,32]. If present, the characteristic central stellate scar with dystrophic

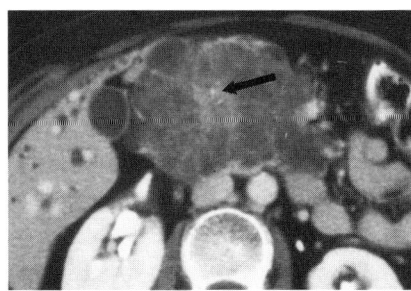

Fig. 4. Serous cystic tumor. Contrast-enhanced axial CT image demonstrates a well-defined cystic mass with central stellate scar (*arrow*).

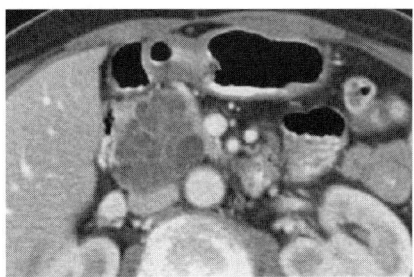

Fig. 5. Serous cystic tumor. Contrast-enhanced axial CT image shows a well-defined mass in the pancreatic head composed of numerous tiny cysts.

calcifications is demonstrated [29]. The amount of fibrous stroma determines the appearance of the tumor on contrast-enhanced CT images. A tumor containing innumerable cysts appears as an irregular heterogeneously enhancing mass, whereas a tumor with microscopic cysts and a dominant fibrous stroma presents as a homogenous mass on postcontrast images [36].

Mucinous cystic tumor

Mucinous cystic tumors (cystadenomas, cystadenocarcinomas, or macrocystic adenomas) range from tumors with malignant potential to frankly malignant mucinous cystadenocarcinomas [3]. In 95% of cases, they occur in women during their fourth to sixth decades of life. Most tumors are located in the tail or body of the pancreas. These encapsulated hypovascular tumors are most frequently multilocular. They may contain internal septations, solid papillary excretions, and occasionally peripheral calcifications (Fig. 6) [37,38].

Unenhanced MDCT studies show a round to slightly lobulated mass that is well delineated and has smooth external margins. Attenuation values are usually similar to that of water [35]. MDCT scans obtained after the intravenous administration of contrast material may demonstrate enhancement of the wall and

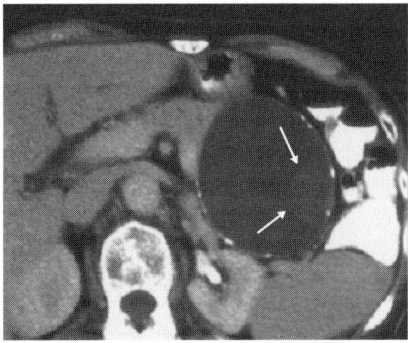

Fig. 6. Mucinous cystic tumor. Contrast-enhanced axial CT image shows a large cystic lesion containing a mural nodule (*arrows*). Note small foci of calcifications within the wall of the tumor.

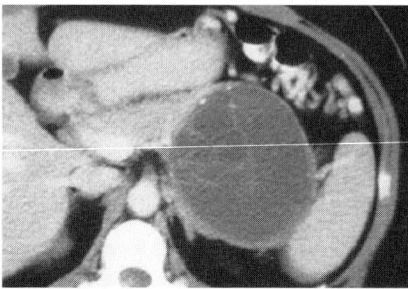

Fig. 7. Mucinous cystic tumor. Contrast-enhanced axial CT image demonstrates septations within the lesion and small peripheral calcifications.

the presence of thin septations [3,29]. On the internal surface of the tumor, nodularities representing papillary projections may be demonstrated (Fig. 7).

Intraductal papillary mucinous tumor

Intraductal papillary mucinous tumors (IPMTs) are newly reclassified and increasingly reported [39,40]. They are cystic pancreatic neoplasms with proliferation of pancreatic ductal epithelium and excess mucin production [35]. These tumors are also known as mucin-producing tumors, intraductal mucin-hypersecreting neoplasms, mucin-hypersecreting tumors, or mucinous ductal ectasias. They are classified into main and branch duct types. The branch duct type mostly presents in the uncinate process or pancreatic head, but it can also involve the body or tail [41,42].

On unenhanced MDCT, branch-duct tumor appears as clusters of multiple small cysts or as a single cystic lesion with irregular, lobulated margins and septations [43]. Diffuse or segmental dilatation of the main pancreatic duct is typical for main-duct type tumors (Fig. 8). Contrast-enhanced, thin-section MDCT images may demonstrate communications between dilated cystic segments and the main pancreatic duct. MDCT may also depict the papilla bulging into the duodenal lumen and hyperdense filling defects secondary to mucin in the dilated duct.

Solid and papillary epithelial neoplasm

Solid and papillary epithelial neoplasms (SPENs) are a benign or low-grade malignant neoplasms occurring predominantly in women 10 to 50 years of age (mean 24 years). These tumors are usually found incidentally or during the work-up for abdominal discomfort. Metastases are rare, but local recurrence is possible. After resection of the tumor, the prognosis is excellent, with a cure rate of 95% [38,44,45].

SPENs are large (range 3–18 cm, mean diameter 10 cm), well-demarcated, solitary masses that can occur in every portion of the pancreas. They are en-

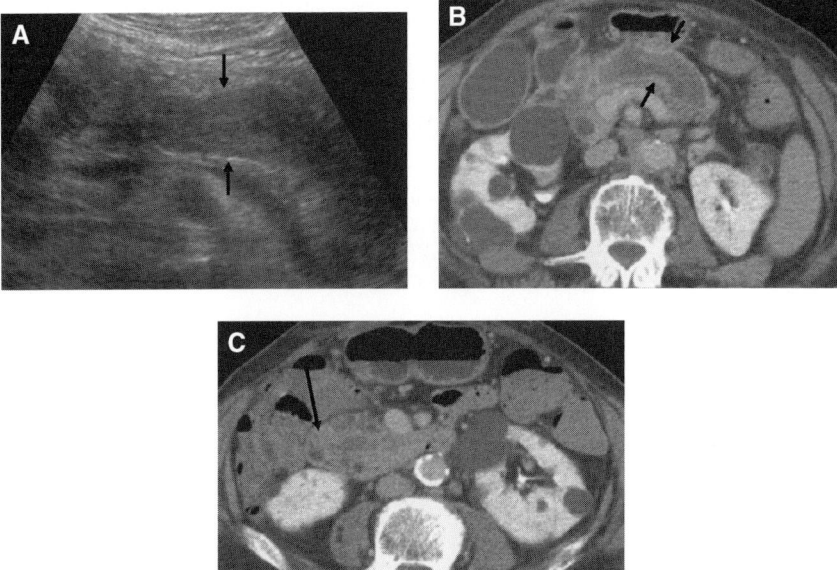

Fig. 8. IPMT, main duct type. Ultrasound (*A*) and contrast enhanced axial CT (*B*) images show marked dilatation of the main pancreatic duct with presence of internal debris within the duct (*arrows*). (*C*) Contrast-enhanced axial CT image demonstrates bulging of the papilla into the duodenum (*arrow*).

capsulated by a thick, fibrous capsule. Therefore, invasion into adjacent organs is rarely seen. The tumor can be entirely solid; however, with increasing tumor size, solid and cystic components are found side by side due to hemorrhage and necrosis.

On MDCT, SPENs present as large, well-defined masses with variable density internally [35,45]. Their fibrous capsule is thick and hypodense on unenhanced

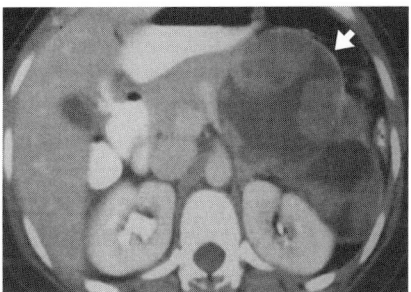

Fig. 9. SPEN. Contrast-enhanced axial CT image shows a large, lobulated mass located in the tail of pancreas. A hypervascular capsule is seen (*arrow*). Note that the tumor is composed of solid and cystic components.

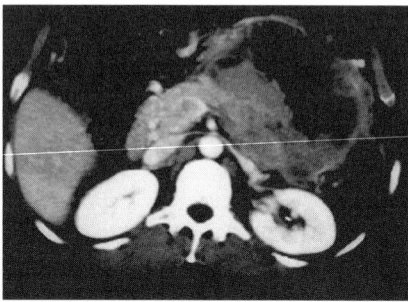

Fig. 10. SPEN. Contrast-enhanced axial CT scan demonstrates a well-defined large mass in the pancreatic tail composed of solid and cystic components.

CT images (Figs. 9 and 10) [29]. After intravenous contrast administration, the capsule enhances. Calcifications, when present, typically are located at the periphery of the tumor.

Endocrine pancreatic tumors

Endocrine pancreatic tumors (EPTs) (formerly known as islet cell tumors) are uncommon neoplasms arising from endocrine cells of the pancreas. In the case of

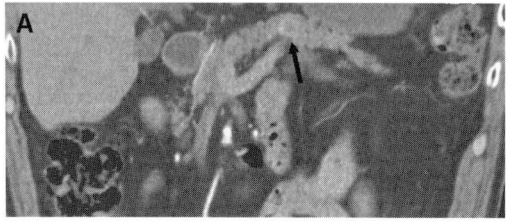

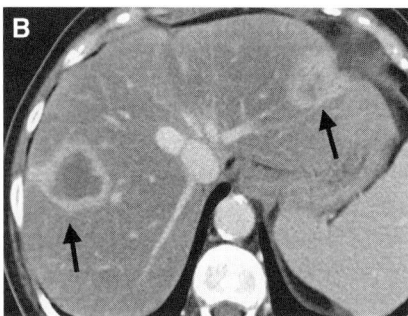

Fig. 11. Insulinoma. (*A*) Contrast-enhanced coronal reformatted CT image shows a small hypervascular lesion in the body of the pancreas (*arrow*). (*B*) Axial contrast-enhanced CT image shows hypervascular hepatic metastases (*arrows*).

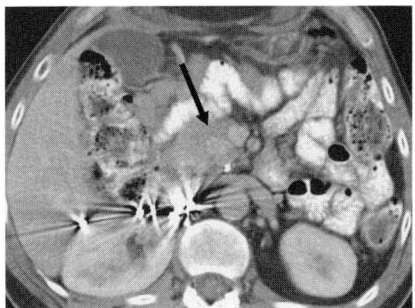

Fig. 12. Insulinoma, MEN I syndrome. CT image shows a hypervascular lesion in the pancreatic head (*arrow*). Note that the patient had a prior right adrenalectomy.

a hyperfunctioning tumor, the diagnosis is almost always established biochemically, when the lesion is small in size [46]. Nonhyperfunctioning EPTs frequently elude diagnosis because clinical symptoms do not typically present until the tumor reaches a particular size.

Due to their rich vascular supply, EPTs appear as hypervascular lesions compared with the pancreatic parenchyma on contrast-enhanced CT images. It is essential to image the tumor during the arterial phase because the attenuation difference between the lesion and the normal parenchyma is often greatest in this phase.

It has been reported that large EPTs with diameters > 5 cm have a high risk to be malignant (Figs. 11–13) [47,48]. In staging malignant EPTs with MDCT,

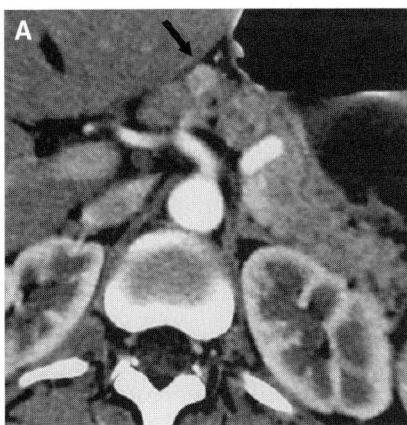
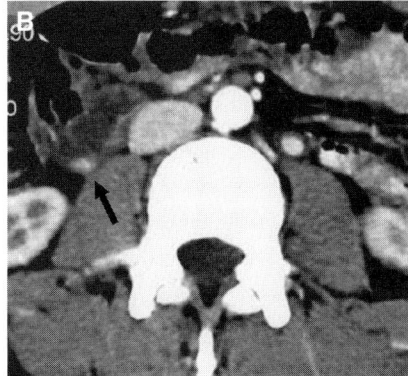

Fig. 13. Gastrinoma. (*A*) Contrast-enhanced axial CT image shows a hypervascular lesion (*arrow*) in the pancreatic neck. (*B*) A second hypervascular lesion (*arrow*) is shown in the duodenal wall.

detection of local extension, encasement of major peripancreatic vessels, and metastases to liver and regional lymph nodes are essential.

Acinar cell carcinoma

Acinar cell carcinoma accounts for <1% of pancreatic malignancies. Elderly men are affected most commonly (range 3–90 years of age, mean 65 years). The tumor is usually large (mean diameter 10 cm) and presents with nonspecific symptoms. In up to 30% of cases, hyperlipasemia syndrome, which is characterized by polyarthralgia, eosinophilia, and disseminated fat necrosis, may be present.

On MDCT, acinar cell carcinoma presents usually as an exophytic, well-demarcated, and hypoattenuated tumor (Fig. 14). It shows minimal enhancement after intravenous contrast material administration. The tumor frequently undergoes changes, such as cystic degeneration or central necrosis, that may be well depicted on MDCT images [46].

Pancreatoblastoma

Pancreatoblastoma is a rare tumor; however, it is the most common pancreatic neoplasm in childhood. The tumor mostly occurs in boys (male/female ratio 2:1) within the first 7 years of life (mean age 4 years).

On MDCT, the tumor typically presents as a large (diameter ranging from 7–18 cm), well-demarcated, heterogenous, and septated mass replacing the pancreas. In the solid parts of the tumor, there may be significant enhancement after intravenous contrast administration. Calcifications, ascites, and metastases may be seen [49–51]. In our experience, the tumor can show an early rim-like contrast enhancement with late washout, indicating its vascular nature.

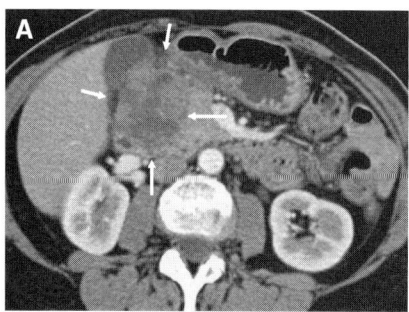 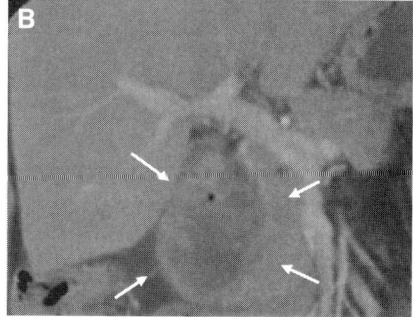

Fig. 14. Acinar cell carcinoma. (*A*) Contrast-enhanced axial CT image demonstrates a large, well defined, exophytic lesion in the pancreatic head composed of solid and cystic parts. (*B*) Corresponding coronal reformatted CT image.

Characterization of pancreatic tumors with multidetector-row computed tomographyy

CT is the most commonly used imaging modality for the initial detection and preoperative staging of pancreatic adenocarcinoma [21]. It has an accuracy rate of about 95% to 97% for detection and of virtually 100% for staging unresectable carcinomas. Recent developments are further improving the diagnostic potential of CT for pancreatic adenocarcinomas. For example, in a recent study of Catalano et al [25], MDCT with a high-resolution, dual-phase protocol correctly demonstrated unresectable neoplasms in 26 of the 27 cases and resectability in 12 of the 14 patients.

In the case of a mucinous cystic neoplasm, the most important distinction to be made is between this tumor and a pseudocyst [52]. Findings such as the absence of radiologic signs of pancreatitis, a solid component within the cystic lesion, and a radiologically normal appearance of the pancreatic tissue adjacent to the lesion favor the diagnosis of a mucinous cystic tumor [53].

It is usually not difficult to differentiate between mucinous cystic tumors and serous ones. Mucinous cystic lesions are generally composed of six or fewer cysts, and each cyst measures >2 cm in diameter, whereas serous cystic lesions tend to have more than six small cysts (diameter <2 cm) [35]. The presence and location of the calcifications are additional features that can be helpful in arriving at an accurate diagnosis. Central calcifications, if present, are characteristic for serous tumors, whereas more than 25% of mucinous tumors show peripheral calcifications [43]. If the lesion is unilocular and small, differentiation can be impossible.

The main challenges in the differential diagnosis of IPMTs are differentiating the main-duct type tumor from chronic pancreatitis, the branch-duct type tumor from other cystic neoplasms of the pancreas, and the segmental dilatation caused by a main-duct tumor from a pseudocyst [35]. Demonstration of intraductal filling defects, communication with the main pancreatic duct, and a herniated papillary orifice into the duodenal lumen favor the diagnosis of IPMT.

The hypervascularity of endocrine pancreatic tumors is the key for correct diagnosis. Most other pancreatic tumors, including adenocarcinomas, are hypovascular. Serous cystadenomas may be hypervascular, but the presence of multiple cysts within these tumors is helpful for the diagnosis.

Magnetic resonance cholangiopancreatography of biliary and pancreatic malignancies

Technique

MRCP is typically performed using heavily T2-weighted sequences that depict the biliary tract and pancreatic duct as high signal intensity structures [7,16]. There are three basic techniques to obtain MRCP images [16,54]. The classic approach creates multiple thin slices with a thickness of 3 to 6 mm using a two-dimensional multisection technique (Fig. 15). The resulting images are best viewed sequentially by means of a cine mode, and maximum intensity projection (MIP) postprocessing is typically performed to create a single overview image. The major limitations of this approach are long acquisition times (sometimes several minutes) and the difficulty in mentally integrating the single images, a problem that can be partially solved by means of a MIP postprocessing. However, MIP projects structures with high signal intensity along an imaginary ray onto a single pixel and may lead to diagnostic errors. If, for example, a part of duodenum and the common bile duct are being projected onto the same pixel, the common bile duct may be obscured because of the high signal intensity of the duodenal fluid [54]. The two-dimensional, thick-slab technique, the second approach that can be used to create MRCP images, is an efficient way to solve this problem [9]. In this technique, several single slices with a thickness of 30 to 70 mm ("thick slabs") are obtained using a breath-hold period of a few seconds for each (Fig. 16). A major advantage of this approach is that it allows dynamic imaging. The third approach is the double-echo or multi-echo half-Fourier-acquisition, single-shot, turbo-spin echo technique. It is used as a complement to

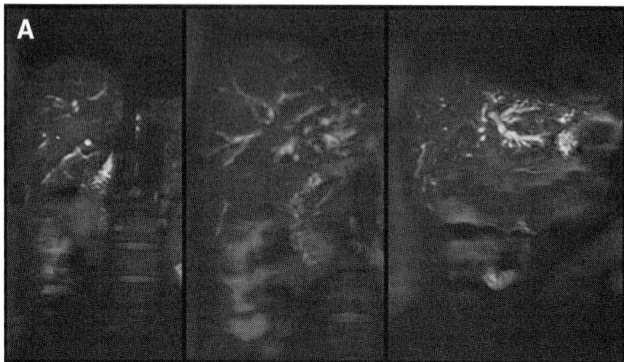

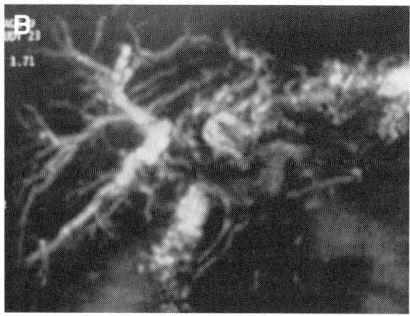

Fig. 15. MRCP, "thin-slice" technique (patient with Klatskin tumor). (*A*) Multiple coronal, fat-saturated, T2-weighted, thin-slice (3 mm thickness) images. (*B*) MIP image obtained from the coronal T2-weighted data set.

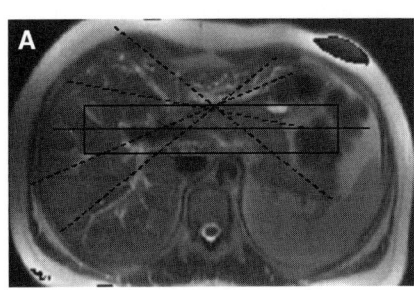 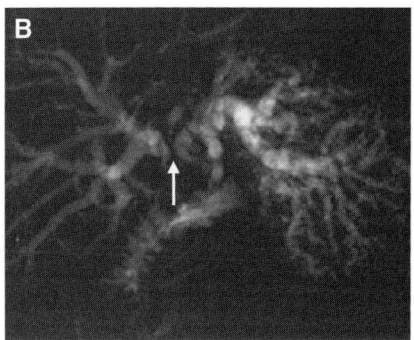

Fig. 16. MRCP, "thick-slab" technique. (*A*) Sequence planning on an axial T2-weighted image. (*B*) "Thick slab" MRCP shows the same Klatskin tumor as in Fig. 15. Note the increased detail of the involvement of the right hepatic duct (*arrow*).

the "thick slab" method and is efficient in detecting subtle pathologies of the ductal system [9,16]. In this technique, a short acquisition time (400 milliseconds) allows obtaining slices during quiet breathing. The slice thickness is typically 2 to 5 mm, and the images are heavily T2 weighted.

One of the important technical limitations of MRCP is the susceptibility artifacts caused by the presence of air, metallic clips, or stents within the field of view. Due to the visual effect of this artifact, aerobilia can be mistaken for intraductal stones. Fortunately, susceptibility artifacts are nearly eliminated with newer techniques [7]. Another problem is the presence of a metallic stent in the immediate proximity of a duct, which may mislead to an impression of ductal stenosis [54].

Extrahepatic cholangiocarcinoma

Extrahepatic cholangiocarcinoma, which accounted for only 0.5% of all new cancer cases in the United States in 2000, represents a relatively rare entity [55]. Histopathologically, it is an adenocarcinoma arising from the ductal epithelium and is the most common primary tumor of the biliary system. Extrahepatic cholangiocarcinomas include biliary adenocarcinomas located at the bifurcation or proximal hepatic duct (Klatskin tumors) and the distal duct types. They are usually seen in older patients presenting with painless jaundice, weight loss, and cholangitis [56]. Most are locally infiltrative; however, in decreasing order of frequency, lymphatic, hepatic, peritoneal and hematogenous spread is possible [57].

Once the diagnosis has been established, an accurate local staging of the tumor is essential for the planning of patient management because few patients are eligible for the surgery at the time of diagnosis [58–60]. The staging system described by Bismuth and Corlette [61] is widely accepted as a guide for the extension of surgery required (options ranging from en bloc resections of the extrahepatic bile duct up to hemi-hepatectomy) [62].

MRCP images typically reveal irregular stenoses of the bile duct segments associated with pre-stenotic dilatations of the intrahepatic bile ducts. They can involve the distal common hepatic duct alone (Bismuth type I), the confluence of the left and right hepatic duct (Bismuth type II), the confluence and the right (Bismuth type IIIa) or the left (Bismuth type IIIb) hepatic duct, or the left and right secondary confluence (Bismuth type IV) (Fig. 17). Macroscopically, hilar cholangiocarcinomas are usually classified into three types, including sclerotic, nodular, and papillary tumors. Papillary tumors have the highest resectability, whereas the sclerotic tumors have the lowest. On MRCP images, the sclerotic type, which is the most frequently encountered type, may be seen as a stretch of narrowed lumen.

The accuracy of MRC in assessing the level and the morphology of the obstruction is comparable to that of ERCP or percutaneous transhepatic cholangiography [55]. Compared with ERCP, MRCP may more accurately depict the suprahilar tumor extension in the case of a severe stenosis of the confluence (because the accuracy of ERCP is impaired due to insufficient contrast filling in such cases) [58]. Another advantage of MRCP is its ability to visualize an undrained bile duct without injection of contrast material. This eliminates the requirement that opacified bile ducts during direct cholangiographies need to be drained to avoid secondary cholangitis [64]. In addition, portal vascular invasion and hepatic metastases in patients can be detected accurately with dynamic contrast-enhanced MR sequences coupled to the MRCP protocol (Fig. 18). It offers significant advantages in the preoperative staging of hilar cholangiocarcinoma because it becomes possible to simultaneously assess the bile duct, the vascular structures, and the liver parenchyma [63]. Furthermore, MRCP can be performed in patients with gastric outlet and duodenal obstruction or with a surgically rearranged anatomy (Billroth II, Roux-en-Y) and is useful in patients in whom ERCP is unsuccessful or provides incomplete information [65]. Because of these reasons, ERCP should not be performed for diagnostic purposes but should be reserved for therapeutic interventions [52].

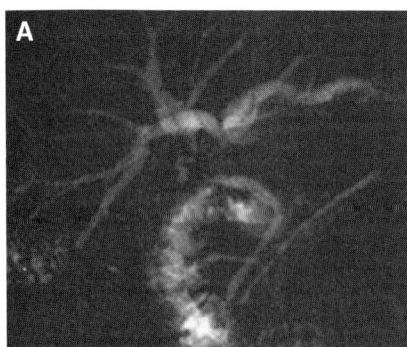 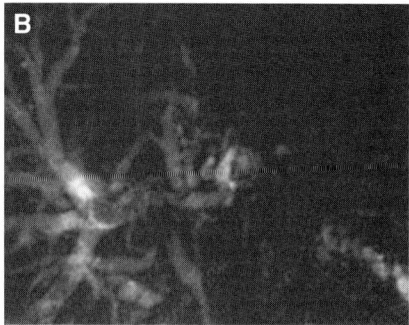

Fig. 17. Hilar cholangiocarcinoma. (A) MRCP image shows involvement of the primary confluence and the right secondary confluence, type IIIa. (B) Involvement of the left and right secondary confluence, type IV.

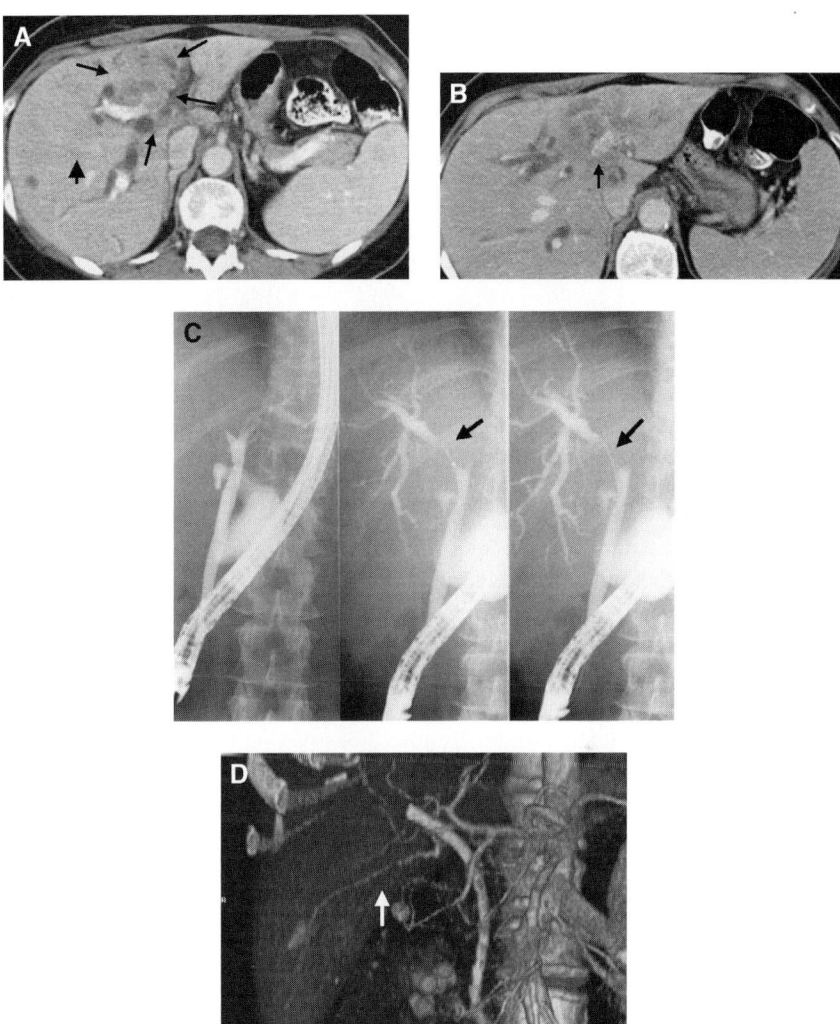

Fig. 18. Hilar cholangiocarcinoma. (*A*) Contrast-enhanced axial CT image shows an ill-defined, heterogenous lesion (*arrows*) in the porta hepatis and heterogenous enhancement of the normal liver parenchyma suggesting vascular invasion (*arrowhead*). (*B*) Attenuated left portal vein is consistent with portal venous invasion (*arrow*). (*C*) ERCP shows obstruction of the right hepatic duct (*arrows*). (*D*) 3D CT angiogram demonstrates involvement of the right hepatic artery (*arrow*). Note the presence of a biliary stent.

Pancreatic adenocarcinoma

On MRCP, an abrupt transition of the intrapancreatic portion of the common bile duct is typical for adenocarcinoma [56]. The stricture usually has a length of several centimeters and usually has irregular contours. In adenocarcinomas involving the pancreatic head, the "double duct" sign representing dilated common

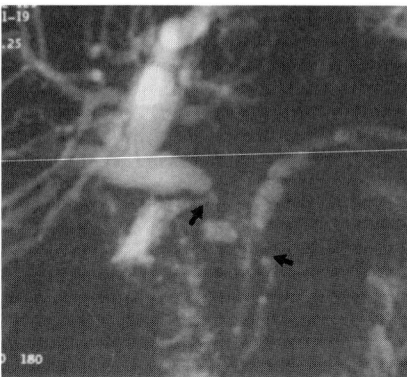

Fig. 19. Pancreatic adenocarcinoma. MRCP image shows dilatation of biliary tree and main pancreatic duct. The distal segments of the bile duct and pancreatic duct are also seen, forming the "four-segment" sign (*arrows*).

bile and pancreatic ducts can be frequently depicted. If the short segments of the biliary and pancreatic ducts distal to the obstruction are visualized, the proximal biliary and pancreatic ducts and their distal parts appear as four separate ducts. This appearance is called as "the four segment sign" and allows differentiation of pancreatic adenocarcinoma from distal cholangiocarcinoma and ampullary carcinoma (Fig. 19) [66,67]. An important advantage of MRCP is that it does not identify only dilated ducts proximally to the obstruction but also ducts that are tumor encased but not obstructed [16,35]. Adamek et al [68] reported that MRCP is more sensitive and specific (84% and 97%) in the diagnosis of pancreatic carcinoma than is ERCP (70% sensitivity and 94% specificity). Adding other MR sequences to the examination protocol further improves the overall sensitivity and specificity of MR imaging for pancreatic adenocarcinoma [4] (Fig. 20). Particularly, when T1- and T2-weighted MR imaging and MR angiography are performed in the same examination setting as MRCP, an assessment for resectability can be made. In patients with unresectable disease, MRCP is critical for planning palliative endoscopic and percutaneous procedures [16,69].

Intraductal papillary mucinous tumors

MRCP patterns include segmental or diffuse involvement of the main pancreatic duct in the main duct tumors and microcystic or macrocystic mass-like lesions in the branch duct tumors [10] (Fig. 21). With progression, branch duct tumors may seed the main pancreatic duct and consequently demonstrate findings consistent with main duct tumors. On MRCP, observation of thick walls and mural nodules helps in the diagnosis of malignancy. The size of the tumor is also important. In a study by Obara et al [70], 83% of the tumors > 4 cm in diameter were found to be malignant. A main duct dilatation > 15 mm [71] and a diffuse main pancreatic duct dilatation associated with the branch type tumors are other MRCP findings associated with malignancy [72]. ERCP has been considered the

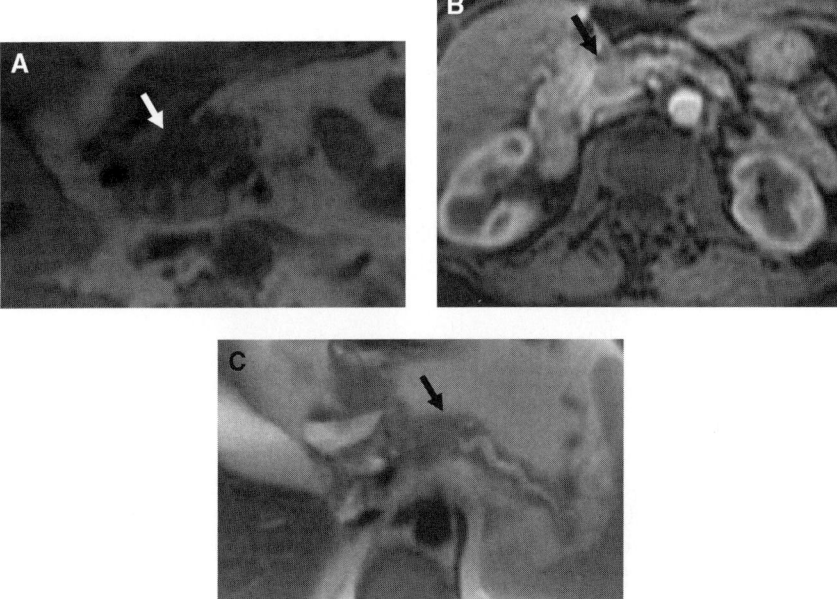

Fig. 20. Pancreatic adenocarcinoma. (*A*) T1-weighted, axial MR image shows a hypointense mass lesion in the pancreatic head (*arrow*). (*B*) Fat-saturated, post-gadolinium, MR image demonstrates the hypovascular nature of the lesion (*arrow*). (*C*) T2-weighted MR image shows the isointense lesion (*arrow*), atrophied pancreatic tail, and dilated main pancreatic duct.

gold standard for IPMTs traditionally [35]; however, there are several studies reporting the superiority of MRCP to ERCP in evaluating intraductal papillary mucinous tumors of the pancreas [39,43,73–75]. When used to look for branch type cystic dilatations, ERCP may be burdened by false negatives due to the inability of contrast to depict ductectesia filled with mucin [39]. This is not a

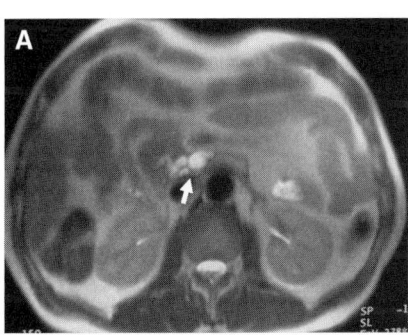
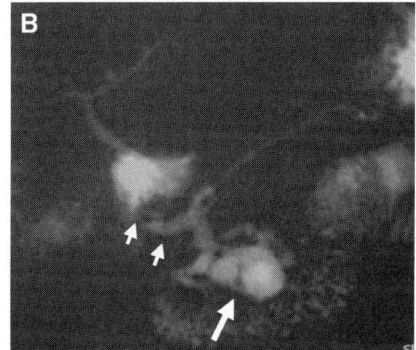

Fig. 21. Intraductal papillary mucinous tumor, side-branch type. (*A*) T2-weighted, axial MR image shows multiloculated cystic lesion in the uncinate process (*arrow*). (*B*) MRCP image shows communication of the tumor with the main pancreatic duct, which is dilated up to the papilla (*arrows*).

problem for MRCP because mucin has a high signal intensity that makes it indistinguishable from pancreatic juice [43]. MRCP was also shown to be more sensitive than ERCP in the visualization of intramural nodules [30] and papillary protrusions [76]. ERCP keeps its important role when biopsy, cytologic, or pancreatic juice sampling is needed.

Computed tomographic colonography (virtual colonoscopy)

Technique

Optimal CT colonography technique requires careful cleansing and distention of the colon. Residual stool causes similar problems encountered at barium enema radiography because it simulates polyps or tumoral masses. Good colonic cleansing is achieved by a 48-hour, low-residue diet and the ingestion of a cathartic or laxative that promotes evacuation of colonic contents. Stool markers (mostly barium) can be administered per os 24 to 48 hours before CT to improve differentiation of soft tissue intraluminal lesions and retained stool. This technique is called fecal tagging (Fig. 22) [77,78]. Colon insufflation is performed with the patient in a lateral decubitus position after gentle placement of a catheter tip (with or without retention cuff) in the rectum. The colon is insufflated with room air to maximum patient tolerance or to a set volume. Most patients retain 1.5 to 2 liters. Carbon dioxide may be preferred to air because it is absorbed by the colon mucosa and reduces discomfort after the procedure [79]. CT is performed in supine and prone positions. If a prone position is impossible for the patient, a left lateral decubitus position is preferred for optimal air redistribution to the segments, which are not optimally distended in supine position. Administration of intravenous contrast can sometimes be helpful in the characterization of detected lesions (Fig. 23) [80], but intravenous contrast is usually not used in the screening setting due to the potential side effects of contrast agents and the increased cost. The use of a MDCT with narrow detector collimation is a prerequisite for an accurate CT colonography and for optimal 3D reconstructions

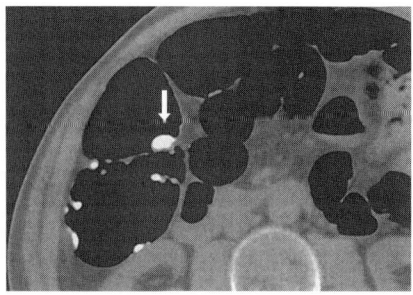

Fig. 22. Fecal tagging. Marked feces due to barium ingestion before examination on the dependent bowel wall (*arrow*) can be differentiated from a polyp.

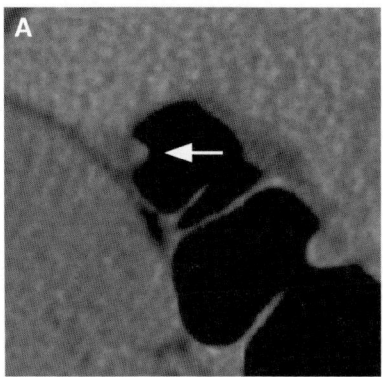
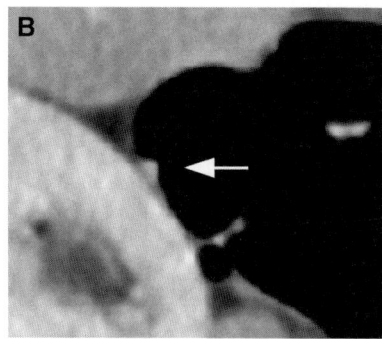

Fig. 23. Colonic polyp. Precontrast (*A*) and postcontrast (*B*) CT images show enhancement of the polyp (*arrows*) after intravenous administration of the contrast material.

[81]. The CT parameters used are a result of the type of scanner, the image quality needed, and the radiation dose one is willing to give. Images are reconstructed as 1.5- to 3-mm-thick sections with a reconstruction interval of 30% to 60%. Coronal and sagittal multiplanar reconstructions are routinely obtained [82–85]. 3D endoluminal images are useful to confirm the presence of a lesion and to improve diagnostic confidence. Most CT manufactures have software for creating 3D endoluminal and multiplanar reformatted views. Workstations equipped with such software display 2-dimensional (2D) and 3D images on a single interactive screen, and this promotes a quick 2D-3D correlation. Most investigators use a primary 2D interpretation with "lumen tracking," starting from the rectum and following the course of the bowel from slice to slice to the cecum [86,87]. 3D imaging is complementary to axial and multiplanar reformatted 2D images and should be used as an adjunct to confirm the 2D observation and improve the characterization of a lesion [88].

Virtual colonoscopy as a diagnostic tool

Colorectal cancer is the fourth most common cancer after breast, lung, and prostate cancers and is the second leading cause of cancer-related deaths in United States [89]. The majority of the colorectal cancers arise from preexisting adenomas through the so-called "adenoma-to-carcinoma" sequence [90,91]. The duration of this sequence is ~10 years [92]. Due to this long interval, it can be suggested that colorectal carcinoma is a potentially preventable disease, as long as these adenomatous polyps are detected and removed before they become malignant. To find and remove polyps larger than 1 cm is important as a colorectal cancer prevention strategy because 99% of the discovered adenomas smaller than 1 cm (they constitute 70% of the detected adenomas in screening studies) do not contain adenocarcinomas [86,93], whereas 10% of adenomas 1 to 2 cm in diameter and more than 40% of adenomas >2 cm in diameter harbor adenocarcinomas.

Until the mid-1990s, colonoscopy and double-contrast barium enema (DCBE) were the methods available for polyp detection. According to the literature, sensitivity of DCBE for the detection of polyps < 1 cm is between 50% and 80% and between 75% and 95% for the detection of polyps >1 cm. The sensitivity of colonoscopy is approximately 75% for the detection of polyps < 1 cm and 90% for polyps larger than 1 cm. The specificity of this technique is assumed to be 100% [89]. The main advantages of conventional colonoscopy are the direct visualization of the colonic mucosa and its potential to remove small polyps. However, it requires an intensive preparation, and in as many as 15% of cases, the endoscopist is unable to reach the cecum [94]. The completion rate for colonoscopy varies from 75% to 99% and depends mainly on the skills of the examiner, anatomic variations, anatomic alterations due to prior abdominal surgery, bowel preparation, and patient's cooperation. Compliance plays a key role in an effective screening program. Compliance is only about 40% in a screening setting for colonoscopy [95]; this low rate is most probably due to the pain experienced during the procedure and the intense bowel-cleansing regimen.

CT colonography (virtual colonoscopy) is a promising new method for detecting colorectal polyps and cancers (Fig. 24) [96]. It uses a rapid CT (preferably a MDCT) to generate data that are converted by computer software into 2D and 3D displays of the colon [97]. It has several advantages: no sedation is needed; it is minimally invasive; and the examination is well tolerated, less expensive, and less time consuming than conventional colonoscopy. There is still a need for bowel cleansing and infusion of air to expand the colon, which are considered the most uncomfortable parts of the examination by the patients. Nevertheless, patients mostly prefer CT colonography to optical colonoscopy [98–102].

It can be assumed that CT colonography is promising for the detection of polyps ≥1 cm in diameter. For polyps with a diameter >1 cm, virtual colonoscopy has sensitivities between 82% and 93% [103,104]. The specificity of the technique varies from 90% to 97.7%. For polyps ≤5 mm, reported sensitivities are 11% to 59%; for polyps 6 to 9 mm, reported sensitivities are 16% to 60%. There are contradictory results in the literature. In a recent multi-centric study, Cotton et al [105] reported a low sensitivity (39%) for detecting polyps sized at least 6 mm with virtual colonoscopy. The sensitivity was not much higher (55%) with a threshold of 10 mm. In their study, the sensitivity of conventional colonoscopy for polyps ≥6 mm was 99%. Although this study is criticized because of the lack of experience of the involved radiologists in evaluating CT colonographics and the relatively outdated CT technique used [106], it constitutes a strong argument against the use of virtual colonoscopy as a primary screening tool. On the other hand, in a more recent study, Pickhardt et al [107] reported CT colonography sensitivities of 85.7% and 92.2% for adenomas at 6 and 10 mm thresholds, respectively. In this study, CT outperformed conventional colonoscopy for lesions over 8 mm.

Although there is no clear consensus about the use of CT colonography as a screening tool, the general trend in medicine is to replace invasive techniques with

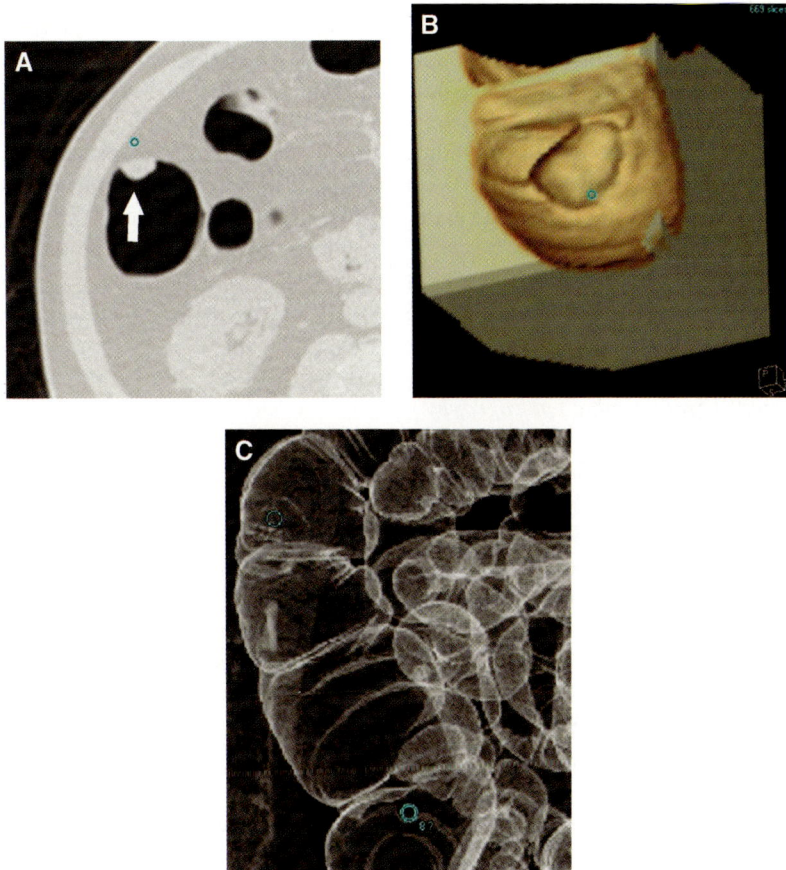

Fig. 24. Polyp on the nondependent wall in the ascending colon (*A*) and corresponding 3D image
(*B*). On surface-shaded 3D image (*C*), the lesion is easily located within the colon.

noninvasive or less invasive ones and to reserve invasive techniques for problem solving and interventions. CT colonography fits in this trend perfectly [88].

Computed tomographic enteroclysis and computed tomographic enterography

Computed tomographic enteroclysis

The cleansing preparation for CT enteroclysis requires, like all other intestinal
endoscopic, fluoroscopic, and virtual "scopic" techniques, a low-residual diet,
ample fluids, and a laxative before the examination. Nothing should be eaten by

mouth on the day of examination. Colonic enemas are generally not recommended [108]. Patients should be given an option of sedation [109]. Positive intraluminal contrast materials (iodinated water-soluble contrast or diluted barium) are used when small bowel obstruction or the possibility of internal extraintestinal fistula are clinical indications. Neutral contrast materials (such as methylcellulose) are the choice in evaluating disease activity in Crohn's disease or in the case of unexplained anemia or GI bleeding [110]. Intravenous nonionic iodinated contrast agents can be used in combination with neutral intraluminal contrast material. According to Maglinte et al [110], a slice thickness of 3.0 mm with a reconstruction increment of 1.5 mm for 16-row MDCTs allows for reformatting multiplanar images with high spatial resolution.

Computed tomographic enterography

With CT enterography, opacification of the small intestine is obtained through orally administered contrast agents (Fig. 25). As in CT enteroclysis, positive or neutral contrast materials including water are used for the visualization of small bowel loops. Positive agents are usually used for routine cases but may cause problems when used during 3D imaging or angiography. In such cases, neutral or negative contrast agents are preferred. Examinations aiming to evaluate inflammatory or neoplastic conditions should be performed with intravenous contrast administration and neutral intraluminal contrast agents. In our daily practice, we prefer a collimation of 0.75 mm and an increment of 3 mm as scan parameters to create routine axial and coronal images of small bowel. In an ongoing study in

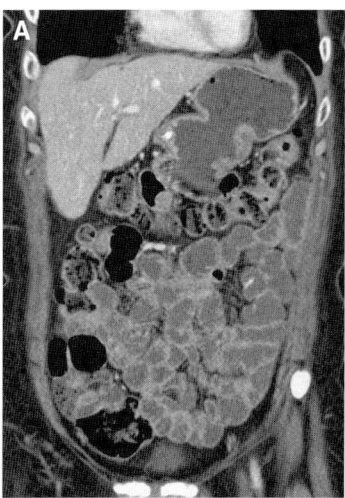 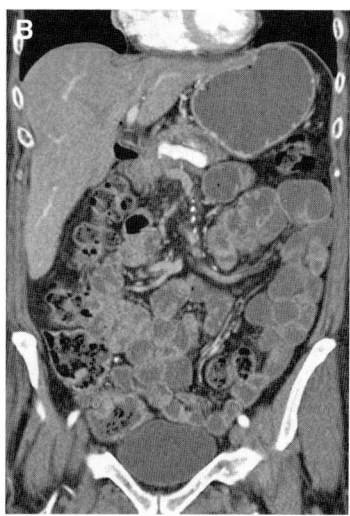

Fig. 25. (*A,B*) Normal CT coronal images with orally administered low density barium (Volumen, EZ-EM) and intravenously administered nonionic contrast material. Low-density barium allows distention of small bowel loops and evaluation of the small bowel wall on postcontrast CT images.

our institution, we perform CT-enterography with oral administration of a low-density barium preparation (Volumen EZ-EM; 1450 mL over 45 minutes).

Imaging of small bowel

The prevalence of small bowel disease is low, and the clinical diagnosis is difficult because of nonspecific symptoms. CT enteroclysis or enterography are

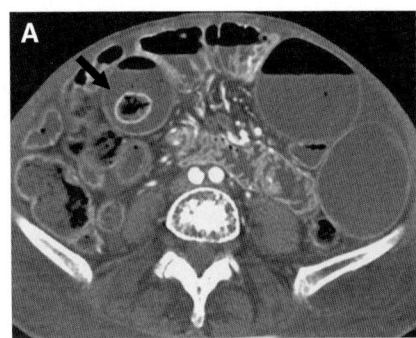
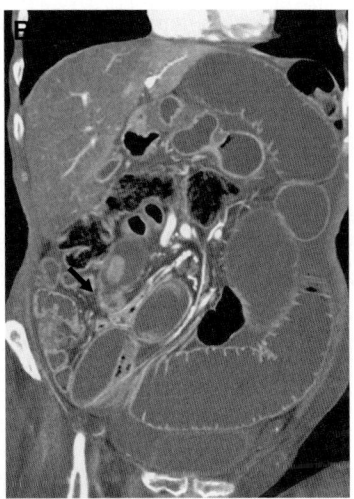
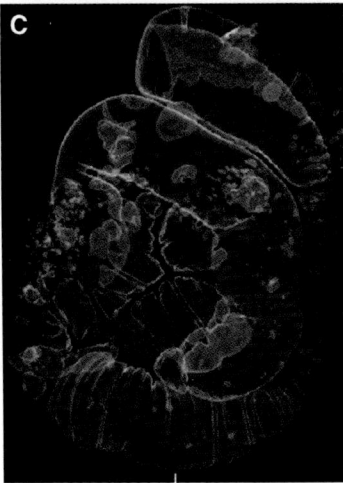

Fig. 26. Low-density barium small bowel study with axial (*A*) and coronal (*B*) images shows an adhesion as cause of small bowel obstruction and presence of an enterolith (*arrows*) in the dilated small bowel proximal to the transition point. (*C*) Virtual enterography image shows the transition point and location of the enterolith.

especially indicated for patients with symptoms of intermittent small bowel obstruction, for patients with unexplained abdominal pain (particularly if there is a history of previous abdominal surgery), for Crohn's disease and its complications, for GI bleeding, for unexplained anemia, and for small bowel neoplasms (Figs. 26 and 27) [110]. The main disadvantages of conventional enteroclysis are the overlapping bowel loops and its inability to provide extraintestinal information, whereas in axial CT imaging of the small bowel, volume challenge is lacking. CT enteroclysis combines the advantages of enteral volume challenge and the ability of cross-sectional imaging and reformatting [111]. CT enterography is an elegant alternative for CT enteroclysis. Its main advantage is that it does not require catheterization. New developments in 3D imaging techniques are consistently improving the diagnostic ability of this noninvasive technique. High-resolution 3D images and reformats of small bowel can be obtained routinely in daily practice.

The diagnostic potential and quality of these techniques are, with the introduction of MDCT, dramatically improved. MDCT allows faster scanning, which results in improved temporal resolution due to fewer motion artifacts and decreased image noise due to the chance of using increased tube currents. The other important advantage of MDCT is its ability to scan with thinner slice thickness, which improves spatial resolution and allows reformatting of multiplanar high-quality images.

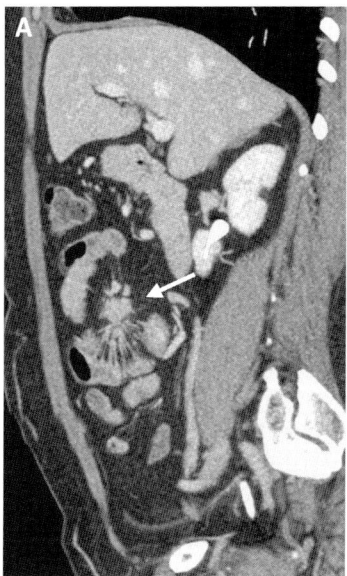
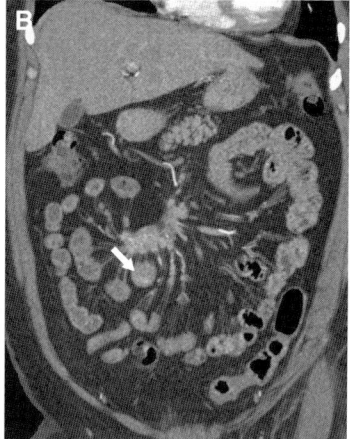

Fig. 27. Small bowel carcinoid tumor. Contrast-enhanced, sagittal and coronal CT images show desmoplastic reaction and mesenteric metastases (*A*, *arrow*) and the presence of a small tumor in an ileal bowel loop (*B*, *arrow*).

Magnetic resonance imaging in rectal cancer

Technique

Pelvic MR imaging for rectal carcinoma uses a phased-array coil (PA-MRI), a set of "parallel-working" surface coils, to reach a high signal-to-noise ratio and spatial resolution. A common examination approach is to obtain sagittal T2-weighted images through the pelvis initially. These images demonstrate the relationship of the tumor and rectum. The second step is to image the pelvis with a T2-weighted sequence in the axial plane using a smaller FOV (usually 16 cm instead of 24 cm), a higher matrix (usually 512 × 512 instead of 256 × 256), and a thin slice thickness (3 mm) [112]. These high-resolution images demonstrate local tumor stage. Scanning the entire pelvis using T1-weighted and T2-weighted conventional sequences may be helpful in detecting distant lymphadenopathy.

In endorectal MR imaging (ER-MRI), a rectal coil with an inflatable balloon is used. The optimal imaging sequences for endoluminal MR imaging of the ano-rectum have not been determined. In our experience, multiplanar T2-weighted, turbo, spin-echo and axial T1-weighted, spin-echo MR imaging give optimal results. The T2-weighted images clearly demonstrate normal anatomy and allow differentiation of the rectal wall layers. T1-weighted imaging is helpful in determining the extent of the lesion in the mesorectum and lymph nodes. The use of intravenously administered gadolinium may be helpful in determining tumor extent and in differentiating T2 from T3 tumors.

Rectal cancer and magnetic resonance imaging

The preoperative evaluation of a patient with rectal cancer determines the type of surgical approach and the need for chemotherapy and radiotherapy. Tumor size, local stage, presence of distant metastases, and proximity to the anal sphincter decide which individuals are eligible for local excision and which require transanal resection or abdominoperineal or low anterior resection. An accurate preoperative assessment of the patient is valuable for the centers administrating neoadjuvant chemoradiotherapy before the surgery. Because pelvic radiation may result in anal sphincter injury, anorectal functional problems, cystitis, impotence, and sterility in premenopausal women, accurate staging to avoid unnecessary radiotherapy is important. MR imaging was first introduced for staging of rectal cancer in 1986 [113]. It has been performed using body coils [112]. Modern MR imaging techniques use phased-array surface coils or endo-rectal coils to reach a better spatial resolution and thus an improved accuracy for predicting the tumor stage.

With phased-array coils and high-resolution imaging techniques, it is possible to discriminate the five concentric layers of the rectal wall [114]. The current literature [114,115] suggests that high-resolution, phased-array techniques can accurately predict the depth of any extramural penetration and, more importantly, can predict the relationship between the tumor and the mesorectal fascia.

According to our experience, endorectal MR imaging can be combined with conventional MR imaging to provide complete abdominal and pelvic imaging (Fig. 28). Because of the high signal-to-noise ratios, images with excellent spatial resolution allowing optimal identification of the rectal wall layers are created. Preliminary results from our institution demonstrate an overall accuracy of 88% in staging distal tumors by means of endorectal MR imaging. On this basis, we are able to recommend preoperative chemoradiation therapy for patients with stage II and III cancer and a local excision rather than a radical resection for stage I patients with appropriate tumors. Like in transrectal ultrasonography (TRUS), stenotic tumors constitute the major limitation of endorectal MR imaging, and in some cases it may be impossible to traverse the stenosis. In our experience, endorectal MR imaging is less operator dependent than TRUS.

In a recent study by Matsuoka et al [116], ER-MRI and PA-MRI examinations yielded the same accuracy (80% each) for diagnosing the depth of tumor invasion. Two patients were understaged with both of the modalities due to technical limitations. In one patient, slice and gap intervals did not allow detection of a microscopic invasion. In the other patient, who had a tumor in the anal canal, discrimination between the tumor and adjacent anal canal structures was not possible.

TRUS has been applied to the staging of rectal cancer for many years [112]. Its ability to visualize the different layers of the rectal wall was its main strength. Many investigators have attempted to assess the accuracy of TRUS for staging rectal tumors. In a recent study, the overall accuracy of this technique for staging rectal tumors was 69% [117]. There are also studies reporting accuracies of 97%

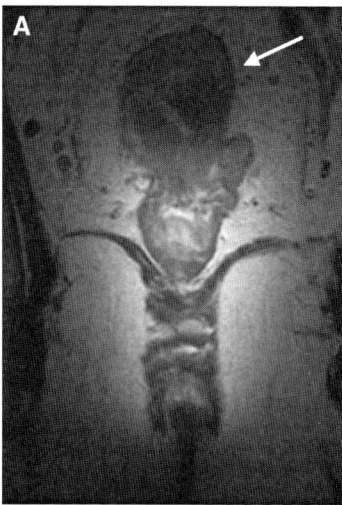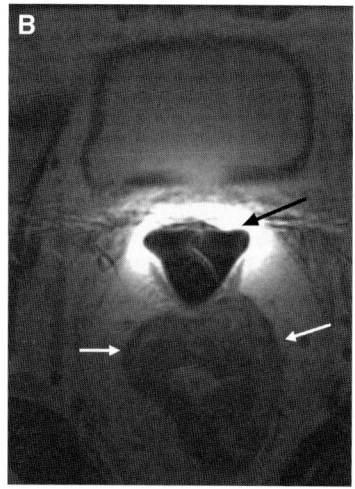

Fig. 28. Rectal cancer (T2N0Mx). Coronal (*A*) and axial (*B*) T2-weighted MR images show a large mass (*white arrows*) with involvement of the muscularis propria. No tumor is seen in the mesorectal fat. Note the presence of an endorectal coil (*black arrow*).

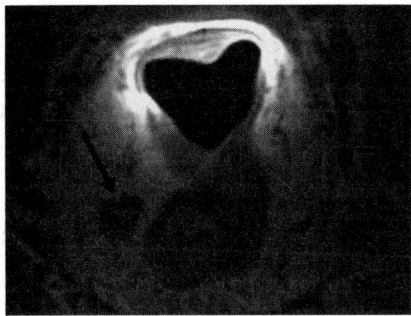

Fig. 29. Rectal cancer (T3N1Mx). Axial T1-weighted MR image shows an enlarged lymph node in the mesorectal fat (*arrow*).

[118]. The main problem of TRUS is the overstaging of T2 tumors due to the extensive peritumoral tissue reaction surrounding the growing tumor. Differentiating between T2 and T3 tumors is also a critical issue for MR imaging, and Brown et al [113] reported that MR correctly predicted the T stage in every case (five T2, 18 T3, and two T4 tumors). TRUS has some limitations, such as operator dependency, limitation to tumors located 8 to 10 cm from the anal verge when a rigid probe is used, and no assessment of stenotic tumors. Moreover, TRUS cannot identify the mesorectal fascia. This is an important issue in determining the spread of stage T3 tumors considered for total mesorectal excision and classifying lymph nodes. This may explain the more recent widespread use of MR imaging because these limitations do not apply to MR imaging with external coils [119].

In preoperative staging, accurate diagnosis of metastatic lymph nodes is an issue that needs improvement like with all other neoplastic entities (Fig. 29). None of the existing imaging modalities have satisfactory and consistent results for the detection and characterization of lymph node involvement.

Summary

Developments in imaging technology in recent years have led to many improvements in the field of diagnostic GI radiology. With its fast and thin-section scanning abilities, MDCT strengthens the place of CT as the most efficient tool to diagnose, characterize, and preoperatively stage pancreatic neoplasms. MRCP has widely replaced ERCP in the diagnosis and staging of pancreato-biliary malignancies. MR imaging, using phased-array or endorectal coils, demonstrates local tumor invasion accurately in rectal cancers and thus allows improved surgical planning. Virtual colonoscopy with MDCTs is an efficient screening method for colon cancer, and MDCT enterography is becoming the standard imaging technique for many small bowel disorders. The continuing developments in CT and MR technology will most probably further improve accuracies of these and other imaging applications in the near future.

References

[1] McNulty NJ, Francis IR, Platt JF, et al. Multi-detector row helical CT of the pancreas: effect of contrast-enhanced multiphasic imaging on enhancement of the pancreas, peripancreatic vasculature, and pancreatic adenocarcinoma. Radiology 2001;220:97–102.

[2] O'Malley ME, Boland GW, Wood BJ, et al. Adenocarcinoma of the head of the pancreas: determination of surgical unresectability with thin-section pancreatic-phase helical CT. AJR Am J Roentgenol 1999;173:1513–8.

[3] Mortele KJ, Ji H, Ros PR. CT and magnetic resonance imaging in pancreatic and biliary tract malignancies. Gastrointest Endosc 2002;56(Suppl):S206–12.

[4] Wallner BK, Schumacher KA, Weidenmaier W, et al. Dilated biliary tract: evaluation with MR cholangiography with a T2-weighted contrast-enhanced fast sequence. Radiology 1991; 181:805–8.

[5] Soto JA, Barish MA, Yucel EK, et al. MR cholangiopancreatography: findings on 3D fast spin-echo imaging. AJR Am J Roentgenol 1995;165:1397–401.

[6] Barish MA, Yucel EK, Soto JA, et al. MR cholangiopancreatography: efficacy of three-dimensional turbo spin-echo technique. AJR Am J Roentgenol 1995;165:295–300.

[7] Jara H, Barish MA, Yucel EK, et al. MR hydrography: theory and practice of static fluid imaging. AJR Am J Roentgenol 1998;170:873–82.

[8] Soto JA, Barish MA, Yucel EK, et al. Pancreatic duct: MR cholangiopancreatography with a three-dimensional fast spin-echo technique. Radiology 1995;196:459–64.

[9] Soto JA, Barish MA, Alvarez O, et al. Detection of choledocholithiasis with MR cholangiography: comparison of three-dimensional fast spin-echo and single- and multisection half-Fourier rapid acquisition with relaxation enhancement sequences. Radiology 2000;215: 737–45.

[10] Fayad LM, Kowalski T, Mitchell DG. MR cholangiopancreatography: evaluation of common pancreatic diseases. Radiol Clin N Am 2003;41:97–114.

[11] Barish MA, Ferrucci JT. MR cholangiopancreatography challenges invasive methods. Diagn Imaging (San Franc) 1998;20:32–6.

[12] Barish MA, Yucel EK, Ferrucci JT. Magnetic resonance cholangiopancreatography. N Engl J Med 1999;341:258–64.

[13] Soto JA, Yucel EK, Barish MA, et al. MR cholangiopancreatography after unsuccessful or incomplete ERCP. Radiology 1996;199:91–8.

[14] Soto JA, Barish MA, Yucel EK, et al. Magnetic resonance cholangiography: comparison with endoscopic retrograde cholangiopancreatography. Gastroenterology 1996;110:589–97.

[15] Barish MA, Soto JA. MR cholangiopancreatography: techniques and clinical applications. AJR Am J Roentgenol 1997;169:1295–303.

[16] Fulcher AS, Turner MA. MR cholangiopancreatography. Radiol Clin N Am 2002;40:1363–76.

[17] Mortele KJ, Ros PR. Magnetic resonance imaging of the exocrine pancreas. Rays 2001; 26:117–26.

[18] Warshaw AL, Fernandez-del Castillo C. Pancreatic carcinoma. N Engl J Med 1992;326:455–65.

[19] Steele Jr GD, Osteen RT, Winchester DP, et al. Clinical highlights from the National Cancer Data Base: 1994. CA Cancer J Clin 1994;44:71–80.

[20] Vellet AD, Romano W, Bach DB, et al. Adenocarcinoma of the pancreatic ducts: comparative evaluation with CT and MR imaging at 1.5 T. Radiology 1992;183:87–95.

[21] Choi BI, Chung MJ, Han JK, et al. Detection of pancreatic adenocarcinoma: relative value of arterial and late phases of spiral CT. Abdom Imaging 1997;22:199–203.

[22] Bluemke DA, Cameron JL, Hruban RH, et al. Potentially resectable pancreatic adenocarci-

noma: spiral CT assessment with surgical and pathologic correlation. Radiology 1995;197: 381–5.

[23] Freeny PC, Traverso LW, Ryan JA. Diagnosis and staging of pancreatic adenocarcinoma with dynamic computed tomography. Am J Surg 1993;165:600–6.

[24] Freeny PC, Marks WM, Ryan JA, et al. Pancreatic ductal adenocarcinoma: diagnosis and staging with dynamic CT. Radiology 1988;166:125–33.

[25] Catalano C, Laghi A, Fraioli F, et al. Pancreatic carcinoma: the role of high-resolution multislice spiral CT in the diagnosis and assessment of resectability. Eur Radiol 2003;13:149–56.

[26] Graf O, Boland GW, Warshaw AL, et al. Arterial versus portal venous helical CT for revealing pancreatic adenocarcinoma: conspicuity of tumor and critical vascular anatomy. AJR Am J Roentgenol 1997;169:119–23.

[27] Boland GW, O'Malley ME, Saez M, et al. Pancreatic-phase versus portal vein-phase helical CT of the pancreas: optimal temporal window for evaluation of pancreatic adenocarcinoma. AJR Am J Roentgenol 1999;172:605–8.

[28] Horton KM, Fishman EK. Adenocarcinoma of the pancreas: CT imaging. Radiol Clin N Am 2002;40:1263–72.

[29] Ros PR, Mortele KJ. Imaging features of pancreatic neoplasms. JBR-BTR 2001;84:239–49.

[30] Soriano A, Castells A, Ayuso C, et al. Preoperative staging and tumor resectability assessment of pancreatic cancer: prospective study comparing endoscopic ultrasonography, helical computed tomography, magnetic resonance imaging, and angiography. Am J Gastroenterol 2004; 99:492–501.

[31] Rosch T, Dittler HJ, Strobel K, et al. Endoscopic ultrasound criteria for vascular invasion in the staging of cancer of the head of the pancreas: a blind reevaluation of videotapes. Gastrointest Endosc 2000;52:469–77.

[32] Ahmad NA, Kochman ML, Lewis JD, et al. Can EUS alone differentiate between malignant and benign cystic lesions of the pancreas? Am J Gastroenterol 2001;96:3295–300.

[33] Muller MF, Meyenberger C, Bertschinger P, et al. Pancreatic tumors: evaluation with endoscopic US, CT, and MR imaging. Radiology 1994;190:745–51.

[34] Ros PR, Hamrick-Turner JE, Chiechi MV, et al. Cystic masses of the pancreas. Radiographics 1992;12:673–86.

[35] Hammond N, Miller FH, Sica GT, et al. Imaging of cystic diseases of the pancreas. Radiol Clin N Am 2002;40:1243–62.

[36] Itai Y, Ohhashi K, Furui S, et al. Microcystic adenoma of the pancreas: spectrum of computed tomographic findings. J Comput Assist Tomogr 1988;12:797–803.

[37] Mitchell DG, Shapiro M, Schuricht A, et al. Pancreatic disease: findings on state-of-the-art MR images. AJR Am J Roentgenol 1992;159:533–8.

[38] Ohtomo K, Furui S, Onoue M, et al. Solid and papillary epithelial neoplasm of the pancreas: MR imaging and pathologic correlation. Radiology 1992;184:567–70.

[39] Sugiyama M, Atomi Y, Hachiya J. Intraductal papillary tumors of the pancreas: evaluation with magnetic resonance cholangiopancreatography. Am J Gastroenterol 1998;93:156–9.

[40] Taouli B, Vilgrain V, Vullierme MP, et al. Intraductal papillary mucinous tumors of the pancreas: helical CT with histopathologic correlation. Radiology 2000;217:757–64.

[41] Shimizu M, Manabe T. Mucin-producing pancreatic tumors: historical review of its nosological concept. Zentralbl Pathol 1994;140:211–23.

[42] Procacci C, Megibow AJ, Carbognin G, et al. Intraductal papillary mucinous tumor of the pancreas: a pictorial essay. Radiographics 1999;19:1447–63.

[43] Sahani D, Prasad S, Saini S, et al. Cystic pancreatic neoplasms evaluation by CT and magnetic resonance cholangiopancreatography. Gastrointest Endosc Clin N Am 2002;12:657–72.

[44] Choi BI, Kim KW, Han MC, et al. Solid and papillary epithelial neoplasms of the pancreas: CT findings. Radiology 1988;166:413–6.

[45] Cantisani V, Mortele KJ, Levy A, et al. MR imaging features of solid pseudopapillary tumor of the pancreas in adult and pediatric patients. AJR Am J Roentgenol 2003;181:395–401.

[46] Sheth S, Fishman EK. Imaging of uncommon tumors of the pancreas. Radiol Clin N Am 2002;40:1273–87.

[47] Buetow PC, Miller DL, Parrino TV, et al. Islet cell tumors of the pancreas: clinical, radiologic, and pathologic correlation in diagnosis and localization. Radiographics 1997;17:453–72.

[48] Furukawa H, Mukai K, Kosuge T, et al. Nonfunctioning islet cell tumors of the pancreas: clinical, imaging and pathological aspects in 16 patients. Jpn J Clin Oncol 1998;28:255–61.

[49] Herman TE, Siegel MJ, Dehner LP. CT of pancreatoblastoma derived from the dorsal pancreatic anlage. J Comput Assist Tomogr 1994;18:648–50.

[50] Mergo PJ, Helmberger TK, Buetow PC, et al. Pancreatic neoplasms: MR imaging and pathologic correlation. Radiographics 1997;17:281–301.

[51] Robey G, Daneman A, Martin DJ. Pancreatic carcinoma in a neonate. Pediatr Radiol 1983;13: 284–6.

[52] Buetow PC, Rao P, Thompson LD. From the Archives of the AFIP. Mucinous cystic neoplasms of the pancreas: radiologic-pathologic correlation. Radiographics 1998;18:433–49.

[53] Shyr YM, Su CH, Tsay SH, et al. Mucin-producing neoplasms of the pancreas: intraductal papillary and mucinous cystic neoplasms. Ann Surg 1996;223:141–6.

[54] Van Hoe L, Mermuys K, Vanhoenacker P. MRCP pitfalls. Abdom Imaging 2004;29:360–87.

[55] Zech CJ, Schoenberg SO, Reiser M, et al. Cross-sectional imaging of biliary tumors: current clinical status and future developments. Eur Radiol 2004;14:1174–87.

[56] Mortele KJ, Wiesner W, Cantisani V, et al. Usual and unusual causes of extrahepatic chole-stasis: assessment with magnetic resonance cholangiography and fast MRI. Abdom Imaging 2004;29:87–99.

[57] Yeh TS, Jan YY, Tseng JH, et al. Malignant perihilar biliary obstruction: magnetic resonance cholangiopancreatographic findings. Am J Gastroenterol 2000;95:432–40.

[58] Cha JH, Han JK, Kim TK, et al. Preoperative evaluation of Klatskin tumor: accuracy of spiral CT in determining vascular invasion as a sign of unresectability. Abdom Imaging 2000;25: 500–7.

[59] Lygidakis NJ, Sgourakis GJ, Dedemadi GV, et al. Long-term results following resectional surgery for Klatskin tumors: a twenty-year personal experience. Hepatogastroenterology 2001; 48:95–101.

[60] Bathe OF, Pacheco JT, Ossi PB, et al. Management of hilar bile duct carcinoma. Hepato-gastroenterology 2001;48:1289–94.

[61] Bismuth H, Corlette MB. Intrahepatic cholangioenteric anastomosis in carcinoma of the hilus of the liver. Surg Gynecol Obstet 1975;140:170–8.

[62] Khan SA, Davidson BR, Goldin R, et al. British Society of Gastroenterology. Guidelines for the diagnosis and treatment of cholangiocarcinoma: consensus document. Gut 2002;51(Suppl 6): VI1–9.

[63] Manfredi R, Masselli G, Maresca G, et al. MR imaging and MRCP of hilar cholangiocarci-noma. Abdom Imaging 2003;28:319–25.

[64] Nichols DA, MacCarty RL, Gaffey TA. Cholangiographic evaluation of bile duct carcinoma. AJR Am J Roentgenol 1983;141:1291–4.

[65] Varghese JC, Farrell MA, Courtney G, et al. Role of MR cholangiopancreatography in patients with failed or inadequate ERCP. AJR Am J Roentgenol 1999;173:1527–33.

[66] Kim JH, Kim MJ, Chung JJ, et al. Differential diagnosis of periampullary carcinomas at MR imaging. Radiographics 2002;22:1335–52.

[67] Ly JN, Miller FH. MR imaging of the pancreas: a practical approach. Radiol Clin N Am 2002; 40:1289–306.

[68] Adamek HE, Albert J, Breer H, et al. Pancreatic cancer detection with magnetic resonance cholangiopancreatography and endoscopic retrograde cholangiopancreatography: a prospective controlled study. Lancet 2000;356:190–3.

[69] Barish M, Soto J, Ferrucci J. Magnetic resonance pancreatography. Endoscopy 1997;29:487–95.

[70] Obara T, Maguchi H, Saitoh Y, et al. Mucin-producing tumor of the pancreas: surgery or follow-up? Nippon Shokakibyo Gakkai Zasshi 1994;91:66–74.

[71] Terris B, Ponsot P, Paye F, et al. Intraductal papillary mucinous tumors of the pancreas confined to secondary ducts show less aggressive pathologic features as compared with those involving the main pancreatic duct. Am J Surg Pathol 2000;24:1372–7.

[72] Irie H, Honda H, Aibe H, et al. MR cholangiopancreatographic differentiation of benign and malignant intraductal mucin-producing tumors of the pancreas. AJR Am J Roentgenol 2000; 174:1403–8.

[73] Yamaguchi K, Chijiwa K, Shimizu S, et al. Comparison of endoscopic retrograde and magnetic resonance cholangiopancreatography in the surgical diagnosis of pancreatic diseases. Am J Surg 1998;175:203–8.

[74] Koito K, Namieno T, Ichimura T, et al. Mucin-producing pancreatic tumors: comparison of MR cholangiopancreatography with endoscopic retrograde cholangiopancreatography. Radiology 1998;208:231–7.

[75] Fukukura Y, Fujiyoshi F, Sasaki M, et al. HASTE MR cholangiopancreatography in the evaluation of intraductal papillary-mucinous tumors of the pancreas. J Comput Assist Tomogr 1999;23:301–5.

[76] Onaya H, Itai Y, Niitsu M, et al. Ductectatic mucinous cystic neoplasms of the pancreas: evaluation with MR cholangiopancreatography. AJR Am J Roentgenol 1998;171:171–7.

[77] Pickhardt PJ. Three-dimensional endoluminal CT colonography (virtual colonoscopy): comparison of three commercially available systems. AJR Am J Roentgenol 2003;181:1599–606.

[78] Lefere PA, Gryspeerdt SS, Dewyspelaere J, et al. Dietary fecal tagging as a cleansing method before CT colonography: initial results polyp detection and patient acceptance. Radiology 2002; 224:393–403.

[79] Yee J. CT colonography: examination prerequisites. Abdom Imaging 2002;27:244–52.

[80] Oto A, Gelebek V, Oguz BS, et al. CT attenuation of colorectal polypoid lesions: evaluation of contrast enhancement in CT colonography. Eur Radiol 2003;13:1657–63.

[81] Wessling J, Fischbach R, Meier N, et al. CT colonography: protocol optimization with multi-detector row CT study in ananthropomorphic colon phantom. Radiology 2003;228:753–9.

[82] Iannaccone R, Laghi A, Catalano C, et al. Feasibility of ultra-low-dose multislice CT colonography for the detection of colorectal lesions: preliminary experience. Eur Radiol 2003;13: 1297–302.

[83] Van Gelder RE, Venema HW, Serlie IW, et al. CT colonography at different radiation dose levels: feasibility of dose reduction. Radiology 2002;224:25–33.

[84] McCollough CH. Optimization of multidetector array CT acquisition parameters for CT colonography. Abdom Imaging 2002;27:253–9.

[85] Pickhardt PJ, Choi JR, Hwang I, et al. Computed tomographic virtual colonoscopy to screen for colorectal neoplasia in asymptomatic adults. N Engl J Med 2003;349:2191–200.

[86] Macari M, Bini EJ, Jacobs SL, et al. Colorectal polyps and cancers in asymptomatic average-risk patients: evaluation with CT colonography. Radiology 2004;230:629–36.

[87] Ferrucci JP. Colon cancer screening with virtual colonoscopy: promise, polyps, politics. AJR Am J Roentgenol 2001;177:975–88.

[88] Johnson CD, Dachman AH. CT-colonography: the next colon screening examination? Radiology 2000;216:331–41.

[89] Geenen RW, Hussain SM, Cademartiri F, et al. CT and MR colonography: scanning techniques, postprocessing, and emphasis on polyp detection. Radiographics 2004;24:E18.

[90] Morson BC. The evolution of colorectal carcinoma. Clin Radiol 1984;35:425–31.

[91] Toribara NW, Sleisenger MH. Screening for colorectal cancer. N Engl J Med 1995;332:861–7.

[92] Bond JH. Clinical evidence for the adenoma-carcinoma sequence, and the management of patients with colorectal adenomas. Semin Gastrointest Dis 2000;11:176–84.

[93] Muto T, Bussey HJ, Morson BC. The evolution of cancer of the colon and rectum. Cancer 1975;36:2251–70.

[94] Anderson ML, Heigh RI, McCoy GA, et al. Accuracy of assessment of the extent of examination by experienced colonoscopists. Gastrointest Endosc 1992;38:560–3.

[95] Angtuaco TL, Banaad-Omiotek GD, Howden CW. Differing attitudes toward virtual and conventional colonoscopy for colorectal cancer screening: surveys among primary care physicians and potential patients. Am J Gastroenterol 2001;96:887–93.

[96] Chaoui AS, Blake MA, Barish MA, et al. Virtual colonoscopy and colorectal cancer screening. Abdom Imaging 2000;25:361–7.

[97] Ji H, Rolnick JA, Haker S, et al. Multislice CT colonography: current status and limitations. Eur J Radiol 2003;47:123–34.

[98] Svensson MH, Svensson E, Lasson A, et al. Patient acceptance of CT colonography and conventional colonoscopy: prospective comparative study in patients with or suspected of having colorectal disease. Radiology 2002;222:337–45.

[99] Thomeer M, Bielen D, Vanbeckevoort D, et al. Patient acceptance for CT colonography: what is the real issue? Eur Radiol 2002;12:1410–5.

[100] Ristvedt SL, McFarland EG, Weinstock LB, et al. Patient preferences for CT colonography, conventional colonoscopy, and bowel preparation. Gastroenterol 2003;98:578–85.

[101] Gluecker TM, Johnson CD, Harmsen WS, et al. Colorectal cancer screening with CT colonography, colonoscopy, and double-contrast barium enema examination: prospective assessment of patient perceptions and preferences. Radiology 2003;227:378–84.

[102] Fenlon HM, Nunes DP, Schroy III PC, et al. A comparison of virtual and conventional colonoscopy for the detection of colorectal polyps. N Engl J Med 1999;341:1496–503.

[103] Macari M, Bini EJ, Xue X, et al. Colorectal neoplasms: prospective comparison of thin-section low-dose multi-detector row CT colonography and conventional colonoscopy for detection. Radiology 2002;224:383–92.

[104] Gluecker T, Dorta G, Keller W, et al. Performance of multidetector computed tomography colonography compared with conventional colonoscopy. Gut 2002;51:207–11.

[105] Cotton PB, Durkalski VL, Pineau BC, et al. Computed tomographic colonography (virtual colonoscopy): a multicenter comparison with standard colonoscopy for detection of colorectal neoplasia. JAMA 2004;291:1713–9.

[106] Ferrucci J, Barish M, Choi R, et al. Virtual colonoscopy. JAMA 2004;292:431–2.

[107] Pickhardt PJ, Choi JR, Hwang I, et al. Nonadenomatous polyps at CT colonography: prevalence, size distribution, and detection rates. Radiology 2004;232:784–90.

[108] Maglinte DD, Lappas JC, Heitkamp DE, et al. Technical refinements in enteroclysis. Radiol Clin N Am 2003;41:213–29.

[109] Maglinte DD, Cordell WH. Strategies for reducing the pain and discomfort of nasogastric intubation. Acad Emerg Med 1999;6:166–9.

[110] Maglinte DD, Bender GN, Heitkamp DE, et al. Multidetector-row helical CT enteroclysis. Radiol Clin N Am 2003;41:249–62.

[111] Bender GN, Maglinte DD, Kloppel VR, et al. CT enteroclysis: a superfluous diagnostic procedure or valuable when investigating small-bowel disease? AJR Am J Roentgenol 1999;172:373–8.

[112] Goh V, Halligan S, Bartram CI. Local radiological staging of rectal cancer. Clin Radiol 2004;59:215–26.

[113] Hodgman CG, MacCarty RL, Wolff BG, et al. Preoperative staging of rectal carcinoma by computed tomography and 0.15T magnetic resonance imaging: preliminary report. Dis Colon Rectum 1986;29:446–50.

[114] Brown G, Richards CJ, Newcombe RG, et al. Rectal carcinoma: thin-section MR imaging for staging in 28 patients. Radiology 1999;211:215–22.

[115] Beets-Tan RG, Beets GL. Rectal cancer: review whith emphasis on MR imaging. Radiology 2004;232:335–46.

[116] Matsuoka H, Nakamura A, Masaki T, et al. Comparison between endorectal coil and pelvic phased-array coil magnetic resonance imaging in patients with anorectal tumor. Am J Surg 2003;185:328–32.

[117] Garcia-Aguilar J, Pollack J, Lee SH, et al. Accuracy of endorectal ultrasonography in preoperative staging of rectal tumors. Dis Colon Rectum 2002;45:10–5.

[118] Lindmark G, Elvin A, Pahlman L, et al. The value of endosonography in preoperative staging of rectal cancer. Int J Colorectal Dis 1992;7:162–6.

[119] Bipat S, Glas AS, Slors FJ, et al. Rectal cancer: local staging and assessment of lymph node involvement with endoluminal US, CT, and MR imaging. A meta-analysis. Radiology 2004;232:773–83.

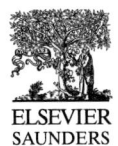

ELSEVIER
SAUNDERS

Gastrointest Endoscopy Clin N Am
15 (2005) 615–629

GASTROINTESTINAL
ENDOSCOPY CLINICS
OF NORTH AMERICA

Emerging Endoscopic Techniques in Oncology

Kyung W. Noh, MD[a], Timothy A. Woodward, MD[a], Michael B. Wallace, MD, MPH[a,b,*]

[a]Division of Gastroenterology and Hepatology, Mayo Clinic, 4500 San Pablo Road, Jacksonville, FL 32224, USA
[b]Division of Endoscopic Research, Mayo Clinic, 4500 San Pablo Road, Jacksonville, FL 32224, USA

New techniques have expanded the role of endoscopy in the diagnosis, staging, therapy, and palliation of malignancies. In this article, we cover three major areas of emerging technologies: endoscopic ultrasound (EUS), luminal stent technology, and photodynamic therapy (PDT). Although EUS and PDT have been used for more than two decades, they have only recently emerged as established integral methods in the armamentarium of the gastrointestinal (GI) endoscopist. Because both have become "mainstream," many new applications continue to emerge. The advantage of EUS over all other noninvasive imaging modalities is its ability to acquire images in real time from within the GI tract and to place needles for diagnosis and therapy directly into tumors, lymph nodes, and other structures with precision. One of the most exciting aspects of EUS is its expansion into therapeutics. Palliation of pancreatic cancer pain using EUS-guided celiac plexus neurolysis (CPN) and relief of malignant pancreaticobiliary strictures through EUS-guided biliary drainage have been achieved. Other potential therapies include pancreatic tumor ablation with locally delivered radiofrequency energy, brachytherapy, and immunotherapy or gene therapy.

PDT has long been used for palliation of obstructing cancer but has only recently been approved by the FDA for ablation of dysplasia in Barrett's esophagus. Many other applications, such as ablation of cholangiocarcinoma, are emerging.

---

* Corresponding author. Division of Gastroenterology and Hepatology, Mayo Clinic, 4500 San Pablo Road, Jacksonville, FL 32224.
  E-mail address: wallace.michael@mayo.edu (M.B. Wallace).

1052-5157/05/$ – see front matter © 2005 Elsevier Inc. All rights reserved.
doi:10.1016/j.giec.2005.03.001

giendo.theclinics.com

Endoscopic ultrasound diagnosis

Pancreatic cancer

In the United States, pancreatic cancer is the fifth leading cause of cancer-related death [1]. Its prognosis after diagnosis is poor, with a 5% 5-year survival [2]. Surgical resection is the only option for a cure. Due to its late presentation, resection is possible only in 15% to 20% of cases. Pancreatic cancer is usually refractory to conventional chemotherapy. An understanding of the biology and pathogenesis of pancreatic cancer and early detection is paramount in the management of this disease.

EUS has been used in the evaluation of pancreatic masses and in the diagnosis and staging of pancreatic cancer. In a meta-analysis, EUS has a sensitivity of 98% in detecting pancreatic cancer. This was superior to other modalities including ultrasound, CT, and angiography [3]. Initially, the specificity of EUS in pancreatic cancer was suboptimal because it was less able to differentiate between focal chronic pancreatitis and cancer. EUS-guided fine needle aspiration (EUS-FNA) has increased the specificity [4–8]. In a large, single-center study of 233 patients, EUS-FNA of suspected pancreatic cancer masses had a sensitivity of 91%, a specificity of 100%, and an accuracy of 92% [9]. Because CT and MRI technology has improved, these technologies may supplant EUS for the staging of many pancreatic cancers. There are still several areas where EUS plays a key role in this disease.

For tissue confirmation of suspected tumors, especially in unresectable tumors, EUS remains the most accurate and reliable method. Resectable tumors do not require tissue confirmation; however, many surgeons and patients prefer to have a definitive diagnosis to aid in surgical planning, patient preparation, and rapid palliation in the event that laparotomy identifies unresectable disease. Although needle track seeding is rare, recent reports [10] of needle track seeding warrant caution in performing FNA of resectable tumors in the body and tail of the pancreas. Tumors in the head can generally be sampled via the duodenum, which is resected (along with the needle path) in a standard Whipple operation.

EUS plays a vital role in the detection of tumors when cross-sectional imaging is equivocal. The high degree of resolution allows imaging of tumors as small as 3 to 4 mm and commonly detects tumors that are not seen or are only vaguely seen by CT.

To further improve diagnostic accuracy, analysis of tumor markers in pancreatic juice has been evaluated. Mutations in codon 12 of the K-*ras* oncogene can be found in 75% to 100% of pancreatic ductal carcinomas. The mutation seems to occur early in the tumorigenesis of pancreatic cancer [11–15]. The high incidence of K-*ras* mutations in the pancreatic cancer has led to efforts to use it as a tool for the early diagnosis of pancreatic cancer. Several studies have evaluated the presence of K-*ras* mutations in the pancreatic juice and EUS-FNA specimens as a marker of pancreatic cancer. The incidence of K-*ras* mutation in the pancreatic juice of patients with pancreatic cancer ranges from 50% to 89%

[16–18]. In EUS-FNA samples, K-*ras* mutations were detected in 77% of specimens in cases of pancreatic carcinoma [19].

The ability to use K-*ras* mutation detection in the early diagnosis of pancreatic cancer is uncertain. Complicating factors include the detection of K-*ras* mutations in cases of chronic pancreatitis and older individuals without evidence of pancreatic disease [15,16,20]. K-*ras* mutations have been found in up to 40% of patients with chronic pancreatitis [21]. There is preliminary evidence that K-*ras* mutations in patients with chronic pancreatitis may detect microscopic cancer or predict progression to cancer [21]. Overall, K-*ras* mutation seems to be an early and integral event in the pathogenesis of pancreatic cancer. The poor specificity of the test limits its use as a lone screening tool. Combining K-*ras* detection with other molecular markers (eg, p53 [22,23] and telomerase [24,25]) and imaging tools (eg, EUS) should improve the diagnostic yield of pancreatic cancer [18,19,26].

Pancreatic cysts

Cystic lesions of the pancreas are being detected but remain poorly understood. They are broadly divided into mucinous and nonmucinous lesions. Mucinous lesions (mucinous cystic neoplasms and intraductal papillary mucinous neoplasms) are considered to be premalignant or malignant, and surgical resection is generally recommended for appropriate candidates. Nonmucinous lesions (serous cystadenomas and pseudocysts) have low or no malignant potential. Resection is indicated only in the setting of uncontrollable symptoms [27]. Accurate methods to diagnose and determine the malignant potential of cystic lesions of the pancreas are highly desirable, but current methods are limited.

EUS is a valuable tool for the evaluation of the pancreatic cystic lesions. It offers the highest resolution available for imaging the entire pancreatic parenchyma and duct. EUS provides detailed information regarding the wall and septations of the cyst, which can be helpful in the diagnosis of cystic lesions of the pancreas.

EUS-FNA and cyst fluid analysis have been valuable in differentiating cystic lesions of the pancreas. Cytology is considered to be a poor marker. It has a specificity approaching 100% but a sensitivity ranging from 27% to 64% [28–30]. Cytology of cyst fluid is often nondiagnostic [31] due to low cellularity of the aspirated fluid and therefore leads to a high false-negative rate. Thus, investigators have evaluated the use of tumor markers in the cyst fluid. CEA and CA 72-4 were found in high concentrations in mucinous cystic neoplasms [32–35]. Various series have demonstrated that the cyst fluid CEA of benign cystic lesions is low. The mean values ranged from 1.1 to 7.5 ng/mL in pseudocysts and serous cystadenomas [29,32,36]. In contrast, the mean CEA values of mucinous cystadenoma and cystadenocarcinoma ranged from 5607 to 22,239 ng/mL [32,37,38].

The Cooperative Pancreatic Cyst Study evaluated the cystic fluid of 341 patients who underwent EUS-FNA of cystic lesions of the pancreas. One hundred twelve of these patients had surgical confirmation of the diagnosis. The receiver-operator characteristic curves were plotted for each tumor marker (CEA, CA 72-4, CA 125, CA 19-9, and CA 15-3) to predict a mucinous or nonmucinous cystic lesion. The accuracy was greatest for CEA and CA 72-4. The CEA cutoff value of 192 ng/mL provided the greatest accuracy of 0.79 (1.0 is perfect), with a moderate sensitivity of 0.73 and a specificity of 0.84. For CA 72-4, the cutoff value of 7 ng/mL provided an accuracy of 0.72, a sensitivity of 0.80, and a specificity of 0.61. This study confirmed that mucinous cystic lesions have a much higher concentration of CEA (mean CEA 5607 ng/mL) as compared with nonmucinous cystic lesions (mean CEA 284 ng/mL) [38].

The study evaluated the ability of EUS to differentiate mucinous and non-mucinous lesions based on morphology because mucinous lesions generally are unilocular and macrocystic and have a thickened cyst wall [39,40]. The results revealed a sensitivity of 56%, a specificity of 45%, and an accuracy of 51% [38]. Thus, the overall accuracy of CEA was significantly better than EUS morphology or cytology alone. When the three tests were used together (eg, calling the lesion mucinous if any one of three were positive), the sensitivity increased to 91%, but the specificity and accuracy dropped to 31% and 62%, respectively. The study concluded that the use of cyst fluid CEA concentration alone was more accurate than combination testing. The clinician using these tests in practice must take into account other factors, such as surgical risk and co-morbid disease. In young healthy patients, it may be preferable to maximize the sensitivity (ie, consider surgery if any of the three tests is positive), whereas in higher-risk older patients, high specificity may be preferable (ie, requiring two or three features to consider surgery). Another practical implication of this study is what test to order when only a limited fluid sample is available (eg, in very small cysts). In our practice, we use the first sample for CEA (a minimum of 0.5 mL is required) and use additional fluid for cytologic analysis.

Lung cancer

One of the most important emerging fields of endoscopy and EUS is the staging of nonsmall cell lung cancer (NSCLC). NSCLC is the single most common cause of cancer death in the United States and in many developed countries. The most common site of metastasis in NSCLC is the mediastinal lymph nodes, and their status dictates therapy. Patients with no mediastinal metastases (stage I or II) are treated with surgery alone. Patients with ipsilateral mediastinal metastases are treated with chemoradiotherapy with or without surgery. Patients with contralateral or distant metastases are treated palliatively.

Traditional methods of mediastinal lymph node staging include transbronchial needle aspiration (TBNA), which is a "blind" procedure because the bronchoscopist is not able to directly visualize the target. The bronchoscopist must use information from CT scanning to locate the lymph node; thus, small lymph nodes may be missed. Furthermore, TBNA is not able to access the aorto-pulmonary window or inferior mediastinal lymph nodes [41]. EUS has the advantage of direct visualization of the lymph node for FNA targeting and is capable of sampling a wide range of lymph node locations that bronchoscopy cannot, such as the inferior mediastinal lymph nodes and the left adrenal gland.

Mediastinoscopy is widely considered the gold standard for staging the mediastinum but has limited access to key locations, such as the aorto-pulmonary window and inferior mediastinum. Mediastinoscopy is also a more invasive procedure that requires surgical incision, general anesthesia, and typically overnight hospitalization. A recent comprehensive review of invasive staging modalities by the American College of Chest Physicians found EUS-FNA comparable to mediastinoscopy [42]. Mediastinoscopy is best seen as complementary to EUS because it is better suited to evaluating the anterior mediastinum, and EUS is better suited to the posterior and inferior mediastinum.

The endoscopist can access lymph nodes lateral to the trachea, the posterior aorto-pulmonary window, subcarina, and inferior mediastinum along the esophagus with EUS (Fig. 1). In addition, samples of suspected metastases to the liver and adrenal gland can be obtained. The classic features of malignant lymph nodes include hypoechogenicity, round shape, size >1 cm, and sharply demarcated borders [42]. These criteria are not perfect, and it is our practice to sample at least one lymph node in the subcarinal and aorto-pulmonary window. In more than seven large trials, compared with surgical staging, EUS with FNA was reported to have a sensitivity of 93% and a specificity of 98% [43]. The procedure is safe and has an overall complication rate of <0.5% [43].

The major limitations or EUS-FNA for lung cancer staging are the inability to see image in front of the air-filled trachea and the inability to detect small "micrometastases" in lymph nodes. Two emerging technologies seem to offer promise in these areas. Endobronchial ultrasound (EBUS) is a technique nearly identical to EUS but uses a prototype small-caliber echoendoscope passed into the airway to image and direct real-time guided FNA in the anterior mediastinum (Fig. 2). Preliminary work with this instrument by our and other groups suggests that the combination of EUS and EBUS provides the most comprehensive method available for minimally invasive staging of the mediastinum.

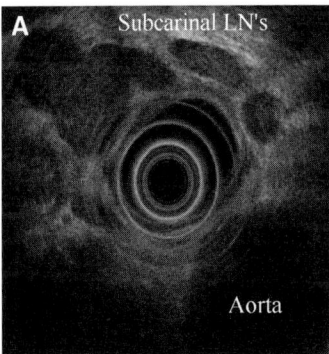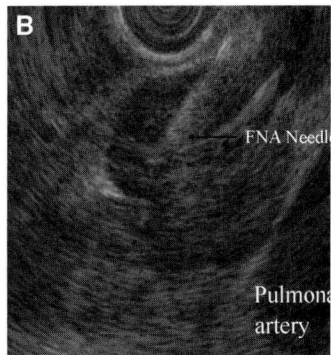

Fig. 1. (*A*) Radial EUS view of subcarinal lymph nodes. (*B*) EUS-FNA of mediastinal lymph node.

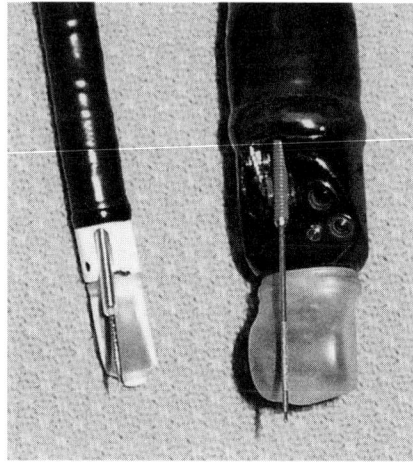

Fig. 2. EBUS scope (*left*) and linear array EUS scope (*right*).

The detection of micrometastases can be facilitated by the use of high-output, sensitive technologies such as real-time polymerase chain reaction. Using these methods, we have identified several markers, such as telomerase [44] and KS 1/4, which can accurately identify signatures of metastatic disease in approximately 20% of cytopathology negative lymph nodes [45]. Studies are underway to determine if these micrometastases confer a worse prognosis and to identify a group that may benefit from systemic chemotherapy. Perhaps the most promising aspect of this technology is the broad applicability to other tumors. Combining EUS-FNA access to tissue with modern genomic and proteomic methods offers a rich area for further research and clinical applications.

Endoscopic ultrasound therapy

Pancreatic tumor ablation

The ability of EUS to precisely localize and place needles into pancreatic tumors has sparked interest in pancreatic tumor ablation. Because most pancreatic cancer is not curable at the time of diagnosis, palliation of symptoms is the primary goal of therapy. The cause of morbidity in pancreatic cancer is largely due to mass effect and local invasion of the tumor, leading to pain, biliary obstruction, and duodenal obstruction. Chemotherapy is generally ineffective, and external beam radiation is associated with significant collateral damage to the adjacent organs. EUS-guided ablation of pancreatic tumor through local delivery of radiofrequency energy, brachytherapy, immunotherapy, or gene therapy is under investigation.

Radiofrequency ablation of the pancreas has been performed in a porcine model. A 19-gauge RFA needle was used to cause thermal ablation of the pancreas in 13 pigs. This caused a 1 cm, round area of necrosis that was confirmed by necropsy. One pig developed signs of pancreatitis, with a fluid collection and elevated lipase. Radiofrequency ablation has the potential to be used in the ablation of small pancreatic tumors and in the palliation of unresectable pancreatic adenocarcinoma [46].

It is feasible to use EUS-targeted delivery of an anti-tumor agent directly into pancreatic cancers. Eight patients with unresectable pancreatic cancer had implantation of allogenic mixed lymphocyte culture (cytoimplant) through EUS-guided fine needle injection (EUS-FNI). The results showed the procedure to be safe with mild side effects. Median life expectancy in the study was >13 months [47], A multicenter, randomized, controlled trial of cytoimplant versus gemcitabine chemotherapy was completed in 2000 but has not been reported. Several other EUS-injectable agents are also under investigation, including an attenuated adenovirus (ONYX-015) that preferentially replicates in and kills malignant cells. Twenty-one patients with locally advanced pancreatic adenocarcinoma underwent weekly EUS-FNI of ONYX-015 over an 8-week period. The final four treatments were given in conjunction with gemcitabine. Three patients showed a minor response to treatment. The complications of this therapy included two patients who developed sepsis and two patients who had duodenal perforations [48]. Although neither of these studies has identified a clearly efficacious agent, both proved the feasibility of directly injectable therapy and have opened the door to new, potentially more effective agents.

Surgically placing brachytherapy seeds in patients with unresectable tumors has been shown to provide pain relief in a significant proportion of patients with few complications [49]. However, this requires a laparotomy, which is a significant deterrent to its use. EUS has been used to guide placement of inert brachytherapy seeds in pigs (Fig. 3) but not in humans [50]. A major hurdle to this technology is the inability to precisely place seeds at the rigid space intervals necessary for effective brachytherapy. Other agents, such as colloidal P32, may allow more even and feasible EUS-directed brachytherapy.

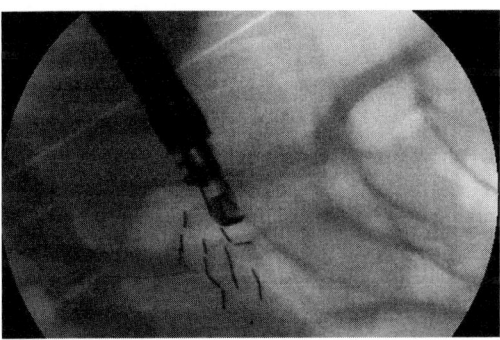

Fig. 3. EUS-guided placement of inert brachytherapy seeds in pigs.

Celiac plexus blockade/neurolysis

Pain is a significant source of morbidity in patients with unresectable pancreatic cancer and chronic pancreatitis. EUS-guided celiac plexus blockade (CPB) and celiac plexus neurolysis (CPN) provide pain relief without the significant side effects of narcotic use. CPN is a chemical splanchnicectomy of the celiac plexus to ablate the nerves that transmit pain [51]. This procedure can be performed under CT or fluoroscopic guidance, surgically or endoscopically. In a prospective study, EUS-guided CPN provided pain relief that was durable for 24 weeks in 78% of patients. No significant procedure-related complications were reported [51]. A prospective, randomized controlled trial evaluating the efficacy of EUS-guided CPN versus placebo in the relief of pancreatic cancer associated pain is underway.

CPB is a method of temporary pain control using an anesthetic agent (eg, bupivacaine) and a long-acting corticosteroid (eg, triamcinolone). It is typically used to control flares of pain in chronic pancreatitis. The rationale for avoiding CPN in this group is the potential for retroperitoneal scarring caused by the ethanol injection of CPN, which could interfere with subsequent surgery (eg, Puestow procedure) in chronic pancreatitis patients. Multiple trials have demonstrated the efficacy of CPB, with pain control lasting approximately 3 months [52]. A randomized controlled trial of EUS CPB compared with CT-guided CPB showed the EUS approach to be superior for pain relief [53]. Given the temporary nature of this procedure and chronic nature of the disease, our practice is to restrict its use to controlling only severe flares of pain that cannot be controlled with typical outpatient analgesics.

Biliary obstruction is a frequently encountered problem in pancreatic cancer. Endoscopic retrograde cholangiopancreatography (ERCP) with stent placement is the standard therapy for these patients. In some patients, endoscopic placement is not possible due to duodenal obstruction or difficulty in cannulating the duct. In addition, stent occlusion or tumor ingrowth remains a significant problem. EUS-guided hepaticogastrostomy was proposed to overcome these problems. EUS-guided hepaticogastrostomy was first performed in pigs. Stent placement was successful in three out of five pigs with relief of jaundice [54]. EUS-guided palliative drainage was attempted in four patients with malignant pancreaticobiliary strictures. Technical success was achieved in three patients, and cholestasis was relieved. No major complications were reported [55]. These techniques may become an option for failed ERCP [56].

Luminal stent technology

Self-expanding metal stents (SEMS) were introduced in the early 1990s and have been used as an alternative to surgery in the palliation of luminal obstruction due to GI cancer. The major sites of use include the esophagus, the gastroduodenum, and the colon [57]. SEMS can be placed through the scope under fluoroscopic or endoscopic guidance [58].

In the esophagus, the small caliber of the SEMS allows for easier deployment without aggressive dilation. In a retrospective trial of 120 patients comparing SEMS with plastic stents, the technical success rate was the same at 94%, and functional success rates were comparable at 89% and 85%. There were three procedure-related deaths in the plastic stent group [59].

A systematic review of the use of SEMS for gastroduodenal malignancies reviewed published data on 606 patients. Technical success in SEMS placement was achieved in 589 patients (97%). Functional relief of symptoms was achieved in 89% of the patients in whom the SEMS was deployed. Acute complications, including bleeding and perforation, were reported in seven patients (1.2%). Long-term complications included stent obstruction mainly due to tumor ingrowth (18%) and stent migration (5%). The median survival was 12 weeks.

The use of SEMS in colorectal cancer is becoming more commonplace. It can be placed across an obstructing colonic mass for preoperative decompression or palliation [57]. The success rates for stent deployment and clinical decompression ranged from 70% to 95% [60]. In addition to relief of colonic obstruction, preoperative stent placement allows for adequate staging of disease and bowel preparation before surgery. The ability to cleanse the bowel proximal to the obstruction may allow for a one-stage colonic resection without the need for diverting colostomy. In addition, preoperative chemoradiation is possible because the stent allows for decompression of the bowel and adequate nutrition during adjuvant therapy [60]. In the case of an unresectable tumor, the SEMS can be left in place for relief of symptoms.

Multiple studies suggest that endoscopic placement of SEMS is a safe and effective method to relieve luminal obstruction due to GI malignancies. Emerging issues in stent technology include the development of removable stents; drug-eluting stents; and improved stent design to optimize patency, reduce gastro-esophageal reflux, and minimize stent migration.

Removable stents are appealing for therapy of nonmalignant strictures that do not respond to routine dilation. Potential applications include post-photodynamic therapy (PDT) strictures, anastomotic strictures, and radiation strictures. One such stent device is available. Preliminary experience suggests that this device is effective and safe, but larger studies are needed [61]. Drug-eluting stents have had a profound effect on cardiovascular disease. The market for drug-eluting stents in GI disease is much smaller than in cardiovascular disease, which has limited industry incentives for development. Potential applications include malignant and benign strictures, including Crohn's disease-related bowel strictures. New stent design and manufacturing methods have allowed development of anti-reflux stents and other custom stent shapes using laser etching of solid metal tubes. These technologies have the capability of producing more precise shape and mechanical properties for difficult locations, such as the upper esophagus.

Photodynamic therapy

Barrett's esophagus is a long-term consequence of acid reflux disease and is thought to be a risk factor for the development of esophageal adenocarcinoma [62]. The risk is increased in the setting of dysplasia. High-grade dysplasia is an indication for esophagectomy in suitable candidates. Esophagectomy carries a considerable risk of mortality and morbidity, and many patients are unwilling or unable to tolerate such an operation. PDT offers an alternative to surgery for the treatment of Barrett's esophagus with high-grade dysplasia and superficial esophageal adenocarcinoma.

PDT is based on the concept that specific photosensitizers, such as porphyrins, accumulate preferentially into dysplastic or malignant cells [63]. After the photosensitizing agent is administered, the drug is concentrated into tumor tissue. At 48 hours, the ratio of photosensitizer concentration in neoplastic and non-neoplastic tissue is 2:1. It remains inactive until it is exposed to a specific wavelength of (typically red) light. This induces a photodynamic reaction and destruction of the tumor tissue. The most commonly used photosensitizing agent (and the only one approved by the FDA for this indication) is porfimer sodium (Photofrin; Axcan Scandipharm, Quebec, Canada). Newer agents include aminolevulinic acid, a prodrug that stimulates the production of the endogenous photosensitizer, protoporphyrin IX, within the mucosal cells of the gut. It has the advantage of specific mucosal photosensitization and therefore does not damage the underlying muscle layer, reducing the risk of stricture formation. Meta-tetrahydroxyphenyl chlorin is a powerful photosensitizer that has been associated with severe strictures and tissue necrosis. This drug is not available in the United States [63].

The differentiation between superficial lesions (eg, high-grade dysplasia and carcinoma limited to the mucosa) and more invasive lesions is paramount in determining whether a patient is suitable candidate for endoscopic therapies such as PDT and endoscopic mucosal resection (EMR) [64]. EUS aids in the selection of patients because it allows for a detailed evaluation of the esophageal wall and lymph node involvement. A number of studies have shown the accuracy of EUS in the T and N staging to be approximately 85% and 75%, respectively. The N-staging accuracy has improved with EUS-FNA [64,65]. EUS cannot distinguish between high-grade dysplasia and early carcinoma [66,67]. Whether this is important is not known because PDT seems to be affective for both lesions. It is critical to identify deeply invasive (T2 or higher) tumors or nodal metastasis because these do not respond well to PDT and are better suited for surgery or combined therapy (chemoradiotherapy + surgery).

PDT for Barrett's esophagus with high-grade dysplasia has been reported to eliminate Barrett's esophagus in 0% to 61% and to eliminate high-grade dysplasia in 88% to 100%, with a mean follow-up ranging from 9.9 to 50.6 months [68–76]. The PHO-BAR study, an international, multicenter, randomized controlled trial, randomized 200 patients with Barrett's esophagus with high-grade dysplasia into PDT with omeprazole (20 mg twice a day) and omeprazole alone.

At 1 year, the PDT group had elimination of Barrett's mucosa in 41% of patients and elimination of high-grade dysplasia in 72% of patients. This was a statistically significant improvement over drug therapy alone. In addition, there was a significant reduction in the development of esophageal adenocarcinoma [63,77]. In the series with the longest follow-up time, 103 patients underwent PDT using porfimer sodium with a mean follow-up of 50.65 months. In 65 patients with Barrett's esophagus with high-grade dysplasia, 94% of patients had eradication of high-grade dysplasia [76].

EUS-guided EMR has been proposed for the treatment of superficial adenocarcinoma arising from an area of Barrett's esophagus, but EMR of an entire area of cancer and susceptible regions may be difficult due to its large surface area [78]. Recent efforts to perform widespread esophageal mucosectomy in animal models highlight the technical challenges [79]. PDT and EMR have been used to complement each other in the treatment of superficial esophageal cancer in the setting of Barrett's esophagus [80]. A retrospective review comparing combined PDT and EMR versus esophagectomy of early esophageal carcinoma revealed that 20 out of 24 patients undergoing combined PDT and EMR remained disease free over a follow-up period of 12 months, and all 64 patients undergoing surgery remained disease free at 19 months. The PDT and EMR group had significantly fewer procedure-related complications and a lower mortality rate [81]. This illustrates that combination therapy of PDT and EMR may be an option for suboptimal surgical candidate with early esophageal adenocarcinoma.

Summary

New endoscopic techniques have allowed for less invasive, safer, and more effective means of diagnosing and treating disease. Advances in diagnostic endoscopy will aid in the earlier detection of cancers through the use of tumor markers and more advanced endoscopes with higher resolution. Therapeutic endoscopic methods, such as PDT and EMR, have achieved clinical success in the cases in superficial GI tumor. Current therapies requiring surgical intervention or pancreaticobiliary cannulation may be replaced by less invasive methods, such as EUS. The key to developing these techniques will be through creative use of endoscopy and careful experimentation.

References

[1] National Cancer Institute. Annual cancer statistics review 1973–1988. Bethesda (MD): US Department of Health and Human Service; 1991 [NIH publication no 91-2789].
[2] Ahmad NA, Lewis JD, Ginsberg GG, et al. Long term survival after pancreatic resection for pancreatic adenocarcinoma. Am J Gastroenterol 2001;96:2609–15.
[3] Yasuda K, Mukai H, Nakajima M. Endoscopic ultrasonography diagnosis of pancreatic cancer. Gastrointest Endosc Clin North Am 1995;5:699–712.

[4] Brugge WR. Endoscopic ultrasonography: the current status. Gastroenterology 1998;115: 1577–83.

[5] Wiersema MJ, Vilmann P, Giovannini M, et al. Endosonography-guided fine-needle aspiration biopsy: diagnostic accuracy and complication assessment. Gastroenterology 1997;112:1087–95.

[6] Chang KJ, Nguyen P, Erickson RA, et al. The clinical utility of endoscopic ultrasound-guided fine-needle aspiration in the diagnosis and staging of pancreatic carcinoma. Gastrointest Endosc 1997;45:387–93.

[7] Bhutani MS, Hawes RH, Baron PL, et al. Endoscopic ultrasound guided fine needle aspiration of malignant pancreatic lesions. Endoscopy 1997;29:854–8.

[8] Williams DB, Sahai AV, Aabakken L, et al. Endoscopic ultrasound guided fine needle aspiration biopsy: a large since center experience. Gut 1999;44:720–6.

[9] Raut CP, Grau AM, Staerkel GA, et al. Diagnostic accuracy of endoscopic ultrasound-guided fine needle aspiration in patients with presumed pancreatic cancer. J Gastrointest Surg 2003;7: 118–28.

[10] Micames C, Jowell PS, White R, et al. Lower frequency of peritoneal carinomatosis in patients with pancreatic cancer diagnosed by EUS-guided FNA vs percutaneous FNA. Gastrointest Endosc 2003;58:690–5.

[11] Tada M, Omata M, Ohto M. Clinical application of *ras* gene mutation for diagnosis of pancreatic adenocarcinoma. Gastroenterology 1991;100:233–8.

[12] Villanueva A, Reyes G, Cuatrecasas M, et al. Diagnostic utility of K-*ras* mutations in fine-needle aspirates of pancreatic masses. Gastroenterology 1996;110:1587–94.

[13] Almoguera C, Shibata D, Forrester K, et al. Most human carcinomas of the exocrine pancreas contain mutant c K-*ras* genes. Cell 1988;53:549–54.

[14] Inoue S, Tezel E, Nakao A. Molecular diagnosis of pancreatic cancer. Hepatogastroenterology 2001;48:933–8.

[15] Wong T, Howes N, Threadgold J, et al. Molecular diagnosis of early pancreatic ductal adenocarcinoma in high-risk patients. Pancreatol 2001;1:486–509.

[16] Boadas J, Mora J, Urgell E, et al. Clinical usefulness of K-*ras* gene mutation detection and cytology in pancreatic juice in the diagnosis and screening of pancreatic cancer. Eur J Gastroenterol Hepatol 2001;13:1153–9.

[17] Ha A, Watanabe H, Yamaguchi Y, et al. Usefulness of supernatant of pancreatic juice for genetic analysis of K-*ras* in diagnosis of pancreatic carcinoma. Pancreas 2001;23:356–63.

[18] Okai T, Watanabe H, Yamaguchi Y, et al. EUS and K-*ras* analysis of pure pancreatic juice collected via a duodenoscope after secretin stimulation for diagnosis of pancreatic mass lesion: a prospective study. Gastrointest Endosc 1999;50:797–803.

[19] Tada M, Komatsu Y, Kawabe T, et al. Quantitative analysis of K-*ras* gene mutation in pancreatic tissue obtained by endoscopic ultrasonography-guided fine needle aspiration: clinical utility for diagnosis of pancreatic tumor. Am J Gastroenterol 2002;97:2263–70.

[20] Kimura W, Zhao B, Futakawa N, et al. Significance of K-*ras* codon 12 point mutation in pancreatic juice in the diagnosis of carcinoma of the pancreas. Hepatogastroenterology 1999; 46:532–9.

[21] Queneau PE, Adessi GL, Thibault P, et al. Early detection of pancreatic cancer in patients with chronic pancreatitis: diagnostic utility of a K-*ras* point mutation in the pancreatic juice. Am J Gastroenterol 2001;96:700–4.

[22] Wang Y, Yamaguchi Y, Watanabe H, et al. Detection of p53 gene mutations in the supernatant of pancreatic juice and plasma from patients with pancreatic carcinoma. Pancreas 2004;28:13–9.

[23] Yamaguchi Y, Watanabe H, Yrdiran S, et al. Detection of mutation of p53 tumor suppressor gene in pancreatic juice and its application to diagnosis of patients with pancreatic cancer: comparison of patients with pancreatic cancer: comparison with K-*ras* mutation. Clin Cancer Res 1999;5: 1147–53.

[24] Myung SJ, Kim MH, Kim YS, et al. Telomerase activity in pure pancreatic juice for the diagnosis of pancreatic cancer may be complementary to K-*ras* mutation. Gastrointest Endosc 2000;51:708–13.

[25] Uehara H, Nakaizumi A, Tatsuta M, et al. Diagnosis of pancreatic cancer by detecting telome-

rase activity in pancreatic juice: comparison with K-*ras* mutations. Am J Gastroenterol 1999; 94:2513–8.

[26] van Heek T, Rader AE, Offerhaus GJ, et al. K-*ras*, p53, and DPC4 (MAD4) alterations in fine-needle aspirates of the pancreas: a molecular panel correlates with and supplements cytologic diagnosis. Am J Clin Pathol 2002;117:755–65.

[27] Levy MJ, Clain JE. Evaluation and management of cystic pancreatic tumors: emphasis on the role of EUS FNA. Clin Gastroenterol Hepatol 2004;2:639–53.

[28] Sedlack R, Affi A, Vazquez-Sequeiros E, et al. Utility of EUS in the evaluation of cystic pancreatic lesions. Gastrointest Endosc 2002;56:543–7.

[29] Pinto MM, Meriano FV. Diagnosis of cystic pancreatic lesions by cytologic examination and carcinoembryonic antigen and amylase assays of cyst contents. Acta Cytol 1991;35:456–63.

[30] Mallery S, Quirk D, Lewandrowski K, et al. EUS-guided FNA with cyst fluid analysis in pancreatic cystic lesions. Gastrointest Endosc 1998;47:AB504.

[31] Centeno BA, Warshaw AL, Mayo-Smith W, et al. Cytologic diagnosis of pancreatic cystic lesions: a prospective study of 28 percutaneous aspirates. Acta Cytol 1997;41:972–80.

[32] Lewandrowski KB, Southern JF, Pins MR, et al. Cyst fluid analysis in the differential diagnosis of pancreatic cysts: a comparison of pseudocysts, serous cystadenomas, mucinous cystic neoplasms, and mucinous cystadenocarcinoma. Ann Surg 1993;217:41–7.

[33] Hammel P, Levy P, Voitot H, et al. Preoperative cyst fluid analysis is useful for the differential diagnosis of cystic lesions of the pancreas. Gastroenterology 1995;108:1230–5.

[34] Sperti C, Pasquali C, Guolo P, et al. Serum tumor markers and cyst fluid analysis are useful for the diagnosis of pancreatic cystic tumors. Cancer 1996;78:237–43.

[35] Sand JA, Hyoty MK, Mattila J, et al. Clinical assessment compared with cyst fluid analysis in the differential diagnosis of cystic lesions in the pancreas. Surgery 1996;119:275–80.

[36] Tatsuta M, Iishi H, Ichii M, et al. Values of carcinoembryonic antigen, elastase 1, and carbohydrate antigen determinant in aspirated pancreatic cystic fluid in the diagnosis of cysts in the pancreas. Cancer 1986;57:1836–9.

[37] Hammel P. Role of tumor markers in the diagnosis of cystic and intraductal neoplasm. Gastrointest Endosc Clin North Am 2002;12:791–801.

[38] Brugge WR, Lewandrowski K, Lee-Lewandrowski E, et al. Diagnosis of pancreatic cystic neoplasm: a report of the cooperative pancreatic cyst study. Gastroenterology 2004;126:1330–6.

[39] Fickling WE, Wallace MB. Endoscopic ultrasound and upper gastrointestinal disorders. J Clin Gastroenterol 2003;36:103–10.

[40] O'Toole D, Palazzo L, Hammel P, et al. Macrocystic pancreatic cystadenoma: the role of EUS and cyst fluid analysis in distinguishing mucinous and serous lesions. Gastrointest Endosc 2004;59:823–9.

[41] Fickling W, Wallace MB. EUS in lung cancer. Gastrointest Endosc 2002;56:S18–21.

[42] Catalano MF, Sivak MV, Rice M, et al. Endosonographic features predictive of lymph node metastasis. Gastrointest Endosc 1994;40:442–6.

[43] Wallace MB, Fritscher-Ravens A, Savides TJ. Endoscopic ultrasound for the staging of non-small-cell lung cancer. Endoscopy 2003;35:606–10.

[44] Wallace MB, Block M, Hoffman BJ, et al. Detection of telomerase expression in mediastinal lymph nodes of patients with lung cancer. Am J Respir Crit Care Med 2003;167:1670–5.

[45] Wallace MB, Block MI, Gillanders W, et al. Accurate molecular detection of non-small cell lung cancer metastases in mediastinal lymph nodes sampled by endoscopic ultrasound-guided needle aspiration. Chest 2005;127:430–7.

[46] Goldberg SN, Mallery S, Gazelle GS, et al. EUS-guided radiofrequency ablation in the pancreas: results in a porcine model. Gastrointest Endosc 1999;50:392–401.

[47] Chang KJ, Nguyen PT, Thompson JA, et al. Phase I clinical trial of allogeneic mixed lymphocyte culture (cytoimplant) delivered by endoscopic ultrasound-guided fine needle injection in patients with advanced pancreatic carcinoma. Cancer 2000;88:1325–35.

[48] Hecht JR, Bedford R, Abbruzzese JL, et al. A phase I/II trial of intratumoral endoscopic ultrasound injection of ONYX-015 with intravenous gemcitabine in unresectable pancreatic carcinoma. Clin Can Res 2003;9:555–61.

[49] Nori D, Merimsky O, Osin AD, et al. Palladium-103: a new radioactive source in the treatment of unresectable carcinoma of the pancreas. J Surg Oncol 1996;61:300–5.

[50] Wallace MB, Hawes RH. Emerging indications for EUS. Gastrointest Endosc 2000;52:S55–60.

[51] Gunaratnam NT, Sarma AV, Norton ID, et al. A prospective study of EUS-guided celiac plexus neurolysis for pancreatic cancer pain. Gastrointest Endosc 2001;54:316–24.

[52] Levy MJ, Wiersema MJ. EUS-guided celiac plexus neurolysis and celiac plexus block. Gastrointest Endosc 2003;57:923–30.

[53] Gress F, Schmitt C, Sherman S, et al. A prospective randomized comparison of endoscopic ultrasound- and computed tomography-guided celiac plexus block for managing chronic pancreatitis pain. Am J Gastroenterol 1999;94:900–5.

[54] Sahai AV, Hoffman BJ, Hawes RH. Endoscopic ultrasound-guided hepaticogastrostomy to palliate obstructive jaundice: preliminary results in pigs. Gastrointest Endosc 1998;47:AB52.

[55] Burmester E, Niehaus J, Leineweber T, et al. EUS-cholangio-drainage of the bile duct: report of 4 cases. Gastrointest Endosc 2003;57:246–51.

[56] Kahaleh M, Yoshida C, Kane L, et al. Interventional EUS cholangiography: a report of five cases. Gastrointest Endosc 2004;60:138–42.

[57] Baron TH. Expandable metal stents for the treatment of cancerous obstruction of the gastrointestinal tract. N Engl J Med 2001;344:1681–7.

[58] Dormann A, Meisner S, Verin N, et al. Self-expanding metal stents for gastroduodenal malignancies: systematic review of their clinical effectiveness. Endoscopy 2004;36:543–50.

[59] Mosca F, Consoli A, Stracqualursi A, et al. Comparative retrospective study on the use of plastic prostheses and self-expanding metal stents in the palliative treatment of malignant strictures of the esophagus and cardia. Dis Esophagus 2003;16:119–25.

[60] Adler DG, Young-Fadok TM, Smyrk T, et al. Preoperative chemoradiation therapy after placement of a self-expanding metal stent in a patient with an obstructing rectal cancer: clinical and pathologic findings. Gastrointest Endosc 2002;55:435–7.

[61] Pungpapong S, Raimondo M, Wallace MB, et al. Problematic esophageal strictures: emerging indications for self-expandable silicone stents. Am J Gastroenterol 2004;99:AB363.

[62] Cameron AJ, Ott BJ, Payne WS. The incidence of adenocarcinoma in columnar-lined (Barrett's) esophagus. N Engl J Med 1985;313:857–9.

[63] Prosst RL, Wolfsen HC, Gahlen J. Photodynamic therapy for esophageal diseases: a clinic update. Endoscopy 2003;35:1059–68.

[64] Scotiniotis IA, Kochman ML, Lewis JD, et al. Accuracy of EUS in the evaluation of Barrett's esophagus and high grade dysplasia or intramucosal carcinoma. Gastrointest Endosc 2001;54:689–96.

[65] Rosch T. Endosonographic staging of esophageal cancer: a review of literature results. Gastrointest Endosc Clin North Am 1995;5:549–57.

[66] Falk GW, Catalano MF, Sivak MV, et al. Endosonography in the evaluation of patients with Barrett's esophagus and high-grade dysplasia. Gastrointest Endosc 1994;40:207–12.

[67] Owens MM, Kimmey MB. The role of endoscopic ultrasound in the diagnosis and management of Barrett's esophagus. Gastrointest Endosc Clin North Am 2003;13:325–34.

[68] Wolfsen HC, Woodward TA, Raimondo M. Photodynamic therapy for dysplastic Barrett esophagus and early esophageal adenocarcinoma. Mayo Clin Proc 2002;77:1176–81.

[69] Overholt BF. Results of photodynamic therapy in Barrett's esophagus: a review. Can J Gastroenterol 1999;13:393–6.

[70] Beejay U, Ribeiro A, Hourigan L, et al. Photodynamic therapy of high grade dysplasia/intramucosal carcinoma in Barrett's esophagus-30 months follow up [abstract]. Gastrointest Endosc 2001;53:AB4116.

[71] Wang KK. Current status of photodynamic therapy of Barrett's esophagus. Gastrointest Endosc 1999;49:S20–3.

[72] Gossner L, May A, Sroka R, et al. Photodynamic destruction of high grade dysplasia and early carcinoma of the esophagus after the oral administration of 5-aminolevulinic acid. Cancer 1999;86:1921–8.

[73] Gossner L, Stolte M, Sroka R, et al. Photodynamic ablation of high grade dysplasia and early cancer in Barrett's esophagus by means of 5-aminolevulinic acid. Gastroenterology 1998;114: 448–55.

[74] Barr H, Shepherd NA, Dix A, et al. Eradication of high-grade dysplasia in columnar-lined (Barrett's) oesophagus by photodynamic therapy with endogenously generated protoporphyrin IX. Lancet 1996;348:584–5.

[75] Ackroyd R, Brown NJ, Davis MF, et al. Aminolevulinic acid-induced photodynamic therapy in the treatment of dysplastic Barrett's oesophagus and adenocarcinoma. Lasers Med Sci 1999;14: 278–85.

[76] Overholt BF, Panjehpour M, Halberg DL. Photodynamic therapy for Barrett's esophagus with dysplasia and/or early stage carcinoma: long-term results. Gastrointest Endosc 2003;58:183–8.

[77] Wolfsen HC. Photodynamic therapy for mucosal esophageal adenocarcinoma and dysplastic Barrett's esophagus. Dig Dis 2002;20:5–17.

[78] Buttar NS, Wang KK, Lutzke LS, et al. Combined endoscopic mucosal resection and photodynamic therapy for esophageal neoplasia within Barrett's esophagus. Gastrointest Endosc 2001; 54:682–8.

[79] Rajan E, Gostout CJ, Feitoza AB, et al. Widespread EMR: a new technique for removal of large areas of mucosa. Gastrointest Endosc 2004;60:623–7.

[80] Wolfsen HC, Hemminger LL, Raimondo M, et al. Photodynamic therapy and endoscopic mucosal resection for Barrett's dysplasia and early esophageal adenocarcinoma. South Med J 2004;97:827–30.

[81] Pacifico RJ, Wang KK, Wongkeesong LM, et al. Combined endoscopic mucosal resection and photodynamic therapy versus esophagectomy for management of early adenocarcinoma in Barrett's esophagus. Clin Gastroenterol Hepatol 2003;1:252–7.

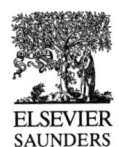

ELSEVIER
SAUNDERS

Gastrointest Endoscopy Clin N Am
15 (2005) 631–651

GASTROINTESTINAL
ENDOSCOPY CLINICS
OF NORTH AMERICA

New Frontiers in Endoscopic Imaging

Linda S. Lee, MD, John M. Poneros, MD*

*Division of Gastroenterology, Brigham and Women's Hospital, Harvard Medical School,
75 Francis Street Boston, MA 02114, USA*

Gastrointestinal (GI) tract malignancies have a tremendous impact on society. Colorectal cancer is the second leading cause of cancer death in the United States and accounts for 10% of all cancer deaths. It is estimated to have affected 148,000 people in 2002 in the United States, and over 57,000 deaths due to colorectal cancer are expected in the United States in 2003 [1,2]. Although esophageal adenocarcinoma is less common than colorectal cancer, its incidence in the United States has increased dramatically over the past two decades [3]. The overall 5-year survival rate is less than 10%. Colonic and esophageal adenocarcinomas arise from pre-malignant lesions; any success in their early detection could significantly reduce their mortality rates.

Significant research efforts are being directed toward using the interaction of light and tissue to detect pre-cancerous lesions of the GI tract. The interaction between light and tissue can be used to study the chemical and physical properties of the tissue being analyzed. The principles being studied could theoretically be applied to the early surveillance of many different types of cancer.

This article reviews the current status of various experimental optical technologies to detect pre-cancerous changes in the GI tract and focuses on the clinical applications of these technologies for the practicing gastroenterologist.

Light-induced fluorescence spectroscopy

Light-induced fluorescence spectroscopy uses characteristic light emission spectra to help differentiate benign from malignant or pre-malignant tissue.

---

* Corresponding author.

E-mail address: jponeros@partners.org (J.M. Poneros).

1052-5157/05/$ – see front matter © 2005 Elsevier Inc. All rights reserved.
doi:10.1016/j.giec.2005.04.006   *giendo.theclinics.com*

Ultraviolet or short-wavelength light from a laser or filtered lamp source is typically used to illuminate the tissue being studied. Endogenous substances in the tissue, known as fluorophores, absorb light of a specific wavelength and emit fluorescent light of a longer wavelength; this is known as the tissue's auto-fluorescence [4–6].

Tissue autofluorescence is dominated by the type and proportion of fluorophores it contains. Fluorophores are present in connective tissue (collagen and elastin), respiratory chain co-enzymes (NADH, flavin), amino acids (tryptophan), and by-products of heme synthesis (porphyrin). Table 1 lists common endogenous fluorophores and their excitation and emission wavelengths. The different layers of the GI tract wall (ie, mucosa, submucosa, and muscularis propria) have distinct fluorophore compositions; tissue autofluorescence is the sum fluorescence of these layers.

Malignant and benign tissue have different emission spectra due to several specific characteristics: (1) the different distribution and concentration of fluorophores and chromophores (which absorb light of a specific wavelength without re-emission of fluorescence); (2) the alteration in tissue architecture, such as mucosal thickening in epithelial tumors; (3) changes in the metabolic status of tumor tissue; and (4) the different biochemical microenvironments, such as the microbial activity that occurs in necrotic tumors, which promotes porphyrin synthesis [5,6]. Romer and colleagues [7] studied the morphologic differences in fluorescence between normal colonic mucosa and adenomas and studied specifically which tissue components contributed to fluorescence. They found that fluorescence mainly arose from collagen fibers in the bowel wall and eosinophil granules in the lamina propria. Fluorescent eosinophil granules were more numerous in adenomas, and cytoplasmic fluorescence was detected in adenomas but not in normal colonic epithelial cells. Determining which cellular compo-

Table 1
Common endogenous fluorophores and their excitation and emission wavelengths

Endogenous fluorophore	Biologic source	Wavelength of max. excitation (nm)	Wavelength of max. emission (nm)
Collagen	Connective tissue	330	390
Elastin		350	420
NADH	Respiratory chain co-enzymes	340	450
FAD, flavins		450	515
Tryptophan	Amino acids	280	350
Phenylalanine		260	280
Tyrosine		275	300
Porphyrins	By-products of heme synthesis	400–450	635, 690
Pyridoxine	Vitamin B6 compounds	330, 340	400
Pyridoxal-5'-phosphate		330	400
Ceroid, lipofuscin	Lipopigment granules	340–395	430–460, 540–640

nents are responsible for the differences in polyp fluorescence will help exploit these fluorescence signatures.

The wavelength of excitation light used is critical when studying tissue autofluorescence because different wavelengths excite distinct fluorophores at varying tissue depths. The optimal excitation and emission wavelengths for various tissue types are unknown and are typically determined by ex vivo experimentation. These results may not accurately reflect in vivo tissue properties due to changes in the microenvironment and metabolic state [5].

In 1990, Kapadia and colleagues [8] reported the first use of laser-induced fluorescence spectroscopy in the GI tract. The authors examined ex vivo colonic tissue using a laser with an excitation wavelength of 325 nm to distinguish adenomatous polyps from hyperplastic polyps. Using linear regression analysis and a training set of 70 tissue specimens (35 normal and 35 adenomatous), a quantitative laser-induced fluorescence score was developed to discriminate adenomas from normal tissue. In the validation set, all 34 normal mucosal specimens, 16 adenomas, and 94% of hyperplastic polyps were correctly identified. These results were confirmed in the first in vivo study by Cothren and colleagues [9] who compared the spectra from different colonic tissues. They developed a spectrofluorometry system with an optical probe that could be passed through the accessory channel of a standard colonoscope and placed in direct contact with tissue. Using 460 and 680 nm excitation wavelengths, they distinguished adenomas from nonadenomas (defined as normal mucosa and hyperplastic polyps) with 97% specificity, 100% sensitivity, and 94% positive predictive value (PPV).

Schomacker and colleagues [10] examined the discrimination of adenomas from hyperplastic polyps in vivo. During routine colonoscopy, an optical fiber probe was passed through the colonoscope, and emission spectra were collected from all polyps requiring resection. Similar to the study by Kapadia and colleagues, linear regression analysis was used to develop a laser-induced fluorescence score to distinguish adenomas from hyperplastic polyps. For an excitation wavelength of 390 nm, using histology as the reference standard, the authors reported a slightly lower sensitivity (86%), specificity (80%), and PPV (86%) compared with previous studies. They postulated that the use of a slightly longer excitation wavelength in vivo (390 nm versus 370 nm in previous studies) and the inclusion of mixed morphology polyps might explain the different results.

In the first blinded study published in 1996, Cothren's group [11] prospectively validated a diagnostic algorithm to distinguish normal colonic mucosa from hyperplastic and adenomatous polyps using fluorescence spectra. In vivo emission spectra were collected from 103 polypoid and 104 normal-appearing colonic mucosal sites using an optical probe passed through the colonoscope. The diagnostic algorithm was developed using emission spectra from 41 polyps and 43 normal-appearing colonic mucosal sites. This algorithm was tested in a blinded fashion using the remaining polypoid and normal colonic specimens. With an excitation wavelength of 370 nm, the sensitivity, specificity, and PPV for differentiating adenomas from nonadenomas (normal mucosa and hyperplastic polyps) were 90%, 95%, and 90%, respectively. In distinguishing adeno-mas from hyperplastic polyps, the sensitivity and specificity were 90% and 82%, respectively. The results of several studies using endogenous fluorescence to diagnose colonic adenomas are summarized in Table 2.

Laser-induced fluorescence spectroscopy has been used to examine upper GI tract epithelia. In 1995, Panjehpour and colleagues [12] published the first use of laser-induced fluorescence spectroscopy to identify esophageal malignancy in vivo. Using linear discriminate analysis, the authors developed a diagnostic al-gorithm that they tested on 108 normal and 26 malignant tissue specimens. At an excitation wavelength of 410 nm, the sensitivity and specificity for detecting malignant esophageal tissue were 100% and 98%, respectively. The investigators then examined the use of laser-induced fluorescence spectroscopy to detect dysplasia in Barrett's esophagus (BE) [13]. They used the differential normalized fluorescence index to distinguish high-grade dysplasia (HGD) from low-grade dysplasia (LGD) or nondysplastic mucosa. For emission wavelengths of 480 and 660 nm at an excitation wavelength of 410 nm, 90% of HGD cases were correctly identified; all examples of LGD and 96% of the cases of nondysplas-tic Barrett's epithelium were appropriately classified. One limitation of this study was that only 28% of LGD specimens with areas of focal HGD were cor-rectly recognized. The clinical significance of focal HGD is controversial [14,15].

Light-induced fluorescence spectroscopy has been studied as an alternative to laser excitation. Mayinger and colleagues [16] used violet-blue light as the ex-citation energy in a pilot study of 11 patients (six with esophageal squamous cell carcinoma, three with gastric cancer, and two with gastric adenomas with severe dysplasia). Biopsies were obtained after spectroscopy and used as the reference standard. The illumination and position of the probe dramatically affected the intensity of the observed spectra in this study; therefore, the spectra were nor-malized before comparison. After normalization, the spectra from normal and premalignant tissue were clearly different; the authors found that esophageal

Table 2
Summary of autofluorescence studies to diagnose colonic adenomas

Authors	System studied	Excitation wavelength (nm)	Tissues studied	Results
Kapadia et al, 1990 [8]	Ex vivo	325	Adenoma versus hyperplastic polyp	94% accurate
Cothren et al, 1990 [9]	In vivo	460, 680	Adenoma versus hyperplastic and normal tissue	100% sensitive 97% specific 94% PPV
Schomacker et al, 1992 [10]	In vivo	390	Adenoma versus hyperplastic polyp	86% sensitive 80% specific 86% PPV
Cothren et al, 1996 [11]	In vivo, blinded	370	Adenoma versus hyperplastic and normal tissue	90% sensitive 95% specific 90% PPV

Abbreviation: PPV, positive predictive value.

squamous cell carcinoma and dysplastic gastric adenomas displayed significantly lower intensity compared with normal mucosa. In this study, interpretation of the diagnostic spectrum was possible only after obtaining a reference spectrum from normal mucosa of the same patient. Compared with laser-induced fluorescence, light-induced fluorescence spectroscopy offers the advantage of being a theoretically safer, less expensive technology, which would allow it to be more easily disseminated.

Fluorescence spectroscopy versus fluorescence spectroscopic imaging

Emitted fluorescent light can be analyzed by point spectroscopy or imaging. In spectroscopy, a point measurement of fluorescence is obtained. During endoscopic GI spectroscopy, an optical fiber probe is passed through the biopsy channel of the endoscope to contact the tissue. The probe delivers excitation light, captures and transmits the emission fluorescence for analysis, and blocks scattered excitation light. During each contact and delivery of excitation light, detailed spectroscopic data are collected from a 1 to 3 mm^3 volume of tissue. Conversely, spectroscopic fluorescence imaging analyzes a larger area of tissue. Recent prototypes involve attaching a unit with two light-sensitive cameras to the optical head of a fiberoptic endoscope. The images from these two cameras are combined into a real-time fluorescent image with normal tissue appearing in one color and abnormal tissue in a different color. The endoscopist can switch back and forth between the white-light endoscopic and real-time fluorescent imaging to image large areas of tissue rapidly. Using this system, any suspicious lesions on white-light endoscopy can be quickly examined using fluorescent imaging. Due to the reduced signal-to-noise ratio with fluorescent imaging, the sensitivity and specificity is thought to be less than point spectroscopy.

In 1999, Wang and colleagues [17] studied a prototype endoscopic fluorescence imaging system to diagnose colonic adenomas. Using histology as the reference standard and a fluorescence threshold of 80% of the average intensity of normal mucosa, this imaging system was 83% sensitive for identifying adenomas; all hyperplastic polyps were correctly classified as nondysplastic. A preliminary study in 2001 compared white-light endoscopy with combination white-light endoscopic and fluorescent imaging in differentiating nondysplastic colonic tissue (normal or hyperplastic) from adenomatous polyps [18]. This study demonstrated a higher sensitivity (95% versus 80%), specificity (80% versus 69%), and PPV (71% versus 59%) with fluorescent imaging when examining 62 lesions.

Fluorescence spectroscopy and imaging have several limitations. Fluorescence analyzes a relatively weak signal that results from the interaction between light and tissue fluorophores and, therefore, necessitates sensitive and expensive instrumentation. In addition, fluorescence spectroscopy and imaging require that the optimal excitation and emission wavelength for each tissue first be determined through ex vivo experimentation, which may not accurately reflect in vivo results [4]. Despite these limitations, this optical technology has shown promise and has provided the earliest experience for investigators working in this field.

Exogenous fluorescent agents

The use of exogenous fluorescent agents has been studied as an alternative to tissue autofluorescence in the detection of pre-cancerous changes in the GI tract. These agents are administered before performing fluorescence spectroscopy or imaging and are used to magnify the abnormal signal from dysplastic tissue. Studies have focused on maximizing the diagnostic yield of these agents by determining the optimal dosage, method of delivery, and timing of the endoscopic procedures during which spectroscopic data are measured. Drug toxicity and imperfect localization of the drug to dysplasia are the limitations of these agents [19,20].

One of the most studied exogenous fluorescent agents to date is 5-aminolevulinic acid (ALA), which is the rate-limiting precursor in heme biosynthesis. Exogenous administration of ALA promotes heme synthesis and causes an accumulation of protoporphyrin IX (PPIX), which best absorbs light at 400 nm and emits red light at 650 nm. PPIX preferentially accumulates in the mucosal epithelium of the epidermis, endometrium, urinary and GI tracts, and their malignant counterparts [21–23]. Neoplastic cells have elevated porphobilinogen deaminase levels and decreased ferrochelatase activity, which is thought to lead to excess PPIX accumulation [24]. This mechanism has been exploited by using ALA as a photosensitizer for photodynamic therapy [25–27]. To optimize the ability to detect malignancy and premalignancy, varying the dose of ALA, the mechanism of delivery (ie, intravenous versus topical spray), and the time delay between sensitization and endoscopy have been studied [23].

In 1996, Von Holstein and colleagues [28] completed the first study using an exogenous fluorophore to perform laser-induced fluorescence spectroscopy in the GI tract. The authors injected the photosensitizer dihematoporphyrin ether to help identify adenocarcinoma within Barrett's mucosa. Photofrin is an exogenous fluorophore with prolonged photosensitivity that can last for 6 to 8 weeks. It is less selectively concentrated in the GI mucosa than ALA. ALA-generated PPIX is typically found in its highest concentration in the mucosal epithelium, whereas Photofrin diffuses throughout the entire esophageal wall. This causes a deeper "burn" when using Photofrin to perform photodynamic therapy but also leads to a higher stricture rate [29–31]. In the study by Von Holstein and colleagues, the investigators used emission spectra from endogenous fluorophores (ie, autofluorescence) and Photofrin to create a fluorescence ratio to identify normal mucosa, BE, dysplasia, and adenocarcinoma. The intensity of autofluorescence at 500 nm for normal mucosa was 6.5 times higher than adenocarcinoma or severe dysplasia, whereas Photofrin produced a fluorescence intensity of 630 nm, which is only 1.2 times higher in tumor compared with normal tissue. The authors concluded that autofluorescence was more useful than exogenous fluorescence with Photofrin in distinguishing normal mucosa from esophageal adenocarcinoma.

The first study using ALA-enhanced fluorescence spectroscopy to detect colonic dysplasia was published by Eker and colleagues [32] in 1999. An oral dose of ALA of 5 mg/kg body weight was administered approximately 2 to 3 hours before colonoscopy and spectroscopy. Linear regression analysis was used to create an algorithm for classifying normal mucosa, hyperplastic polyps, and adenomas. At an excitation wavelength of 337 nm, ALA did not significantly improve the ability to differentiate between adenoma and normal or hyperplastic tissue compared with autofluorescence, but it did improve discrimination using 405 and 436 nm excitation. Sensitivity was 89% and specificity was 94% at a wavelength of 405 nm; sensitivity (86%) and specificity (100%) were similar using 436 nm excitation.

After these initial studies using ALA-enhanced fluorescence spectroscopy, research has focused on ALA-enhanced fluorescence imaging. Mayinger and colleagues [33] studied 22 patients with known or suspected esophageal malignancy or BE who ingested ALA at a dose of 15 mg/kg body weight. Fluorescence imaging, standard white-light endoscopy, and biopsy were performed 6 to 7 hours after ingestion. Tissue histology was used as the reference standard to determine sensitivity and specificity. Although the sensitivity for accurately diagnosing biopsy sites was greater with ALA-enhanced fluorescence imaging compared with white-light endoscopy (85% versus 25%), the specificity was diminished (53% versus 94%) due to PPIX accumulation in inflamed mucosa. An example of ALA-enhanced fluorescence imaging is demonstrated in Fig. 1.

In 2001, Endlicher and colleagues [34] investigated the optimal dose and route of administration of ALA in fluorescence imaging to detect biopsy-proven LGD and HGD within BE. ALA was orally ingested at doses of 5, 10, 20, or 30 mg/kg body weight or sprayed onto Barrett's epithelium using a special spray catheter at a previous endoscopy. Imaging was performed 4 to 6 hours after systemic or 1 to 2 hours after local sensitization. At 20 and 30 mg/kg, the technique was limited by increased side effects such as nausea, vomiting, and elevated liver

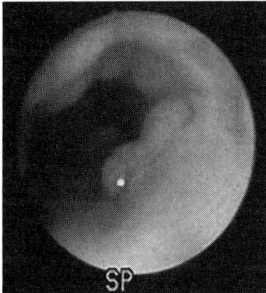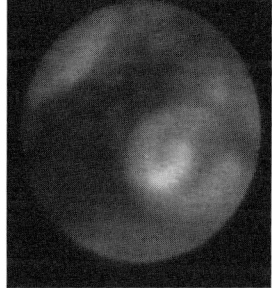

Fig. 1. Endoscopic image of nodule with HGD and corresponding ALA-enhanced fluorescence imaging of an identical nodule. (Courtesy of N. Nishioka, MD, Boston, MA.)

enzymes. The lowest dose of 5 mg/kg failed to detect dysplasia. Sensitivity and specificity for detecting dysplasia were similar for 10 mg/kg (80% and 56%) and 20 mg/kg (100% and 51%). Local sensitization with a spray catheter improved specificity (69%) but reduced sensitivity (60%) and was limited by the need to perform two endoscopies. The overall high rate of false-positive fluorescence in this study resulted from incorrectly classifying inflammatory mucosa, ulcer margins, and bile as malignant.

Brand and colleagues [35] performed the first study to use quantitative ALA-enhanced fluorescence point spectroscopy to differentiate nondysplastic from dysplastic Barrett's epithelium. Oral ALA at a dose of 10 mg/kg body weight was administered 3 hours before endoscopy. A standardized fluorescence intensity value was calculated by accounting for the contribution of autofluorescence at emission wavelengths of 635 and 750 nm. Sensitivity and specificity for distinguishing HGD from nondysplastic and LGD Barrett's mucosa were 77% and 71%, respectively.

The use of ALA-fluorescence imaging to identify colonic dysplasia in ulcerative colitis was studied by Messmann and colleagues [36]. Previous studies had established that a higher dose of ALA is required to sensitize the colon compared with the esophagus [37]. Messmann and colleagues used an oral dose of 20 mg/kg, a 3 g ALA enema, or a spray catheter to detect LGD and HGD in ulcerative colitis. Endoscopy was performed 4 to 6 hours after systemic sensitization and 1 to 2 hours after local sensitization. A total of 481 biopsies were examined from 37 patients with 42 biopsies showing dysplasia (40 with LGD, two with HGD). Using histology as the reference standard, the sensitivity for detecting dysplasia ranged from 43% with oral ALA, to 87% with enema, to 100% with the spray catheter. Oral ALA had a higher specificity of 73% compared with the enema (51%) and spray catheter (62%).

The use of ALA as an exogenous fluorescent agent has shown promise in detecting dysplasia in the upper and lower GI tract with relatively few side effects at the appropriate dose. Further studies with ALA and other exogenous fluorescent agents and improved fluorescent imaging techniques when using these agents are required.

Light-scattering spectroscopy

Fluorescence analyzes the biochemical properties of tissue; light-scattering spectroscopy (LSS) interrogates structural information. The wavelength of the illuminating light and the properties of the scattering particle determine the scattering pattern. Cell nuclei are predominantly responsible for light scattering when tissue is analyzed, specifically the nuclear size and number. Photons are typically scattered multiple times within tissue before being emitted. LSS measures the wavelength and intensity of back-reflected light. It subtracts the diffuse background caused by multiple scattering to allow the analysis of the small amount of back-scattered light from cell nuclei. Dysplastic cells typically have an increased nuclear-to-cytoplasmic ratio and are more crowded together. LSS is a quantitative equivalent to the histologic markers for dysplasia of hyperchromasia and nuclear enlargement. One advantage of LSS compared with laser-induced fluorescence is that the signal intensity of light scattering dominates the fluorescent absorption signal when examining biologic tissue (ie, higher signal-to-noise ratio) [19,38,39].

LSS of the GI tract involves inserting an optical probe through the accessory channel of the endoscope. The tip of the probe contacts the epithelium and emits and collects the white light from about a 1 mm^2 area of tissue. In the first study of LSS in Barrett's epithelium with and without dysplasia, dysplastic epithelium was defined as at least 30% of the nuclei being larger than 10µm [40]. Using this definition and histology as the gold standard, the sensitivity and specificity of LSS for correctly identifying HGD and LGD was approximately 90%; all HGD samples and 87% of LGD samples were correctly classified. The appeal of this technique is that a stronger signal is collected in real-time using white light instead of a laser source.

Raman spectroscopy

When light interacts with tissue, incident photons cause electrons in the tissue to oscillate and emit photons. If the emitted photons have the same energy as the incident photons, no energy transfer occurs, and the scattering is termed "elastic." Although most light–tissue interactions are elastic, some are inelastic, which refers to an energy transfer between the photon and the molecule being illuminated. The phenomenon of inelastic light scattering is termed Raman scattering. The energy transfer causes molecules to vibrate, which results in slight shifts in energy and wavelength of the emitted light relative to the excitation light. Approximately one photon out of 1 million scatters at a wavelength slightly shifted from the original incident wavelength. Thus, Raman scattering is much weaker than elastic scattering, but the signal is highly specific to the molecular composition of the tissue [19,39].

Visible, UV, or near-infrared light may be used to induce Raman scattering, which is measured as a difference in wavelength from the excitation wavelength. When visible light is used for excitation, autofluorescence causes severe interference with the Raman signal, which is typically much weaker than the fluorescent signal. UV light is not optimal for Raman spectroscopy because it can cause tissue injury and does not penetrate tissue to the same depth as visible or near-infrared light. Near-infrared light for Raman spectroscopy has the advantages of minimizing autofluorescence, penetrating more deeply (to a depth of approximately 500 µm), and being nonmutagenic [19,39].

Ex vivo studies using Raman spectroscopy to examine BE reported a sensitivity of 77% and a specificity of 93% for differentiating nondysplastic from dysplastic Barrett's epithelium [41]. Shim and colleagues [42] designed and built a near-infrared device for in vivo Raman spectroscopy. In the first in vivo report using this device, the authors demonstrated the feasibility of in vivo measurements, but the spectral differences between normal tissue and HGD in the esophagus and colon were subtle.

In 2003, Shim and colleagues authors used near-infrared Raman spectroscopy to identify colonic adenomas in vivo [43]. They classified 19 Raman spectra from nine polyps in three patients as hyperplastic or adenomatous using diagnostic algorithms. These algorithms were developed from principal component and linear discriminant analyses in a "leave-one-out," cross-validation method. In this small sample, the diagnostic algorithms were 100% sensitive and 89% specific for differentiating hyperplastic from adenomatous polyps. Raman spectroscopy is a potentially powerful tool for evaluating pre-malignant GI conditions but requires further improvements given its low signal-to-noise ratio.

Trimodal spectroscopy

In 2001, Georgakoudi and colleagues [44] combined several spectroscopic techniques in an attempt to increase the accuracy of detecting dysplasia within BE. They used a combination of fluorescence, reflectance, and light-scattering spectroscopies to analyze the biochemical, architectural, and morphologic characteristics of Barrett's epithelium, with and without dysplasia. The simultaneous use of all three techniques was named "trimodal spectroscopy." The combination of fluorescence and reflectance spectroscopies was applied to remove the distortions introduced into the measured tissue fluorescence spectrum by scattering and absorption. Undistorted fluorescence was then used to analyze the tissue biochemistry, and reflectance and light-scattering spectroscopies were used to analyze the tissue architecture and epithelial cell nuclei.

Data were collected from 40 sites in 16 patients with known BE undergoing standard surveillance endoscopy. Principal component and logistic regression analyses were used to correlate the spectral features and histopathologic diagnosis. In this data set, trimodal spectroscopy classified HGD versus LGD and nondysplastic Barrett's epithelium with 100% sensitivity and 100% specificity. HGD and LGD versus nondysplastic Barrett's epithelium was identified with 100% sensitivity and 93% specificity. This study was not conducted in real time and used "leave-one-out" cross-validation to establish the classification algorithms. Nonetheless, trimodal spectroscopy carries great promise for the detection of dysplastic epithelial changes by combining information regarding the biochemical and architectural characteristics of tissue.

Optical coherence tomography

Optical coherence tomography (OCT) is a novel imaging technique that provides high resolution, two-dimensional, cross-sectional imaging of the GI tract. OCT is analogous to B-mode ultrasound imaging but uses light rather than sound waves. The use of light rather than sound leads to differences in the depth of penetration and resolution of images. With the use of light, tissue resolution is increased by nearly 10 times from ~110 μm to ~10 μm, but the depth of penetration is sacrificed [45–47].

During OCT imaging, backscattered light provides information on the spatial organization of the tissue. OCT measures the echo time delay and magnitude of the backscattered light signal from microstructures within the tissue. Echo time delay refers to the time difference between the signal leaving from and returning to the detector. Because light travels too quickly for the electronic detection of its echo time delay, OCT uses a technique called interferometry to measure the delay. Light from a low coherence light source is split evenly into two separate pathways with one beam directed to the tissue being imaged and the other beam delivered to a reference arm. At the end of the reference arm is a mirror that oscillates at a known distance away from the detector. Each beam of light is reflected from the tissue and the reference mirror and recombined at the detector. The interference created by these two recombined light beams is measured. Interference occurs only when the path lengths of both light beams are matched to within the coherence length of the light source. The axial resolution of an OCT image is determined by the coherence length of the light source used and is approximately 10 μm in the infrared OCT systems. The lateral or transverse resolution is determined by the spatial width of the light source and is approximately 30 μm. As the position of the mirror is moved, information is collected from different tissue levels. By scanning the optical beam across the tissue surface, a two-dimensional picture is created [48,49].

Several in vitro studies have demonstrated the feasibility of OCT imaging in the GI tract [45,49–51]. The clinical value of in vitro studies is limited because the optical properties of nonliving tissue are different from in vivo tissue. In 1997, Sergeev and colleagues [52] published the first in vivo OCT images of normal esophageal epithelium. They imaged four patients and demonstrated five esophageal wall layers composed of mucosa, lamina propria, muscularis mucosa, submucosa, and muscularis propria. Using the same OCT system, Jäckle and colleagues [53,55] presented data from 48 patients, including nine esophageal images, and confirmed their findings. Bouma and colleagues [54] studied 32 patients using a linear scanning device that produces cross-sectional images similar to those of Jäckle and colleagues. By comparing ex vivo measurements of layer thickness by OCT and histology in the same specimen of normal esophagus, they were able to define precisely which OCT image layers corresponded to each esophageal wall component.

The OCT system used by Sivak and colleagues [56] differs from other endoscopic OCT systems in that it acquires images with a radial scanning device similar to high-frequency ultrasound. Sivak and colleagues included 72 OCT images from 38 patients taken from the upper and lower GI tract. Zuccaro and colleagues [57] acquired 477 images of the esophagus and stomach in 69 patients, and Li and colleagues [58] published a descriptive study of eight patients using linear- and radial-scanning OCT catheter probes and spectroscopic OCT.

BE is characterized by the development of specialized intestinal metaplasia above the esophago-gastric junction. The hallmark histologic feature of specialized intestinal metaplasia is the presence of goblet cells. Visualization of individual goblet cells is beyond the resolution of currently available endoscopic OCT devices. However, OCT images of Barrett's epithelium have shown distinct morphologic features that enable the differentiation of Barrett's epithelium from other tissue types. Fig. 2 demonstrates OCT images of normal esophageal squamous epithelium, gastric mucosa, and specialized intestinal metaplasia.

In 2001, Poneros and colleagues [59] developed and prospectively validated the first objective OCT image criteria for diagnosing BE. These criteria were developed by examining 166 OCT-correlated biopsy specimens, which served as the training set. The presence of two or more of the following OCT findings was considered diagnostic for Barrett's epithelium: absence of normal esophageal layering, disorganized architecture, and the presence of submucosal glands that look like areas of low reflectance below the tissue surface or invaginations through the epithelium. An experienced blinded observer used these criteria to analyze 122 OCT images prospectively in the validation set. Using histology as the standard, the OCT criteria were 97% sensitive and 92% specific for Barrett's mucosa with or without dysplasia.

This same group studied the use of OCT in identifying dysplasia in Barrett's mucosa [60]. Because the degree of light reflectivity depends on nuclear size, OCT may be able to characterize dysplasia within Barrett's epithelium by quantifying the OCT signal as a function of depth (ie, higher degrees of dysplasia characterized by larger nuclei would be expected to cause more light scattering). This alteration in the light reflection characteristics of dysplastic tissue may be more reliable than morphologic criteria in identifying dysplasia.

To differentiate specialized intestinal metaplasia from dysplasia, the authors used two parameters that are calculated from the OCT images: slope reflectivity and layer ratio. In a preliminary retrospective study of 11 images of LGD, four of HGD, and 23 of nondysplastic Barrett's epithelium, sensitivity for HGD was 100%, and was specificity 82% to 85%.

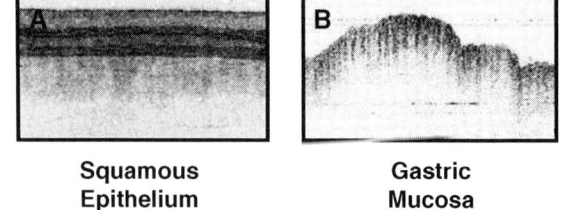 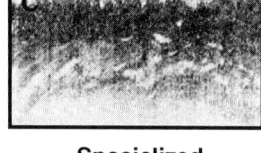

**Squamous   Gastric   Specialized
Epithelium   Mucosa   Intestinal
                                   Metaplasia**

Fig. 2. OCT images of upper GI tract tissues. (*A*) Squamous epithelium typically shows a five-layered appearance. (*B*) Gastric mucosa demonstrates a "pit-and-crypt" morphology. (*C*) Barrett's epithelium, or specialized intestinal metaplasia, reveals an inhomogeneous tissue contrast, an irregular mucosal surface, and submucosal glands. (Courtesy of B. Bouma, PhD, and G. Tearney, MD, Boston, MA.)

Isenberg and colleagues [61] recently published a study in abstract form using OCT to diagnose dysplastic Barrett's epithelium. They used morphologic rather than quantitative criteria to identify dysplasia. Four endoscopists independently reviewed 152 images from 23 patients and rated them from 1 (dysplasia absent) to 5 (dysplasia present). A score of 2 or higher was considered positive for dysplasia. A pathologist blinded to the OCT images reviewed the corresponding biopsies. OCT was 69% sensitive and 71% specific with a PPV of 36% and a negative predictive value (NPV) of 91%. The authors concluded that the high NPV suggested that OCT could be used to target biopsies to areas of higher suspicion for dysplasia in Barrett's epithelium.

OCT images of malignant GI tissue have been published by several groups. Jäckle and colleagues [55] studied six patients with esophageal adenocarcinoma arising from Barrett's mucosa. They described a complete loss of layering and increased heterogeneity in esophageal adenocarcinoma when imaged by OCT. Bouma and colleagues [54] confirmed these results in two patients and described a cellular stroma with large pockets of mucin. Fig. 3 demonstrates an OCT image of esophageal adenocarcinoma. Because of the limited depth of penetration with OCT, the role of OCT in staging esophageal tumors is unclear. EUS accurately stages most endoscopically apparent tumors, but superficial esophageal squamous cell carcinomas in which the tumor echogenicity does not differ significantly from the surrounding normal squamous mucosa are poorly staged by EUS. OCT may be useful in this situation, but experience with OCT in esophageal squamous carcinoma is limited. Jäckle and colleagues [53] and Pitris and colleagues [45] each reported one case of squamous carcinoma identified by loss of normal esophageal layering using OCT.

OCT images of colonic adenomas were examined in a recent study by Pfau and colleagues [62]. During routine colonoscopy, OCT images were obtained from 44 polyps (30 adenomas, 14 hyperplastic polyps) and nearby normal-appearing mucosa in 24 patients. Real-time subjective assessments of the degree of organization and light scattering were performed by the endoscopists who rated the images from 0 (least organization or scattering) to 5 (most organization or scattering). Digital imaging analysis was performed to quantify the degree of

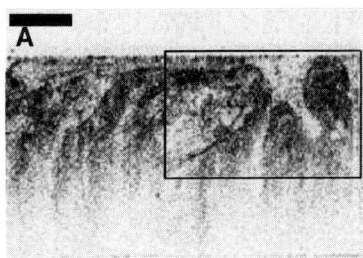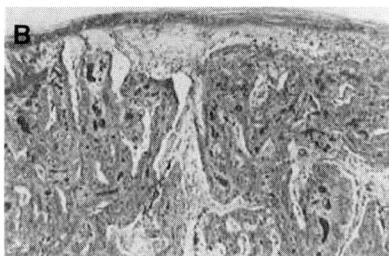

Fig. 3. (A) OCT image of esophageal adenocarcinoma. Scale bar, 500 μm. (B) Corresponding histopathology (hematoxylin-eosin, original magnification ×40). (Courtesy of B. Bouma, PhD, and G. Tearney, MD, Boston, MA.)

light scattering, and histology was used as the reference standard. Adenomas were significantly more disorganized, with less light scattering compared with hyperplastic polyps; normal colonic mucosal specimens were similar to hyperplastic polyps.

OCT images of the biliary tree obtained during ERCP were published in 2002 in a "proof of principle" feasibility study [63]. OCT images of normal bile duct, cholangiocarcinoma, and a malignant biliary stricture due to metastatic colon cancer were acquired from five patients. If proven sensitive for cholangiocarcinoma, OCT would be useful in this disease given the frequent difficulty in obtaining diagnostic tissue.

OCT is an exciting technology that allows real-time tomographic visualization of tissue structures at a higher resolution than any other available endoscopic modality. During OCT, an optical probe is passed down the accessory channel of the endoscope without the need for a conducting medium. OCT is an evolving technology with several limitations, which include the length of time required to obtain images, a shallow depth of visualization, and the inability to visualize subcellular structures. High-resolution OCT imaging that can compare with histology is closer to becoming a reality with the development of ultrashort pulse laser technology. Drexler and colleagues [64] have published OCT images taken with a Ti:sapphire laser system, which achieves a longitudinal resolution of ~1 μm and transverse resolution of 3 μm in vitro. Subcellular structures such as

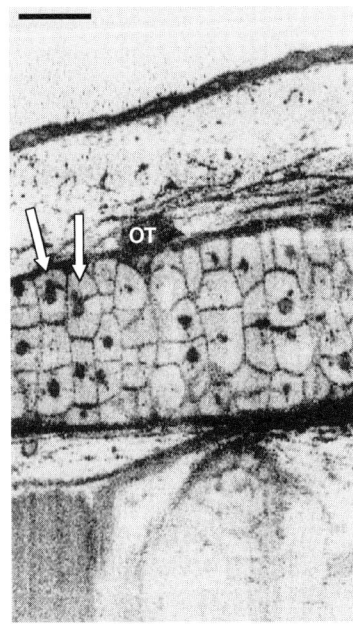

Fig. 4. In vivo OCT image of *X laevis*. Scale bar, 100 μm. The olfactory tract (OT) and mitosis of two cell pairs (*arrows*) are shown. (*From* Drexler W, Morgner U, Kaertner FX, et al. In vitro ultra-high resolution of optical coherence tomography. Opt Lett 1999;24:1221–3; with permission.)

nuclei are readily seen at these resolutions. This system as currently configured is somewhat limited in that it is not catheter based or readily portable, and safety data regarding its interrogating light beam are lacking. Once these limitations are overcome, high-resolution OCT could provide a significant advancement in optical imaging. Fig. 4 demonstrates an in vivo OCT image of an African frog tadpole (*Xenopus laevis*) using this system.

Molecular beacons

Recently, exciting work has been published on the use of optically based, enzyme-activated fluorescent sensors for the in vivo monitoring of protease activity. Proteolytic enzymes have been shown to play an essential role during tumor progression, specifically during high cell turnover, invasion, and angiogenesis [65]. Cathepsin B, a cysteine protease, has been demonstrated to be upregulated in areas of inflammation, necrosis, angiogenesis, and focal invasion of colorectal carcinomas and dysplastic adenomas [66–68]. Fluorescent sensors that operate in the near-infrared (NIR) region have been developed to allow noninvasive monitoring of enzyme activity [69,70]. These targeted NIR fluorochromes have an advantage over other reporters (eg, isotopes) in that they can be "silenced" and "activated" by the enzymes they are used to identify. In their native state, the enzymes are essentially nonfluorescent, but upon enzymatic cleavage they become fluorescent in the near-infrared.

In 2002, Marten and colleagues reported their work using a fluorescent molecular "beacon" to assess cathepsin B protease activity in adenomatous polyps [71]. They used a mouse model that is heterozygous for the germ-line mutation of the mouse homolog of the human APC gene. These animals develop multiple adenomas in the small and large bowel that simulate adenomatous polyps in humans [72].

Using a control set of mice injected with a nonactivatable fluorochrome, indocyanine green, the authors demonstrated that cathepsin B expression was ubiquitous in adenomatous polyps and highest in larger colonic polyps with high degrees of dysplasia. Immunohistochemistry and fluorescence confocal microscopy were used to examine the resected colonic mucosa. Adenomas as small as 50 μm in diameter could be readily identified with the aid of the fluorescent beacon. To quantify the fluorescence signal, the authors calculated a target (adenoma) to background (mucosa) contrast (TBC contrast). A value of 100 represented a 100% higher fluorescence signal of the adenoma compared with mucosa. Contrast in the large adenomas (TBC = 220% ± 97%) was thought to be caused by the higher amount of converting enzyme per lesion. Adenomas in the mice that received indocyanine green showed a significantly lower TBC contrast compared with those that received the cathepsin B sensing probe (TBC = 34% ± 4% versus 119 ± 71%, $P < .01$).

In humans, cathepsin B-positive tumor cells have been observed in 67% of adenomas and 100% of adenomas with HGD or adenocarcinoma [73]. Optically visible, activatable fluorescent beacons could provide an important technology to screen patients for late-stage adenomas. This technology could eventually be adapted to conventional endoscopy or external NIR imaging of the bowel.

Laser scanning confocal microscopy

Laser scanning confocal microscopy (LCM) is another novel optical method that provides subsurface imaging of tissue. This technology combines confocally placed pinholes at the source and detector to reduce out-of-focus light with laser illumination. Images are formed from a scanning laser beam, which results in optical sections through the sample. These slices can be collected through a specimen to determine its 3-dimensional fluorescence structure.

Several studies have examined the ex vivo use of LCM in the GI tract [74–76]. Sakashita and colleagues [76] studied 100 endoscopically or surgically resected colorectal lesions using LCM with histology as the gold standard. There were seven normal mucosa, five hyperplastic polyps, 68 adenomas, 10 cases of HGD, and 10 adenocarcinomas. Nuclei were more commonly visualized in adenomas with HGD or carcinoma than in normal mucosa or hyperplastic polyps. Using these criteria to distinguish the two groups, sensitivity was 60%, specificity was 91%, and PPV was 63%.

The first confocal laser endomicroscope was examined in a recent study of in vivo colonic lesions by Kiesslich and colleagues [77]. A confocal laser microscope was integrated into the distal tip of a conventional video colonoscope, which used argon ion laser at an excitation wavelength of 488 nm. The optical slice thickness was 7 μm with a lateral resolution of 0.7 μm and a depth of penetration of the laser of 0 to 250 μm. Intravenous administration of fluorescein sodium was found to be superior to topical application of acriflavine hydrochloride in its ability to stain the entire mucosa rather than only the superficial

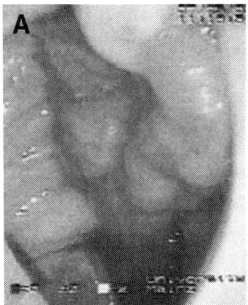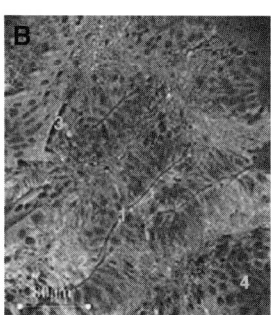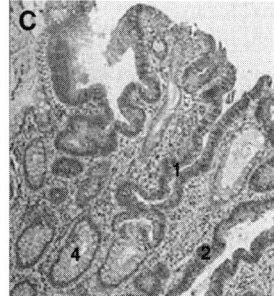

Fig. 5. (*A*) Large colonic polyp seen during endoscopy. (*B*) Confocal laser endomicroscopy shows tubular-shaped crypts with a reduced amount of goblet cells and loss of cellular junctions. (*C*) Corresponding histologic specimen. (*From* Kiesslich R, Burg J, Vieth M, et al. Confocal laser endoscopy for diagnosing intraepithelial neoplasias and colorectal cancer in vivo. Gastroenterology 2004;127:706–13; with permission.)

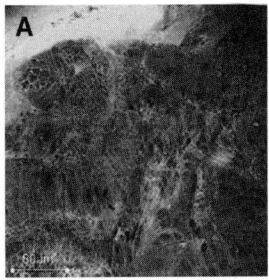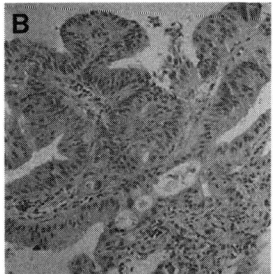

Fig. 6. (*A*) Confocal laser endomicroscopy of colorectal cancer shows irregular cell architecture with total loss of goblet cells. (*B*) Corresponding histologic specimen. (*From* Kiesslich R, Burg J, Vieth M, et al. Confocal laser endoscopy for diagnosing intraepithelial neoplasias and colorectal cancer in vivo. Gastroenterology 2004;127:706–13; with permission.)

epithelial cells. Fluorescein sodium was administered with butylscopolamine during all 45 colonoscopies. The colonic mucosa was classified as normal, regeneration, or neoplasia based on crypt and vessel architecture [78–80], and histology from biopsy specimens was the gold standard. Neoplastic mucosa defined as intraepithelial neoplasms or cancer was diagnosed by LCM with a sensitivity of 97.4% and specificity of 99.4%. Analysis of crypt arrangement and distribution of goblet cells led to a correct prediction of subsequent histologic diagnosis of colonic neoplasias in most patients. Figs. 5 and 6 demonstrate examples of confocal laser endomicroscopy.

Limitations of this technology include the need to place the tip of the endomicroscope vertically against the tissue being examined and the interference of imaging from peristalsis. In the Kiesslich study [77], about 70% of the images from LCM were judged of satisfactory, good, or very good quality. The average procedure time was relatively long at 57 minutes. Finally, after undergoing confocal laser endoscopy, all patients developed a slight yellow coloration of the skin (a side effect of fluorescein sodium), which disappeared in all cases within 60 minutes. No severe side effects were noted.

LCM is a revolutionary new technology that produces virtual histology of the mucosal layer. This technology is limited by the inability to visualize nuclei in vivo due to the use of fluorescein sodium as a fluorescence contrast agent, which is not enriched in the intestinal epithelial cells on systemic administration. Further studies with other fluorescence agents, such as cresyl violet or tetracycline (which potentially have more side effects) are needed. Once this limitation is overcome, LCM could potentially enable the diagnosis of pathology during endoscopic examinations, which would allow immediate therapeutic decisions.

Summary

The optical techniques outlined in this article offer an exciting, potentially powerful means of detecting pre-malignancy in the GI tract. This article provides an overview of the more promising technologies being studied. There are a multitude of others, such as narrow band imaging, that are being investigated. The technologies being developed to detect early GI malignancies could be transferable to other organs. The ultimate goal of optical biopsy refers to the establishment of a tissue diagnosis based on in situ optical measurements without the need for tissue removal. These experimental technologies offer an exciting glimpse into the new frontiers of endoscopic imaging and the ever closer goal of performing an optical biopsy.

References

[1] Grady WM. Genetic testing for high-risk colon cancer patients. Gastroenterology 2003;124: 1574–94.

[2] Jemal A, Murray T, Samuels A, et al. Cancer statistics. Cancer J Clin 2003;53:5–26.

[3] Blot WJ, Devesa SS, Kneller RW, et al. Rising incidence of adenocarcinoma of the esophagus and gastric cardia. JAMA 1991;265:1287–9.

[4] Bohorfoush AG. Tissue spectroscopy for gastrointestinal disease. Endoscopy 1996;28:372–80.

[5] Stepp H, Sroka R, Baumgartner R. Fluorescence endoscopy of gastrointestinal disease: basic principles, techniques, and clinical experience. Endoscopy 1998;30:379–86.

[6] DaCosta RS, Wilson BC, Marcon NE. Light-induced fluorescence endoscopy of the gastrointestinal tract. Gastrointest Endosc Clin N Am 2000;10:37–69.

[7] Romer TJ, Fitzmaurice M, Cothren RM, et al. Laser-induced fluorescence microscopy of normal colon and dysplasia in colonic adenomas: implications for spectroscopic diagnosis. Am J Gastroenterol 1995;90:81–7.

[8] Kapadia CR, Cutruzzola FW, O'Brien KM, et al. Laser-induced fluorescence spectroscopy of human colonic mucosa. Gastroenterology 1990;99:150–7.

[9] Cothren RM, Richards-Kortum R, Sivak MV, et al. Gastrointestinal tissue diagnosis by laser-induced fluorescence spectroscopy at endoscopy. Endoscopy 1990;36:105–11.

[10] Schomacker KT, Frisoli JK, Compton CC, et al. Ultraviolet laser-induced fluorescence of colonic polyps. Gastroenterology 1992;102:1155–60.

[11] Cothren RM, Sivak MV, Van Dam J, et al. Detection of dysplasia at colonoscopy using laser-induced fluorescence: a blinded study. Gastrointest Endosc 1996;44:168–76.

[12] Panjehpour M, Overholt BF, Schmidhammer JL, et al. Spectroscopic diagnosis of esophageal cancer: new classification model, improved measurement system. Gastrointest Endosc 1995; 41:577–81.

[13] Panjehpour M, Overholt BF, Vo-Dinh T, et al. Endoscopic fluorescence detection of high-grade dysplasia in Barrett's esophagus. Gastroenterology 1996;111:93–101.

[14] Buttar NS, Wang KK, Sebo TJ, et al. Extent of high-grade dysplasia in Barrett's esophagus correlates with risk of adenocarcinoma. Gastroenterology 2001;120:1630–9.

[15] Dar MS, Goldblum JR, Rice TW, et al. Can extent of high grade dysplasia in Barrett's esophagus predict the presence of adenocarcinoma at esophagectomy? Gut 2003;52:486–9.

[16] Mayinger B, Horner P, Jordan M, et al. Light-induced autofluorescence spectroscopy for tissue diagnosis of GI lesions. Gastrointest Endosc 2000;52:395–400.

[17] Wang TD, Crawford JM, Feld MS, et al. In vivo identification of colonic dysplasia using fluorescence endoscopic imaging. Gastrointest Endosc 1999;49:447–55.

[18] Song WK, Wilson BC, Marcon NE. Diagnostic potential of light-induced fluorescence endoscopy in the colon. Am J Gastroenterol 2001;96:S167.

[19] Dacosta RS, Wilson BC, Marcon NE. New optical technologies for earlier endoscopic diagnosis of premalignant gastrointestinal lesions. J Gastroenterol Hepatol 2002;17(Suppl):S85–104.

[20] Marcon NE, Wilson BC. The value of fluorescence techniques in gastrointestinal endoscopy-

better than the endoscopist's eye? II: the North American experience. Endoscopy 1998;30: 419–21.

[21] Loh CS, MacRobert AJ, Buonaccorsi G, et al. Mucosal ablation using photodynamic therapy for the treatment of dysplasia: an experimental study in the normal rat stomach. Gut 1996;38:71–8.

[22] van den Boogert J, Houtsmuller AB, de Rooij FWM, et al. Kinetics, localization, and mechanism of 5-aminolevulinic acid-induced porphyrin accumulation in normal and Barrett's-like rat esophagus. Lasers Surg Med 1999;24:3–13.

[23] Messmann H. 5-aminolevulinic acid-induced protoporphyrin IX for the detection of gastrointestinal dysplasia. Gastrointest Endosc Clin N Am 2000;10:497–512.

[24] Hinnen P, de Rooij FW, Velthuysen ML, et al. Biochemical basis of 5-aminolevulinic acid-induced protoporphyrin IX accumulation: a study in patients with (pre)malignant lesions of the esophagus. Br J Cancer 1998;78:679.

[25] Kennedy JC, Pottier RH. Endogenous protoporphyrin IX, a clinically useful photo-sensitizer for photodynamic therapy. J Photochem Photobiol 1992;14:275–92.

[26] Barr H, Shepherd NA, Dix A, et al. Eradication of high-grade dysplasia in columnar-lined (Barrett's) esophagus by photodynamic therapy with endogenously generated protoporphyrin IX. Lancet 1996;348:584–5.

[27] Gossner L, Stolte M, Sroka R, et al. Photodynamic ablation of high-grade dysplasia and early cancer in Barrett's esophagus by means of 5-aminolevulinic acid. Gastroenterology 1998;114: 448–55.

[28] von Holstein CS, Nilsson AMK, Andersson-Engels S, et al. Detection of adenocarcinoma in Barrett's esophagus by means of laser induced fluorescence. Gut 1996;39:711–6.

[29] Nishioka NS. Drug, light and oxygen: a dynamic combination in the clinic. Gastroenterology 1998;114:604–6.

[30] Overholt BF, Panjehpour M, Haydek JM. Photodynamic therapy for Barrett's esophagus: follow-up of 100 patients. Gastrointest Endosc 1999;49:1–7.

[31] Overholt BF, Panjehpour M. Photodynamic therapy for Barrett's esophagus. Gastrointest Endosc Clin N Am 1997;7:207–20.

[32] Eker C, Montan S, Jaramillo E, et al. Clinical spectral characterization of colonic mucosal lesions using autofluorescence and delta aminolevulinic acid sensitization. Gut 1999;44:511–8.

[33] Mayinger B, Neidhardt S, Reh H, et al. Fluorescence induced with 5-aminolevulinic acid for the endoscopic detection and follow-up of esophageal lesions. Gastrointest Endosc 2000;54: 572–8.

[34] Endlicher E, Kneuchel R, Hauser T, et al. Endoscopic fluorescence detection of low and high grade dysplasia in Barrett's esophagus using systemic or local 5-aminolevulinic acid sensitization. Gut 2001;48:314–9.

[35] Brand S, Wang TD, Schomacker KT, et al. Detection of high-grade dysplasia in Barrett's esophagus by spectroscopy measurement of 5-aminolevulinic acid-induced protoporphyrin IX fluorescence. Gastrointest Endosc 2002;56:479–87.

[36] Messmann H, Endlicher E, Freunek G, et al. Fluorescence endoscopy for the detection of low and high grade dysplasia in ulcerative colitis using systemic or local 5-aminolevulinic acid sensitization. Gut 2003;52:1003–7.

[37] Regula J, MacRobert AJ, Gorchein A, et al. Photosensitization and photodynamic therapy of esophageal, duodenal, and colorectal tumors using 5-aminolevulinic acid induced protoporphyrin IX- a pilot study. Gut 1995;36:67–75.

[38] Backman V, Wallace MB, Perlman LT, et al. Detection of preinvasive cancer cells. Nature 2000;406:35–6.

[39] Rollins AM, Sivak MV. Potential new endoscopic techniques for the earlier diagnosis of premalignancy. Best Pract Res Clin Gastroenterol 2001;15:227–47.

[40] Wallace MB, Perelman LT, Backman V, et al. Endoscopic detection of dysplasia in patients with Barrett's esophagus using light-scattering spectroscopy. Gastroenterology 2000;119:677–82.

[41] Shim MG, Wilson BC. The effects of ex vivo handling procedures on the near-infrared Raman spectra of normal mammalian tissues. Photochem Photobiol 1996;63:662–71.

[42] Shim MG, Song LMWK, Marcon NE, et al. In vivo near-infrared Raman spectroscopy: demon-

stration of feasibility during clinical gastrointestinal endoscopy. Photochem Photobiol 2000;72: 146–50.

[43] Molckovsky A, Song LM, Shim MG, et al. Diagnostic potential of near-infrared Raman spectroscopy in the colon: differentiating adenomatous from hyperplastic polyps. Gastrointest Endosc 2003;57:396–402.

[44] Georgakoudi I, Jacobson BC, Van Dam J, et al. Fluorescence, reflectance, and light-scattering spectroscopy for evaluating dysplasia in patients with Barrett's esophagus. Gastroenterology 2001;120:1620–9.

[45] Pitris C, Jesser C, Boppart SA, et al. Feasibility of optical coherence tomography for high-resolution imaging of human gastrointestinal tract malignancies. J Gastroenterol 2000;35:87–92.

[46] Brand S, Poneros JM, Bouma BE, et al. Optical coherence tomography in the gastrointestinal tract. Endoscopy 2000;32:796–803.

[47] Wallace MB, Van Dam J. Enhanced gastrointestinal diagnosis: light-scattering spectroscopy and optical coherence tomography. Gastrointest Endosc Clin N Am 2000;10:71–80.

[48] Tearney GJ, Brezinski ME, Bouma BE, et al. In vivo endoscopic optical biopsy with optical coherence tomography. Science 1997;276:2037–9.

[49] Tearney GJ, Brezinski ME, Southern JF, et al. Optical biopsy in human gastrointestinal tissue using optical coherence tomography. Am J Gastroenterol 1997;92:1800.

[50] Kobayashi K, Izatt JA, Kulkarni MD, et al. High-resolution cross-sectional imaging of the gastrointestinal tract using optical coherence tomography: preliminary results. Gastrointest Endosc 1998;47:515–23.

[51] Tearney GJ, Brezinski ME, Southern JF, et al. Optical biopsy in human pancreatobiliary tissue using optical coherence tomography. Dig Dis Sci 1998;43:1193–9.

[52] Sergeev AM, Gelikonov VM, Gelikonov GV, et al. In vivo endoscopic OCT imaging of precancer and cancer states of human mucosa. Opt Express 1997;1:432–40.

[53] Jäckle S, Gladkova N, Feldchtein F, et al. In vivo endoscopic optical coherence tomography of the human gastrointestinal tract: toward optical biopsy. Endoscopy 2000;32:743–9.

[54] Bouma BE, Tearney GJ, Compton CC, et al. High resolution of the human esophagus and stomach in vivo using optical coherence tomography. Gastrointest Endosc 2000;51:467–74.

[55] Jäckle S, Gladkova N, Feldchtein F, et al. In vivo endoscopic optical coherence tomography of esophagitis, Barrett's esophagus, and adenocarcinoma of the esophagus. Endoscopy 2000;32: 750–5.

[56] Sivak Jr MV, Kobayashi K, Izatt JA, et al. High-resolution endoscopic imaging of the GI tract using optical coherence tomography. Gastrointest Endosc 2000;51:474–9.

[57] Zuccaro G, Gladkova N, Vargo J, et al. Optical coherence tomography of the esophagus and stomach in health and disease. Am J Gastroenterol 2001;96:2633–9.

[58] Li XD, Boppart SA, Van Dam J, et al. Optical coherence tomography: advanced technology for the endoscopic imaging of Barrett's esophagus. Endoscopy 2000;32:921–30.

[59] Poneros JM, Brand S, Bouma BE, et al. Diagnosis of specialized intestinal metaplasia by optical coherence tomography. Gastroenterology 2001;120:7–12.

[60] Poneros JM, Tearney GJ, Bouma BE, et al. Diagnosis of dysplasia in Barrett's esophagus using optical coherence tomography. Gastrointest Endosc 2001;53:AB113.

[61] Isenberg G, Sivak MV, Chak A, et al. Accuracy of endoscopic optical coherence tomography in the detection of dysplasia in Barrett's esophagus. Gastrointest Endosc 2003;57:AB77.

[62] Pfau PR, Sivak Jr MV, Chak A, et al. Criteria for the diagnosis of dysplasia by endoscopic optical coherence tomography. Gastrointest Endosc 2003;58:196–202.

[63] Poneros JM, Tearney GJ, Shiskov M, et al. Optical coherence tomography of the biliary tree during ERCP. Gastrointest Endosc 2002;55:84–8.

[64] Drexler W, Morgner U, Kaertner FX, et al. In vitro ultra-high resolution of optical coherence tomography. Opt Lett 1999;24:1221–3.

[65] Koblinski JE, Ahram M, Sloane BF. Unraveling the role of proteases in cancer. Clin Chim Acta 2000;291:113–35.

[66] Emmert-Buck MR, Roth MJ, Zhuang Z, et al. Increased gelatinase A (MMP-2) and cathep-

sin B activity in invasive tumor regions of human colon cancer samples. Am J Pathol 1994; 145:1285–90.

[67] Hazen LG, Bleeker FE, Lauritzen B, et al. Comparative localization of cathepsin B protein and activity in colorectal cancer. J Histochem Cytochem 2000;48:1421–30.

[68] Herszenyi L, Plebani M, Carraro P, et al. The role of cysteine and serine proteases in colorectal carcinoma. Cancer 1999;86:1135–42.

[69] Weissleder R, Tung CH, Mahmood U, et al. In vivo imaging of tumors with protease-activated near-infrared fluorescent probes. Nat Biotechnol 1999;17:375–8.

[70] Mahmood U, Tung C, Bogdanov A, et al. Near infrared optical imaging system to detect tumor protease activity. Radiology 1999;213:866–70.

[71] Marten K, Bremer C, Khazaie K, et al. Detection of dysplastic intestinal adenomas using enzyme-sensing molecular beacons in mice. Gastroenterology 2002;122:406–14.

[72] Moser AR, Pitot HC, Dove WF. A dominant mutation that predisposes to multiple intestinal neoplasia in the mouse. Science 1990;247:322–4.

[73] Khan A, Krishna M, Baker SP, et al. Cathepsin B and tumor-associated laminin expression in the progression of colorectal adenoma to carcinoma. Mod Pathol 1998;11:704–8.

[74] Inoue H, Igari T, Nishikage T, et al. A novel method of virtual histopathology using laser-scanning confocal microscopy in-vitro with untreated fresh specimens from the gastrointestinal mucosa. Endoscopy 2000;32:439–43.

[75] Inoue H, Cho JY, Satodate H, et al. Development of virtual histology and virtual biopsy using laser-scanning confocal microscopy. Scand J Gastroenterol 2003;237:37–9.

[76] Sakashita M, Inoue H, Kashida H, et al. Virtual histology of colorectal lesions using laser-scanning confocal microscopy. Endoscopy 2003;35:1033–8.

[77] Kiesslich R, Burg J, Vieth M, et al. Confocal laser endoscopy for diagnosing intraepithelial neoplasias and colorectal cancer in vivo. Gastroenterology 2004;127:706–13.

[78] McLaren W, Anikijenko P, Barkla D, et al. In vivo detection of experimental ulcerative colitis in rats using fiberoptic confocal imaging. Dig Dis Sci 2001;46:2263–76.

[79] McLaren WJ, Anikijenko P, Thomas SG, et al. In vivo detection of morphological and microvascular changes of the colon in association with colitis using fiberoptic confocal imaging. Dig Dis Sci 2002;47:2424–33.

[80] Schlemper RJ, Riddell RH, Kato Y, et al. The Vienna classification of gastrointestinal epithelial neoplasia. Gut 2000;47:251–5.

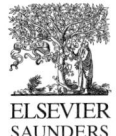

**ELSEVIER
SAUNDERS**

Gastrointest Endoscopy Clin N Am
15 (2005) 653–660

**GASTROINTESTINAL
ENDOSCOPY CLINICS
OF NORTH AMERICA**

Index

Note: Page numbers of article titles are in **boldface** type.

Changing Your Address?

Make sure your subscription changes too! When you notify us of your new address, you can help make our job easier by including an exact copy of your Clinics label number with your old address (see illustration below.) This number identifies you to our computer system and will speed the processing of your address change. Please be sure this label number accompanies your old address and your corrected address—you can send an old Clinics label with your number on it or just copy it exactly and send it to the address listed below.

We appreciate your help in our attempt to give you continuous coverage. Thank you.

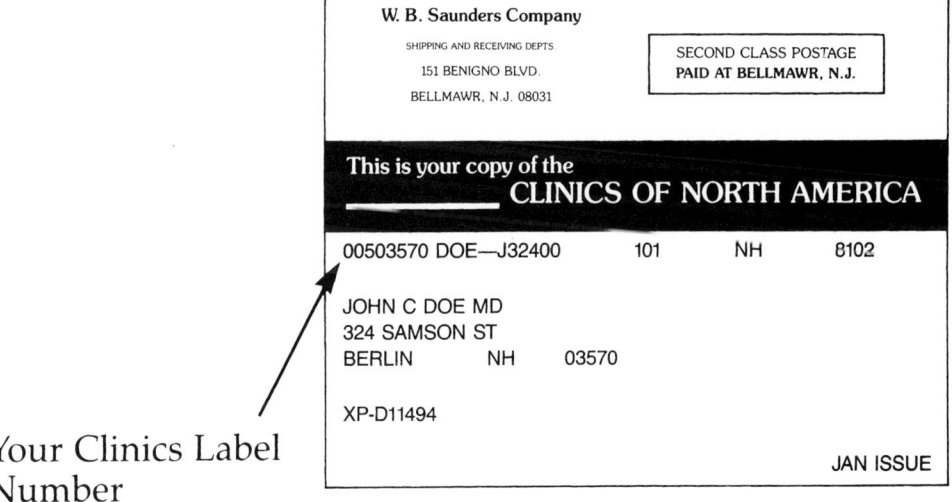

W. B. Saunders Company

SHIPPING AND RECEIVING DEPTS.
151 BENIGNO BLVD.
BELLMAWR, N.J. 08031

SECOND CLASS POSTAGE
PAID AT BELLMAWR, N.J.

This is your copy of the
CLINICS OF NORTH AMERICA

00503570 DOE—J32400   101   NH   8102

JOHN C DOE MD
324 SAMSON ST
BERLIN   NH   03570

XP-D11494

JAN ISSUE

Your Clinics Label Number
Copy it exactly or send your label
along with your address to:
W.B. Saunders Company, Customer Service
Orlando, FL 32887-4800
Call Toll Free 1-800-654-2452

Please allow four to six weeks for delivery of new subscriptions and for processing address changes.

YES! Please start my subscription to the **CLINICS** checked below with the ❏ first issue of the calendar year or ❏ current issues. If not completely satisfied with my first issue, I may write "cancel" on the invoice and return it within 30 days at no further obligation.

Please Print:

Name _____

Address_____

City_____ State _____ ZIP _____

Method of Payment

❏ Check (payable to **Elsevier**; add the applicable sales tax for your area)

❏ VISA   ❏ MasterCard   ❏ AmEx   ❏ Bill me

Card number _____ Exp. date _____

Signature _____

Staple this to your purchase order to expedite delivery

❏ **Adolescent Medicine Clinics**
❏ Individual $95
❏ Institutions $133
❏ *In-training $48

❏ **Anesthesiology**
❏ Individual $175
❏ Institutions $270
❏ *In-training $88

❏ **Cardiology**
❏ Individual $170
❏ Institutions $266
❏ *In-training $85

❏ **Chest Medicine**
❏ Individual $185
❏ Institutions $285

❏ **Child and Adolescent Psychiatry**
❏ Individual $175
❏ Institutions $265
❏ *In-training $88

❏ **Critical Care**
❏ Individual $165
❏ Institutions $266
❏ *In-training $83

❏ **Dental**
❏ Individual $150
❏ Institutions $242

❏ **Emergency Medicine**
❏ Individual $170
❏ Institutions $263
❏ *In-training $85
   ❏ Send CME info

❏ **Facial Plastic Surgery**
❏ Individual $199
❏ Institutions $300

❏ **Foot and Ankle**
Individual $160
Institutions $232

❏ **Gastroenterology**
❏ Individual $190
❏ Institutions $276

❏ **Gastrointestinal Endoscopy**
❏ Individual $190
❏ Institutions $276

❏ **Hand**
❏ Individual $205
❏ Institutions $319

❏ **Heart Failure (NEW in 2005!)**
❏ Individual $99
❏ Institutions $149
❏ *In-training $49

❏ **Hematology/ Oncology**
❏ Individual $210
❏ Institutions $315

❏ **Immunology & Allergy**
❏ Individual $165
❏ Institutions $266

❏ **Infectious Disease**
❏ Individual $165
❏ Institutions $272

❏ **Clinics in Liver Disease**
❏ Individual $165
❏ Institutions $234

❏ **Medical**
❏ Individual $140
❏ Institutions $244
❏ *In-training $70
   ❏ Send CME info

❏ **MRI**
❏ Individual $190
❏ Institutions $290
❏ *In-training $95
   ❏ Send CME info

❏ **Neuroimaging**
❏ Individual $190
❏ Institutions $290
❏ *In-training $95
   ❏ Send CME info

❏ **Neurologic**
❏ Individual $175
❏ Institutions $275

❏ **Obstetrics & Gynecology**
❏ Individual $175
❏ Institutions $288

❏ **Occupational and Environmental Medicine**
❏ Individual $120
❏ Institutions $166
❏ *In-training $60

❏ **Ophthalmology**
❏ Individual $190
❏ Institutions $325

❏ **Oral & Maxillofacial Surgery**
❏ Individual $180
❏ Institutions $280
❏ *In-training $90

❏ **Orthopedic**
❏ Individual $180
❏ Institutions $295
❏ *In-training $90

❏ **Otolaryngologic**
❏ Individual $199
❏ Institutions $350

❏ **Pediatric**
❏ Individual $135
❏ Institutions $246
❏ *In-training $68
   ❏ Send CME info

❏ **Perinatology**
❏ Individual $155
❏ Institutions $237
❏ *In-training $78
   ❏ Send CME info

❏ **Plastic Surgery**
❏ Individual $245
❏ Institutions $370

❏ **Podiatric Medicine & Surgery**
❏ Individual $170
❏ Institutions $266

❏ **Primary Care**
❏ Individual $135
❏ Institutions $223

❏ **Psychiatric**
❏ Individual $170
❏ Institutions $288

❏ **Radiologic**
❏ Individual $220
❏ Institutions $331
❏ *In-training $110
   ❏ Send CME info

❏ **Sports Medicine**
❏ Individual $180
❏ Institutions $277

❏ **Surgical**
❏ Individual $190
❏ Institutions $299
❏ *In-training $95

❏ **Thoracic Surgery (formerly Chest Surgery)**
❏ Individual $175
❏ Institutions $255
❏ *In-training $88

❏ **Urologic**
❏ Individual $195
❏ Institutions $307
❏ *In-training $98
   ❏ Send CME info

*To receive in-training rate, orders must be accompanied by the name of affiliated institution, dates of residency and signature of coordinator on institution letterhead. Orders will be billed at the individual rate until proof of resident status is received.

© Elsevier 2005. Offer valid in U.S. only. Prices subject to change without notice. **MO 10808 DF4184**

Order your subscription today. Simply complete and detach this card and drop it in the mail to receive the best clinical information in your field.

BUSINESS REPLY MAIL

FIRST-CLASS MAIL   PERMIT NO 7135   ORLANDO FL

POSTAGE WILL BE PAID BY ADDRESSEE

PERIODICALS ORDER FULFILLMENT DEPT
ELSEVIER
6277 SEA HARBOR DR
ORLANDO FL 32821-9816

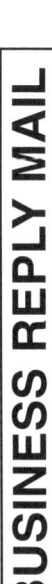